Advances in Vaccine Technology Its Commercial, Social and Economic Impacts

NIPA® GENX ELECTRONIC RESOURCES & SOLUTIONS P. LTD.
New Delhi-110 034

About the Editors

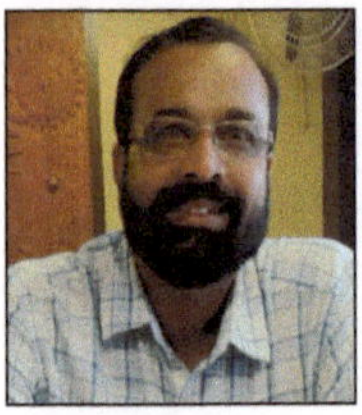

Dr. Snehasish Mishra, PhD, MBA, Associate Professor, is a distinguished faculty member at the School of Biotechnology, KIIT Deemed-to-be University, Bhubaneswar, Odisha, India. With over two decades of research and teaching experience, including international exposure, he has made significant contributions to infection biology, public health, microbial technology, limnology, environmental biotechnology, renewable energy, bioprocess engineering and food sciences. Dr. Mishra leads the Government of India's Ministry of New and Renewable Energy (MNRE) sponsored Biogas Development and Training Centre (BDTC) at KIIT Since 2009, focusing on advancing biogas technologies and promoting sustainable energy solutions. Dr. Mishra has authored over 175 publications, including research articles, popular articles and book chapters, in peer-reviewed journals and books of national and international repute. His scholarly works have garnered more than 2000 citations, reflecting the impact and relevance of his research in the scientific community. Beyond his research, Dr. Mishra is actively involved in skill development and livelihood enhancement initiatives for the farming community through biotechnological interventions. He regularly conducts short-term training programmes funded by the Department of Science and Technology (DST), Department of Biotechnology (DBT) and Ministry of Micro, Small and Medium Enterprises (MSME), on sustainable agricultural practices and renewable energy technologies. Dr. Mishra serves as a reviewer and editorial member for several research journals of international standing, contributing to the advancement of scientific knowledge and maintaining the quality of published research. He actively participates in bioentrepreneurship and industry-academia collaborations, bridging the gap between academic research and practical applications. Dr. Mishra received numerous accolades and recognitions through his career, from academies, societies and associations, acknowledging his continued contributions to science and education. He has successfully guided and continues to mentor numerous PhD, MPhil, MTech, and MSc students, fostering the next-generation scientists and researchers.

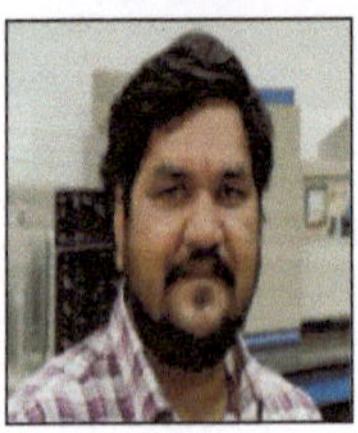

Dr. Puneet Kumar Singh is a researcher at the Bioenergy Lab, School of Biotechnology, KIIT Deemed-to-be University, Bhubaneswar, Odisha, India. Holding a PhD in Biotechnology, his research interests span across microbiology, bioprocess engineering, environmental biotechnology and renewable energy, focusing on waste management and bioenergy generation. A key focus of his work is enhancing biomethanation processes, thermo-alkali combined lignocellulose pretreatments. His research significantly improved biogas yields and provided molecular-level insights, addressing challenges in waste-to-energy conversion and contributing to the development of sustainable energy solutions. His doctoral research centered on circular bioeconomy zero-waste systems, optimising processes to convert organic substrates into renewable energy. Beyond bioenergy, Dr. Singh's research extends to environmental remediation, human and environmental health, with particular focus on the use of materials and metals. Dr. Singh gained valuable experience through collaborations with national and international laboratories, which have enhanced his expertise in environmental microbiology and bioprocess engineering. His ability to integrate diverse methodologies and technologies reflects his commitment to address global sustainability challenges and ensuring the health and wellbeing of one and all through scientific interventions. Dr. Singh has published over 40 research papers and five book chapters in esteemed international journals and publications. Dr. Singh actively contributes to academic and research development at KIIT Deemed-to-be University. He mentors MTech, MSc and PhD students and supports the Bioenergy Lab's mission of advancing renewable and sustainable energy technologies.

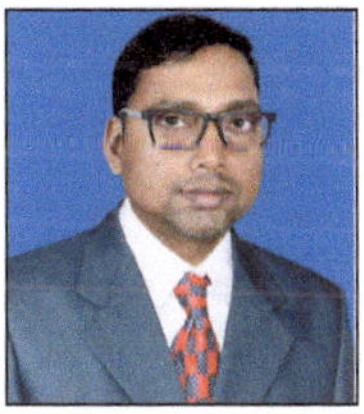

Dr. Ranjan Kumar Mohapatra, an esteemed inorganic chemist specialising in coordination chemistry, works in the Department of Chemistry at the Government College of Engineering, Keonjhar, Odisha, India. He obtained his PhD in 2011 and has since built a remarkable academic and research career. Dr. Mohapatra has published over 300 research and review papers in prestigious national and international journals, 13 books and 25 book chapters, as his significant contributions to the scientific community. He has filed 12 patents, five of which have already been granted, highlighting his focus on practical, innovative solutions. His research interests are broad and interdisciplinary, encompassing bioinorganic chemistry, medicinal chemistry, *in silico* drug design, public health and infectious diseases. His expertise in *in silico* methodologies is particularly noteworthy, enabling him to design and optimise potential drug candidates, which contributes to advancements in medicinal chemistry and development of therapeutics. With nearly two decades of teaching and research experience, Dr. Mohapatra has consistently demonstrated academic excellence. He supervises MPhil and PhD students as a mentor of the next generation scientists. His approachable nature and exceptional teaching skills have earned him significant popularity among his students, who greatly benefit from his extensive knowledge and passion. Dr. Mohapatra is listed among the top 2% of global researchers, a testament to the global impact and relevance of his work in the scientific arena.

Advances in Vaccine Technology Its Commercial, Social and Economic Impacts

Snehasish Mishra, PhD, MBA
Associate Professor
School of Biotechnology
KIIT Deemed-to-be University,
Bhubaneswar, Odisha, India

Puneet Kumar Singh
Researcher, Bioenergy Lab
School of Biotechnology,
KIIT Deemed-to-be University
Bhubaneswar, Odisha, India

Ranjan Kumar Mohapatra
Department of Chemistry
Government College of Engineering
Keonjhar, Odisha, India

NIPA® GENX ELECTRONIC RESOURCES & SOLUTIONS P. LTD.
New Delhi-110 034

NIPA® GENX ELECTRONIC
RESOURCES & SOLUTIONS P. LTD.

101,103, Vikas Surya Plaza, CU Block
L.S.C. Market, Pitam Pura, New Delhi-110 034
Ph : +91-11-43860225, Mob.: +91 9717133558, 9540816132
E-mail: newindiapublishingagency@gmail.com
Website: www.nipaersources.com

Print ISBN: 978-93-58874-24-2

ebook ISBN: 978-93-58872-83-5

Composed and Designed by NIPA®.

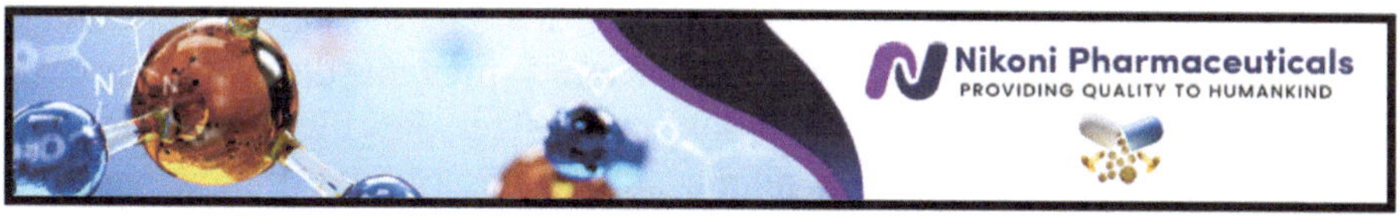

Foreword

Vaccines are not exclusively medical innovations but are powerful tools that have revolutionized public health, reduced the infectious disease burden and have saved millions of lives. The evolution of vaccine technology is a significant accomplishment in medical history, demonstrating a profound intersection of science, society and economy. From the early pioneering work of Edward Jenner with smallpox to the rapid development of the path-breaking mRNA vaccines during the COVID-19 pandemic, vaccinology witnessed remarkable progress that has transformed community health and public healthcare measures. This Edited Volume 'Advances in Vaccine Technology: Its Commercial, Social and Economic Impacts' by Dr. Snehasish Mishra and his Editorial team will undoubtly serve as an essential chronicle in the journey, offering insights into the historical evolution, present-day advancements and the diverse impacts of vaccines on the society. This book thoroughly examines the historical context of vaccine development, emphasizing significant milestones and the unwavering quest for scientific innovation resulting in introducing novel vaccines to combat the diseases once considered invincible. It explores the challenges faced by vaccine developers in early stages and the advancements that have facilitated the development of contemporary vaccines, essential components of global health initiatives now. The advancements of vaccinology transcend traditional scientific endeavors. It includes various commercial, social and economic aspects that profoundly affect individuals, communities and nations. This book evaluates the commercial ramifications of vaccine development, encompassing complex processes of research, production and equitable distribution. It presents the evolution of pharmaceutical industry in response to the increasing demand for vaccinations, and how innovations in vaccine technology have stimulated economic growth and impacted global trade. Societal impact of vaccines is equally profound. The book discusses vaccines in shaping public health policies, enhancing herd immunity and addressing health disparities. It reflects on the ethical implications, public confidence and social responsibilities of stakeholders in vaccine research and delivery. The book explores the economic implications of vaccine technology comprehensively, demonstrating how vaccines prevent disease outbreaks and foster economic stability. The book emphasizes on efficient vaccination programs and the long-term economic advantages of investing in vaccine research and development. To conclude, 'Advances in Vaccine Technology: Its Commercial, Social and Economic Impacts' is a pertinent and essential resource for those seeking to comprehend the intricacies of vaccine research and its extensive societal implications. It is a testament to the enduring power of vaccines to protect, preserve and promote the health and wellbeing of the human population around the world, and beyond. I compliment Dr. Mishra and his team for this commendable endeavor and endorse the book as essential reading and acquisition.

Nrusingh Prasad Mohapatra

(*Dr Nrusingh P. Mohapatra*)

इंडियन इम्यूनोलाजिकल्स लिमिटेड

INDIAN IMMUNOLOGICALS LIMITED

Advances in Vaccine Technology - Its Commercial, Social and Economic Implications

Foreword

The COVID-19 pandemic has highlighted the importance of vaccines, and the social and economic impact vaccines bring. Vaccine development is a long arduous process, but the covid pandemic changed the way vaccines are developed and rolled out. At societal level, people at large understood the value proposition offered by vaccines. It also consolidated an integrated approach to infectious disease management with respect to One Health. At national and international level, covid pandemic stimulated policy on pandemic preparedness and related healthcare interventions. Given the importance of vaccines and their pivotal role in eradicating many infectious diseases over the centuries, it is crucial to understand the challenges and opportunities.

This Edited Volume "Advances in vaccine technology - Its commercial, social and economic impacts" is an exemplary work on medical biotechnology. I applaud Dr. Snehasish Mishra and his co-editors for taking on this arduous work of documenting the historic journey and future expectations in the field of vaccines. With its thorough and perceptive examination of the intricate terrain surrounding COVID-19 vaccine development, this book is an essential resource for scientists, legislators, policy makers, healthcare professionals and the public at large. The meticulous assessment of bioprocesses in vaccine manufacturing underscores the intricate nature of this endeavor and highlights the remarkable achievements of scientists and engineers who worked tirelessly to optimize the operations and production processes. Given the critical role of vaccines in protecting individuals and communities, the integrated focus of the book on public health is particularly timely. By elucidating the epidemiology of the pandemic and the public health strategies implemented to mitigate its impact, this book provides a clear and compelling narrative of the challenges faced and the lessons learnt. The emergence of mRNA technology as a game-changer in vaccine development is a testament to the power of scientific ingenuity. This book explores this groundbreaking platform that offers a fascinating glimpse into the future of vaccine development, as a rapid response platform that has the potential to have vaccines developed within 100 days in future pandemic situations. Showcasing the relentless pursuit of even more effective and affordable vaccines, the chapter on the role of AI in sufficing and advancing the efforts on next-generation vaccine is a beacon of optimism. Examining the latest research and developments, the book provides a roadmap for future vaccine strategies and underscores the importance of continued global investments in this critical area. To conclude, it is a timely and essential contribution to our understanding of the COVID-19 pandemic and the development of vaccines to combat it. It is a testament to the power of human ingenuity and collaboration in the face of adversity. I wholeheartedly recommend this book to anyone seeking a deeper appreciation of the scientific and public health achievements that have brought humanity closer to a world that strives to free itself from the threat of devastating infectious diseases.

Dr. Priyabrata Pattnaik

Preface

This piece of work in its final form had its own share of emotional strain and personal sacrifices. The journey of compiling, researching and articulating the immense complexities of vaccinology demanded a relentless focus that was both intellectually demanding and emotionally taxing. In a world grappled with misinformation and inequity, there were moments of profound self-doubt and pressure, particularly in navigating the ethical and societal dimensions. The responsibility to capture the weight of global health challenges, alongside the inspiring stories of innovation and resilience, often were overwhelming. Yet, the desire to better understanding this critical field was the driving force, providing the determination needed to persevere through the process. All in all, the objective was to provide a 360° view of the world of vaccinology as it has evolved with time.

Immunisation strategies have revolutionised public healthcare significantly, reducing the burden of infectious diseases and saving millions of lives worldwide. Being able to contain pathogenic diseases that were earlier unpreventable, vaccines have fundamentally redefined the threats of infectious diseases towards humanity. This piece of work compiles the multifaceted realm of vaccinology, thoroughly exploring its genesis, contemporary advancements and future directions. It details the evolution of vaccine science from early variolation practices to the sophisticated molecular platforms including that of the mRNA, emphasising the critical role of bioprocess engineering in scaling-up vaccine production to meet the increasing global demand. Driven by the emerging and reemerging infectious diseases as global pandemics and challenges to ensure equitable healthcare, the importance of vaccinology research is paramount. Advancements in bioprocess technologies and artificial intelligence (AI) have revolutionised vaccine development and its large-scale production, highlighting the need for sustained research collaboration to address global health challenges. Integration of reverse vaccinology powered by AI and machine learning (ML) further accelerates the efforts, opening new avenues in combating emerging pathogens rapidly and effectively. This work explores not only the technical aspects of vaccine science but also the societal, ethical and policy dimensions that influence vaccination efforts.

In addition to its technical and scientific content, this book highlights the socioeconomic impact of vaccines, including their role in reducing healthcare costs and saving lives, as demonstrated during the COVID-19 pandemic. It dissects the challenges of vaccine hesitancy, misinformation, and inequitable distribution, offering solutions to these issues and strategies to ensure broader access to immunisation. The One Health framework is another key theme that highlights the interconnectedness of the health of humans, animals and environment to address zoonotic diseases and ensure the health and wellbeing of all. This holistic approach is crucial to prevent future pandemics that extend the vaccination strategies beyond humans to include animals, particularly the disease reservoirs.

The book showcases India's global vaccine diplomacy, illustrating how the country's rapid and large-scale vaccine production positively impacted global healthcare. This underscores India's strategic importance in global vaccine landscape and its commitment to advancing public health. The vast improvements in manufacturing capacity, distribution networks and international collaborations have positioned India as a key player in the global effort to combat infectious diseases. This section not only highlights India's contributions but also explores the challenges it faces in ensuring that vaccines reach all populations, particularly those in underserved regions.

Designed for a broad audience, including researchers, healthcare professionals and policymakers, the book offers comprehensive understanding of the scientific, technological and socioeconomic dimensions of vaccine development. It would serve as an invaluable resource for all involved in the field of public health and vaccinology, whether in research, policy designing or clinical practices. By reflecting on past successes and current challenges, it encourages future innovation and collaboration to counter infectious diseases, contributing to the broader goal of ensuring equitable vaccine access worldwide. The inclusion of practical insights into vaccine production, distribution and policy implementation provides a roadmap to address both the existing and the emerging health threats. Ideas and suggestions for future advancements in vaccine science and its equitable application are warmly invited. It is a sincere hope that this work not only informs but also inspires readers to join the ongoing efforts to improve global health through innovation, collaboration and compassion. This book is a testament to the resilience of science and the human spirit, and its evolution will continue to be shaped by the invaluable contributions of its readers.

Editors

Contents

Terms, Terminologies and Abbreviations

3D cell culture: Cells cultured in a three dimensional space
aAPC: Artificial antigen-presenting cell

A
AAV: Adeno-associated virus
Abate: Reduction in intensity or degree
Abide: Follow or accept without questioning
Aboriginal population: Indigenous people of a region/locality/ethnicity
Absenteeism: Frequent absence from active life
Accordance: Agreement or conformity with the laid-down rules
Accountability: Responsibility for actions or decisions
ACE2: Angiotensin converting enzyme 2
Acellular: Lacking a defined cellular structure
Ache: A continuous/constant pain
ACIP: Advisory committee on immunisation practices
Acquisition: The act of obtaining/acquiring something
Acute: Intensity of a symptom
ADE: Antibody dependent enhancement
Adenoviruses: A group of viruses causing respiratory, eye and gastrointestinal infections (gland-specific diseases)
Adherent cells: Cells attached to a surface
Adjuvant: A substance that enhance the efficacy of a vaccine
Adolescent: A person at an early age (young in the developmental stage)
Adorning: Decorating or embellishing
Aerosol droplet: Airborne contaminated liquid particles capable to spread infection
Aetiological agent: Disease causing pathogen
Afflicted: Affected by pain or suffering
Affordability: Economic feasibility
Age-defying: Resisting the age-related effects
Aggregation: Gathering or clustering of elements/substances
Agony: Extreme physical or mental suffering
Agrarian: A matter that relates to agricultural or rural matters
AI: Artificial intelligence
AIDS: Acquired immunodeficiency syndrome
Ailing: Suffering from illness or poor health
Ailment: Minor or chronic illness
AIR: All India Radio
Allele: A gene variant in an organism

AlphaFold: AI model predicting quaternary (final folded) structure of protein
Alum: A compound [K2SO4(Al2SO4)3.24H2O] used as a vaccine adjuvant
Ambivalence: Conflicting emotions
Amphipathic: Molecules with both hydrophilic as well as hydrophobic region
AMR: Antimicrobial resistance
AMS: Antimicrobial stewardship
Analgesic: Pain-relieving medication or substance
Anamnestic response: Quick immune response upon a reexposure
Anaphylactic shock: Severe allergic reaction requiring immediate treatment
Anatomist: Specialist in anatomy
Angiotensin: A protein that regulates blood pressure and balances the fluid
Animal husbandry: Breeding and raising the livestock
Anionic mRNA: Negatively charged messenger RNA
ANN: Artificial neural network
Anomalies: Abnormalities or deviations from the usual/normal/natural
Anomaly: Deviation from an expected pattern
Anthrax: Infectious disease caused by the bacterium Bacillus anthracis
Anthropogenic: An effect caused due to an human activity
Antibody: A protein formed in response to an immunological trigger
Antibodyomics: The study about the antibodies and their interaction dynamics
Anti-clotting: A substance that prevents the formation of blood clots
Antigen: A substance that is capable of inducing an immune response
Antigenic determinant: The antigen part that is recognised by the antibody
Antigenicity: The ability of an antigenic substance to elicit an immune response
Antisepsis: An infection prevention measure
Antitoxin: Toxin-neutralising antibody
Antiviral: A drug that targets a viral infection
AOM: Acute otitis media (infection of the middle ear)
APC: Antigens presenting cell
Apes: The group of primates excluding monkeys and humans
Apoptosis: Programmed cell death
Apprehensive: Fearful or anxious about the future
Arboviral: Related to viruses that are transmitted by arthropods as carriers
ARDS: Acute respiratory distress syndrome
Arguably: Subject to argument (debatable)
Arsenal: Collection of resources
Artefact: Error/distortion of data, images or substances due to technical flaw
Arthus reaction: Localised immune complex mediated inflammation
Artificial intelligence: Mechanical (computerised) process to simulate human intelligence
Assault: Physical attack or offensive action
Asthma: Chronic disease that cause respiratory difficulties
Astounding: Extremely surprising
Atopic dermatitis Chronic inflammation, redness and irritation of the skin
Attenuated: Weakened, usually referring to viruses or pathogens
Augment: To increase or enhance certain thing
Autoimmunity: Self-attacking immune system
Auxiliary proteins: A proteins that assist the primary functioning of others
Avian: Relating to bird

Avian influenza: Bird-flu caused by viruses
AVMA: American veterinary medical association

B

Bactericidal: A substance that is capable of killing obnoxious/harmful bacteria
Bacterins: A vaccine that is made from killed bacteria
Baculovirus: A virus that could infect insect
Badgers: Burrowing mammals, often the carriers of zoonotic diseases
BARDA: Biomedical advanced research and development authority
BBIL: Bharat biotech international limited, Hyderabad
BCG: Bacille Calmette-Guérin
BCIDE: B-cell integrated development environment
Beacon of hope: A sign or symbol of inspiration
BepiPred: A bioinformatics tool to predict B-cell epitopes
BEVS: Baculovirus expression vector system
Bibliometric: Statistical analyses of publications, like books and articles, to measure their impact
Biodegradable: A material that is capable of naturally decomposing/degrading
Biodistribution: Distribution of a bioactive substance within the body
Bioengineered: Biologically modified (biologics)or bio-derived (biosimilars)
Biofoundry: A facility to operate bioprocesses to produce biological products
Bioinformatics: Using computer, database and statistics to analyse biological data
Biologics: Therapeutics derived from a living organism
Biomarker: Biological indicator to assess physicochemical and ecological conditions
Biomaterial: A material derived from biological source
Biomimic: Imitating a biological system
Bioreactor: A device/vessel that supports biological processes or culture conditions
Biosafety: Protection against harmful biological agents
Biosecurity: Preventing biological threats to health
Biosensor: A device that could detect biological substances or conditions
Bioseparation: Methods or techniques to separate and purify a desired biological material
Biosimilars: Biological products similar to an existing synthesised medication
Bivalent vaccine: A vaccine that targets two distinct antigens simultaneously
Black-box: System wherein the internal working is nondecipherable on realtime bases
Blister: A fluid-filled bump on the skin
Bluetongue: A viral disease (caused by arbovirus) that affect the ruminants
Bolster: To support or strengthen something
Booster: Additional vaccine dose to boost the immunity
Bottleneck: Factors that limit or slow-down the progress of an operation
Bovine: Relating to cattle
Bovo-vaccine: The vaccine obtained from the cowpox virus
Brincidofovir: An antiviral drug to treat viral infections
Broadened: Expanded in scope or range
Bronchoalveolar ravage: Damage to the airways and sacs in the lungs
Brucellosis: Bacterial disease from infected animals
BSL-3: Biosafety level 3
Bubonic plague: Severe disease spread by fleas

Bush meat: Locally-consumed meat obtained from wild animals

C

Calibration: Adjusting an equipment to ensure accuracy
Canine parvovirus: A deadly virus that infects the intestines of dogs
Capillary electrophoresis: A technique to separate the molecules based on their charge
Capsular polysaccharide: A protective sugar layer in bacteria
Carcass: Dead bodies of animals, or cadavers
Carcinoma: Malignant tumour
Cardiac: Relating to the heart or its functions
Cardiovascular: Relating to heart and vessels
Catalysed: Accelerated reaction
Catastrophic: Extremely harmful or disastrous
Cater: To provide for or satisfy the needs
Cathepsins: The enzymes that are involved in degrading proteins at a slightly low pH
Catheter: A tube used in medical procedures
Cationic: Positively charged ionic particles
CBD: Convention on biological diversity
CCDB: Cyber cell database
CDC: Centres for disease control and prevention
CDSCO: Central drugs standard control organisation
CE: Capillary electrophoresis
Cell culture: Growth of cells in vitro, within a laboratory environment
Cell detritus: Debris from cellular degradation
Cell viability: The ability of a cell to survive
Cell line: Laboratory cultured cells used in research and development
Centrifugation: A process to separate components by employing centrifugal force
CEPI: Coalition for epidemic preparedness innovations
Cerebral venous sinus thrombosis: A rare blood clotting condition that affect the brain
Cervical cancer: Cancer affecting the cervix (human body part)
CFR: Case fatality rate
cGMP: Current good manufacturing practices
Chemotherapy: A treatment to kill or inhibit cancer cells using drugs
Chicken cholera: A bacterial disease that affect the poultry
Chimera: An organism with mixed genetic material
Chinchillas: The rodents that are bred for fur or research
CHO: Chinese hamster ovary
Chromatography: Technique to separate chemical mixtures
Chronic disease: Persistent illness
CIHR: Canadian institutes for health research
Cilia: Hairlike structures involved in movement or sensation
Circadian rhythm: 24-hours biological activity cycle
Circumsporozoite: Protein found in the malarial parasite
Civic: Relating to citizens or public affairs
Clade: A group of organisms sharing a common ancestor
Cling: Adhere closely or tightly
Clinical trial: Testing new treatments or interventions on living subjects
Cloning: Producing genetically identical organisms

Clostridial disease: Infections caused by the bacterium Clostridium
Clpro: Chymotrypsin-like cysteine protease
Clumping: Formation of aggregates or clusters
CMV: Cytomegalovirus
CNN: Convolutional neural network
CNS: Central nervous system
Cochlear: Related to the structure of inner ear
Codon: Three-nucleotide sequence coding for amino acids
Coelute: Simultaneous elution of substances in chromatography
Cognitive impairment: Reduced ability to think, concentrate or remember
Cohesive: Unified, holding together effectively
Cohort: A group that shares common characteristics/traits
Colloidal: Particles suspended in a fluid medium
Combat: To actively fight or resist something
Comorbidity: Multiple clinical conditions existing simultaneously
Conducive: Contributing to desired outcome
Conflict: Disagreement or struggle
Congenital: Acquired or inherited since birth
Congestion: Overcrowding or obstruction, often referring to the respiratory system
Conjugated vaccine: A vaccine candidate with an attached carrier protein
Constantinople: Historical city Istanbul
Contagious: Capable of spreading an infection to others
Contiguous: Sharing a common border or the regions that touch each other
Convalescent: Recovering from an illness or injury
COPD: Chronic obstructive pulmonary disease
Coronary disease: That condition that affect the heart and blood vessels
Coronaviridae: A virus family that also includes COVID-19-causing SARS-CoV-2 virus
Coronavirinae: A subfamily of Coronaviridae viruses
Corticosteroids: Steroid hormones used against inflammation
COVID-19: Corona virus disease 2019
CoVs: Corona viruses
Coyotes: Wild canines as the reservoir/host of certain zoonotic diseases
CPPs: Critical process parameters
CQAs: Critical quality attributes
CRISPR/Cas9: Genome editing technique using RNA-guided enzymes
Cross-contamination: Transfer of contaminants between materials
Cross-reactivity: Immune response against similar (yet different) antigens
Cryoprotectant: A substance that prevents cell damage due to freezing
Cryptococcus: A fungal infection that affects the lungs and the brain
Cumbersome: Complicated or difficult to handle
Cupids: Cup-shaped circular objects/structures
Curb: To limit or restrain something
Curtailing: Reducing or limiting something
Cutting-edge: Innovative, advanced or at the forefront
cVLP: Capsid virus like particle
Cytokine storm: Overproduction of proteins by the immune system causing inflammation
Cytoskeleton: Structural framework within a cell
Cytotoxic T-Cells: The immune cells that kill the virus

D

DBT: Department of biotechnology
DCGI: Drugs Controller General of India
DD: Deep docking
D-dimer: A blood clot breakdown product, often elevated in clotting disorders
De novo: Starting from beginning, newly synthesised
Deadenylation: Removal of poly-adenylated tail from RNA
Decrement: Gradual reduction
Deep learning: An advanced machine learning that emplys neural networks
Demography: Study of population characteristics
Denuding: Eroding, stripping or removing
Dermatological: A disease condition relating to the skin
Dexterity: Skill or agility in performing tasks
Dictated: Commanded or directed with authority
Dilemmatic: Involving a difficult choice or conflict
Diligently: With careful and persistent efforts
Dimer: A molecule that comprises two similar subunits
Diphtheria: Bacterial infection affecting the respiratory system
Dissemination: The spread or distribution of information or materials
Dizziness: A feeling of light-headedness or loss of balance
DL: Deep learning
DLin-MC3-DMA: Dilinoleylmethyl-4-dimethylaminobutyrate
DMV: Double-membrane vesicle
DNA digestion: Cutting the DNA strand using specific and specialised enzymes
DoE: Design of experiments
Domino: Chain reaction triggered by an initial event
DOTAP: 1,2-dioleoyl-3-trimethylammonium-propane
Dreaded: Feared greatly or causing terror
Dromedary camels: One-humped camels found in the desert (usually domesticated)
dsDNA: Double-stranded DNA
dsDNA-RT: Double-stranded DNA with reverse transcriptase
dsRNA: Double-stranded RNA
DTP: Diphtheria-Tetanus-Pertussis
Dyspnoea: Difficult or laboured breathing

E

E: Envelope
Ebola: A viral disease that causes severe haemorrhagic fever
Ectodomain: Part of a protein that is exposed to outside the cell
ED: Ectodomain
EMA: European medicines agency
Embryonic: Early developmental stage
Emigrants: People who leave their own country to settle elsewhere
Emulsions: Mixtures of two immiscible liquids
Encapsulated: Enclosed in a protective outer layer
Encroachment: Gradual intrusion into a restricted area

Endemic: Found in a specific region
Endocytosis: Process of cells absorbing material from outside
Endogenous: Originating from within an organism or a system
Endorsement: Approval or support for something
Endosome: Cellular vesicle transporting substances inside
Endotoxin: The toxin released by certain bacteria upon its death
Envisaging: Visualising or imagining the future possibilities
EPI: Expanded programme on immunisation
Epicentre: The central point of an outbreak or an event
Epidemic: A disease outbreak that affects a large population in a region
Epidemiology: The study of diseases and their distribution across populations
Epitope: A specific region on an antigen that is recognised by the immune system
Epitweetr: A tool to analyse epitopes from the social media data
ERGIC: ER-Golgi intermediate compartment
Erroneous: Incorrect or containing errors
ETEC: Enterotoxigenic E. coli
EU: European union
EUA: Emergency use authorisation/approval
Evaded: Escaped successfully
Excipient: An inert substance used while formulating a drug
Exosomes: Small vesicles involved in intercellular communication
Extracorporeal: Occurring outside the body
Extraneous: Contextually unrelated or unnecessary

F

Fallout: After-effects of a significant adverse event
FAO: Food and agriculture organisation
Fatality: The occurrence of death, often as a result of a disease (in medical terms)
Fatigue: Extreme tiredness or lack of energy
FCS: Furin cleavage site
FDA: Food and drug administration
Faecal-oral: Transmission route involving faecal contamination and ingestion
Terminology Definition
Fed-batch: A fermentation/bioprocessing mode involving controlled nutrient addition
Feline: Related to the cat family
Fermentation: A biochemical conversion process
Ferret: To search or investigate thoroughly
fHbp: Factor H-binding protein
Filariasis: A mosquito-transmitted parasitic disease
Flaviviridae: A virus family that includes the Dengue and Zika viruses
Fleeting: Lasting for a very short duration
Floated: To suggest or propose an idea
Flu: Contagious viral infection that affects the respiratory system
FMD: Foot-and-mouth disease
Fomite: An inanimate object that could carry infectious agents
Fowl: Domesticated birds like chicken
Frameshifts: Disrupted genetic code reading during translation
Fraternity: A group that shares common interests or goals

Fringe: At the edges or margins
Furin: An enzyme that is involved in activating the viral proteins

G

Gastroenteritis: The inflammation of the stomach and intestines
GAVI: Global alliance for vacancies and immunisation
Gay male: Homosexual men
GCP: Good clinical practice
Gel permeation chromatography: A technique to separate molecules based on size
Gene silencing: Suppression of gene expression in cells
Gene therapy: A method to treat diseases by altering the responsible genes
Genetic code: The nucleotides sequence in DNA that determines genetic information
Genetic make-up: Genetic composition of an organism
Genetic mutation: Permanent change in the DNA sequence
Genetically engineered: Organisms that are modified at genetic level using molecular techniques
Genital herpes: A sexually-transmitted viral infection
Genocide: Deliberate destruction of racial or ethnic group
Genome: A complete set of genetic material in an organism
Genome sequencing: A technique to determine the complete genome sequence of an organism
Genomics: The study of genes and their functions
Geopolitics: Political influence as shaped by geography
Gerbils: Small rodents, often employed in biotechnological research
GMI: Global microbial identifier
GNRCEM: Gamaleya national research centre of epidemiology and microbiology
Goblet cells: Cells that secrete mucus, often found in the respiratory system
Google DeepMind: AI research company focused on solving complex issues
Grapple: To struggle or wrestle with something difficult
GRIEM: Gamaleya research institute of epidemiology and microbiology
Grimmer: More serious or worrying
Groundhogs: Rodents, sometimes carrying zoonotic diseases
Gynaecological ailment: Disorder related to female reproductive organs

H

HACCP: Hazard analysis critical control point
Haemagglutin esterase: A protein that is involved in the binding and entry of virus
Halal: A practice that is permissible under the Islamic law
Hamster: A small rodent that is often employed in medical research
Harmonisation: Standardising a procedure or regulation across systems
Haves: Privileged group of individuals that possess the resources
Terminology Definition
Havoc: Widespread destruction or chaos
Hazard: Potential source of harm or danger
HBV: Hepatitis B virus
HCV: Hepatitis C virus
HE: Haemagglutin esterase
Hedgehog: A form of spiny mammal that carries zoonotic pathogens
Hepatitis: Inflammation of the liver due to infection or toxins
Hepatocellular: Relating to liver cells

Hepatotropic: Targeting the liver
Herculean: Requiring great strength or effort
Herd immunity: Immunity within a population due to widespread immunisation drive
Heterologous: Derived from a different species or origin
Hib: Haemophilus influenzae type b
HICPAC: Healthcare infection control practices advisory committee
Histocompatibility: Compatibility of tissues for transplantation
Histoplasmosis: A fungal infection that originates from bird droppings
Hitherto: Until now or up to this point in time
HIV: Human immunodeficiency virus
hMPV: Human metapneumovirus
Hoarding: Accumulating excessive amounts of something
Homeostasis: Maintenance of stable internal conditions in an organism
Homogeneity: Uniformity in composition
Homology model: Computational model based on the similarity in sequence
Homosexual: An individual that is sexually attracted to the same gender
Horseshoe bat: A bat species that is known for potentially transmitting zoonotic diseases
Hotspot: An area concentrated with diseased cases
hPIV3: Human parainfluenza virus type 3
HPLC: High-performance liquid chromatography
HPV: Human papillomavirus
HSS: Health and human service
HTS: High-throughput screening
Huge toll: A significant negative impact
Human-centric: Focused on human-related concerns
Humanised: Altered to resemble human characteristics
Humanitarian: Concerned with human welfare and rights
Humoral immunity: Antibody-mediated immune response
HVTR: HIV vaccine translational research
Hybridoma: Trained cell that produces monoclonal antibodies
Hydatid disease: Parasitic infection affecting human organs
Hydrodynamic: Relating to forces acting on fluids
Hydrophobic: Repellent to water; non-polar molecules
Hypercoagulation: Increased blood clotting tendency
Hyper-glycosylation: Excessive addition of sugar molecules
Hypersensitivity: Excessive immune response to stimuli
Hypertension: High blood pressure
Hypotheses: Proposed explanations based on limited evidence

I

IAcV: Inactivated vaccine
IC: Intracellular
ICD: International classification of diseases
ICH: International council for harmonisation
ICMR: Indian council of medical research
ICTV: International committee on taxonomy of virus
ICU: Intensive care unit
ICVT: International committee on virus taxonomy

IEDB: Immune epitope database
IFC: indirect fixed capital
IFN: Interferon
IFR: Infection fatality rate
IHR: International health regulations
IIL: Indian immunologicals limited, Hyderabad
Illness: Clinical condition that affects the health of an individual
Immigrant: A person who moves to a new country to live there permanently
Imminent: About to happen or would soon occur
Immunisation: The process of inducing immunity against a specific pathogen
Immunocompetent: Capable of mounting an immune response
Immunocompromised: Weakened immune system/function
Immunodeficiency: Inability to produce adequate immune response in response to an antigen
Immunodominant: Strongly recognised by the immune system
Immunogen: A substance that is capable of inducing an immune response
Immunogenicity: The ability to stimulate immunity
Immunoglobulins: Antibodies produced by the immune system
Immunology: The study of the immune system and the related disorders
Immunosuppression: Reduced immune function
Immunotherapy: Treating a disease through immunity enhancement
Imprecise: Lacking accuracy or exactness
In silico: The procedure to perform a task through computer simulations
In vitro: Experiments conducted in the lab outside a living organism
In vivo: Experiments conducted within the living organism
Inadvertent: Unintentional or accidental in nature
Incapacitate: Deprived of strength or the ability to function
Indigenous: Native to a specific region
Indiscernible: Unable to detect or perceive clearly
Infancy: Early stage of development
Infectivity: The ability of a pathogen to spread and cause an infection
Infer: Deducing conclusions based on the evidence
Inflammasome: Protein complex triggering inflammatory responses
Inflammation: Body's response to injury or infection with swelling and redness
Inflict: Cause or impose
Influenza: A viral infection that affects the respiratory system
Influx: Arrival or incoming flow of certain thing
Inhabitant: Individual or animal living in a designated region
Inhibition: Prevention or reduction of a process
Inhumane: Lacking compassion
Innumerable: Too many to be counted
Inoculation: Introduction of a vaccine or an antigen
Inpatient: A patient staying in a hospital during treatment
Insertional: Relating to the insertion of something
Instilled: Gradually introduced or established
Intellectual: Educated and scholarly individual
Intensive care unit: A specialised hospital unit to handle the critically ill patients
Interdependent species: Species relying on each other for sustenance
Interferon: A protein that is released to help fight an infection or tumour

Interim: Temporary or provisional
Intermediate host: An organism that is involved in transmitting pathogens to humans
Interspecies: Between different species or organisms
Intestinal: Relating to intestine or the digestive tract
Intracellular: Inside a cell or occurring within a cell
Intradermal: Under the skin layer
Intramuscular: Between the muscle tissue
Intranasal: Through the nose
Intranodal: Located or occurring within the lymph nodes
Intraosseous: Administered into bone marrow or cavity
Intraperitoneal: Injected into the peritoneal cavity
Intricate: Complex or detailed
Intrinsic: Naturally occurring within or inherent in something
Intussusception: Telescoping of one part of intestine
Invade: Entering or spreading into something
Invasion: Entry and spread within an organism
Invoked: Called upon for support or action
Ion-exchange chromatography: Separation of proteins based on their ionic charge differences
IP: Intellectual property
IPV: Inactivated polio vaccine
ISM: Immune stimulatory molecule
Itinerary: Planned route or schedule of a programme
IVT: In vitro transcription

J

JCVI: Joint committee on vaccination and immunisation

L

Lansing: Significant research site
Lastmile: The final stage in the delivery of goods or services
LAV: Live-attenuated vaccine
Legislation: Laws enacted by a governing authority
Legitimate: Acceptable or conforming to established rules
Leishmaniasis: A parasitic disease that is transmitted by sandfly
Lentiviral: Relating to viruses like HIV that causes slow infection
Leprosy: A chronic bacterial disease that affects the nerves
Leptospirosis: A bacterial infection that spreads through animals
Lesion: Damaged tissue area
Lethality: The ability to cause death
Lineage: Descendant group from a common ancestor
LION: lipid inorganic nanoparticle
Lipidised: Containing or converted into lipids
Lipidomics: The study of cellular lipid profiles and functions
Liposome encapsulated: Vesicles-based drug delivery system
Liposome: A form of lipid-bilayer vesicle used in drug delivery
LIV: Louping-ill virus
Live attenuated: A weakened live microorganism
Livestock: Domesticated animals raised for the purpose of food

LMIC: Low-and-medium-income country
LNP: Lipid nanoparticle
Lockdown: Restrictions to limit movement and prevent the spread of a disease
Logistics: The management of supply chain operations
Long-haul: Referring to long-term effects, often in the context of illness
Loom: Emerging or prominent threat
LSTM: Long short-term memory
Lull: A temporary period of calm or inactivity
Lungs deformity: Structural abnormality in lungs
LVV: Lentiviral vector
Lyme disease: Bacterial infection from tick bites
Lymph: A fluid that circulates in the lymphatic system
Lymphadenopathy: Swollen or enlarged lymph nodes
Lymphocytes: White blood cells involved in the immune response
Lyophilisation: Freeze-drying process to preserve a substance, usually bioactive material

M

M: Membrane
mAb: Monoclonal antibody
Macaques: A type of monkey often used in research
Machine learning: The field of AI where computers are trained through data-feeding
Macroeconomy: The overall economy, including national and global economic trends
Mainstay: Essential part of something
Malady: An illness or a disease that affect the body
Malignancy: Cancerous growth
Manifestation: Visible signs or symptoms
Manoeuvrability: The quality of being easy to move and direct
MARIA: Multidimensional approach for research impact assessment
Marmots: A form of large rodent inhabiting in mountainous regions
Marsupials: Mammals carrying young in pouches
Mass immunisation: Large-scale vaccination efforts to protect the population in a region
Massachusetts: A state in the New England region of the United States
Matrix: A material or tissue that surrounds and supports the cells in an organism
Measles: A disease caused by a single-stranded RNA Morbillivirus
Melanoma: A type of skin cancer arising from the melanocytes
Memory B cells: Immune cells remembering an antigen to respond fast to a repeat infection
Meningitis: Inflammation of brain and spinal membranes
Meningococcal: Related to meningitis-causing bacteria
MERS-CoV: Middle East respiratory syndrome coronavirus
Metabolism: Routine biochemical processes in an organism to help maintain life
Metabolomics: The study of the role of small functional molecules in a metabolic pathway
Metagenomics: The study of the genetic material in the environment (ecological niche)
Methylotrophic: A group of organisms that utilise methyl compounds as the energy source
Meticulous: Extremely careful and precise in execution
MHC: Major histocompatibility complex
Miasmas: Foul-air believed to be contaminated and capable of causing a disease
Micelles: Small aggregates of molecules in solution
Microeconomy: The economic state of individuals, households or a business house

Microfluidic: The technology to manipulate small volumes of fluid
Microsimulation model: A small-scale predictive simulation technique
Migration: Movement of people or organisms from one place to another
Milieu: Environment or surrounding conditions
Milkmaid: An individual who milks the cow, related to smallpox immunity
Mimic: To imitate or replicate a process
Minigene: A small segment of a gene used in research
Mired: Stuck or entangled in difficulties
Misdemeanor: A criminal act that is not too serious in nature
Mitigate: To reduce the severity of a condition
ML: Machine learning
MMR: Measles, Mumps and Rubella
Mock viral assay: Simulated test for viral detection
Molecular docking: Computational technique to predict molecular binding of two molecules
Monoclonal antibody: Antibody derived from a single cell clone
Monovalent: A vaccine that is effective against a single antigen
Morbidity: The state of the occurrence of a disease
Morphogenesis: Development of shape and structure in an organism
Mortality: The number of deaths in a specified duration or in a specific place
Mortgage: A loan used to purchase, with a property (usually a real estate) as collateral
Mounted: To be put in place or set-up
MoU: Memorandum of understanding
mRNA: Messenger RNA
MRSA: Methicillin-resistant Staphylococcus aureus
MS: Mass spectrometry
Multi-graft: Procedure involving multiple tissue or organ transplants
Multilamellar: Having multiple layers, typically in structures like vesicles
Multi-stakeholders: Multiple parties with shared interest
Multivalent: A vaccine that targets multiple antigens
Mumps: A viral infection that affect the salivary glands
Mutable: Subject to change or variation
Mutagenesis: Process of introducing genetic mutations
Mutants: Organisms with mutated genes
Mutation: Changes or alterations in genetic material or DNA sequence
Myeloma: Cancer of the plasma cells in bone marrow
Myocarditis: Inflammation of the heart muscle

N

N: Nucleocapsid
NACI: National advisory committee on immunisation
NadA: N. meningitidis adhesin A
NADCP: National animal disease control programme
Nano coreshell: Nanoparticle structure with a core and a surrounding shell
Nano-lipid carrier: A tiny lipid-based vehicle for drug delivery
Nanomedicine: Applying nanotechnology in medical sciences
Nanoparticle: A sub-microscopic particle at nanometer scale
Nanovaccines: Vaccines that employ nanoparticles for delivery/administration
Nausea: A feeling of sickness with an urge to vomit

NCBI: National centre for biotechnology information
NDDB: National dairy development board
NEGVAC: National expert group on vaccine administration for COVID-19
Neoantigen: A novel antigen produced by a mutated cell
Neo-epitope: A new antigenic site formed due to a mutation
NetMHCPan4: A bioinformatics tool to predict T-cell epitopes
Neurodegenerative: Causing progressive loss of neuronal functions
Neutropenia: Abnormally low neutrophil count in the blood
Newcastle disease: A viral infection that affects the poultry
Next-gen: Refers to the latest generation of technology or products
NGIP: Next generation immune genome project
NGO: Non-governmental organisation
NHBA: Neisserial heparin binding antigen
NIAID: National institute of allergy and infectious diseases
Niche: Specific or specialised ecosystem for specific group of organisms
Nidovirales: The Order of a group of viruses that also include the coronaviruses
NIH: National institute of health (USA)
Nipped at bud: Stopped early before the situation worsens
NIR: Near-infrared
NIV: National institute of virology
NiV: Nipah virus
Nosocomial: Infections acquired in a hospital or healthcare setting
NSERC: Natural sciences and engineering research council
nsp: Non-structural protein
NTD: Neglected tropical disease
Nuclease: Enzyme that cleaves the nucleic acids
Nucleocapsid: The protein shell that surrounds the genetic material of a virus
Nucleoprotein: The protein associated with the cellular nucleic acids
Nutrigenomics: The study of nutrition functionalities and the associated genetic interaction

O

Oft-cited: Frequently referenced
Oligomer: Short chain of linked molecules
Oligonucleotides: Short DNA or RNA molecules
Omicron: A SARS-CoV-2 viral variant due to mutation
Omics: Large-scale insight of biological system at molecular level (e.g., genomics)
OMV: Outer membrane vesicle
Oncogenic: Cancercausing
Oncology: The study of traits and treatment of cancer
One health: A holistic approach that links human, animal and environmental health
OPV: Oral polio vaccine
Orchestrate: Organise or arrange systematically
ORF: Open reading frame
Organ failure: A condition (state-of-affair) wherein an organ ceases to function properly
Orthopoxvirus: A viral genera that includes the smallpox causing virus
Orthornavirae: A virus group that includes the coronaviruses
Otitis: A state of inflammation in the ear
Outbreak: A sudden rise in the incidence of a disease

Overrun: To exceed or overwhelm something
Over-the-counter: Medication that is made available without the need of a prescription
Overwhelming: Extremely intense or difficult to handle
OWID: Our world in data
Oxygenation: The process of adding oxygen to the body or tissues

P

PAHO: Pan American health organisation
Palpitation: Irregular or rapid heartbeat
Paltry: Too small to be considered important, useful or relevant
Panacea: Universal solution for all health-related issues
Pandemic: Widespread global disease outbreak
Pangolin: A mammal believed to have been involved in COVID-19 transmission
Paradigm: Model or standard of example/instance
Paradigm shift: Fundamental change in approach or perspective
Paramount: Of utmost importance
Parietal: Pertaining to the walls of a body cavity
PASC: Post-acute sequelae of SARS-CoV-2 infection
PAT: Process analytical technologies
Pathogen: A harmful microorganism that causes a disease
Pathogenesis: The process of disease development
Pathogenicity: The ability of a microorganism to cause a disease
Pathology: The study of diseases
Patrolling: Monitoring or surveying an area
Paucity: A scarcity or insufficiency of something
Peasant: Small-scale farmer or labourer
Peculiar: Unusual or distinctive in characteristics
Peer-review: Expert evaluation in a particular field for validation and quality control
PEG: Polyethylene glycol
Pentamer: A structure that is made up of five subunits or molecules
Peptide: Short chain of amino acids
Perfusion: The process of delivering blood or fluid to the tissues
Perinatal: Relating to the period around birth/parturition
Perpetually: Continuing forever or indefinitely
Persistent: Continuing for a long duration
Personalised medicine: Tailor-made treatment for individual patients
Pertussis: A contagious respiratory disease
Pharmacovigilance: Monitoring the effects of a drug for safety assurance
PHEIC: Public health emergency of international concern
Phenotype: Observable traits or characteristics of an organism
Philanthropic: Concerned with promoting human welfare, often through charity
Philanthropist sources: Resources or funding from charitable individuals
Phosphoprotein: Protein that has an attached phosphate group
Phylogenetics: The study of evolutionary relationships
Physicochemical: Relating to both physical and chemical properties
Pilot-scale: Intermediate testing phase before full-scale production
Pisoniviricetes: A class of viruses that includes Coronaviruses
Pisuviricota: A virus phylum that also includes those that cause respiratory infections

Pivotal: Crucial or important for success
PLA: People's liberation army
Placebo: Biologically inactive/inert substance that mimic a medicine, used in trials
Placebo-controlled A study that uses a placebo (pseudomedicine) for comparison purpose
Plague: A severe infectious disease by Yersinia pestis with high mortality
Planetary health: Sustainable health for the humans, animals and the Earth
Plasma B cells: Immune cells producing antibodies during an immune response
Plasmid: Circular DNA molecule used in genetic engineering
Plausible: Reasonable or likely to be true
Plentiful: Abundant or existing in substantial amount
Pleuropneumonia: Infection of lungs and pleural membranes
Plpro: Papain-like protease
Plug-and-play: A system that work immediately and automatically without complex set-up
Pneumococcal: Relating to the bacterium Streptococcus pneumoniae
Pneumonia: Inflammation of the lungs, often caused by an infection
POHA: Prudential one health approach
Poised: Ready for action or change
Polio: A viral disease that could lead to paralysis
PolypharmDB: A database of polypharmacology and drug interactions
Polyproteins: Long proteins that are cleaved into functional units
Polysaccharide: Carbohydrate made up of numerous forms of sugar molecules
Terminology Definition
Polyvalent vaccine: A vaccine that is effective against multiple pathogenic strains
Posed: Presented or suggested
Postcommercialisation: After a product is introduced in the market
Post harvest Activities after the act of harvesting a crop
Postulate: Suggest or assume as a hypothesis
Poultry: Domesticated birds raised for meat or eggs
Power outage: Interruptions in supply of the electricity supply
Prairie dog: A rodent that is linked to zoonotic diseases
Precautionary: Preventive measures for risk reduction
Precision: Accuracy and consistency in measurements or actions
Pre-clinical: The trials performed before the clinical trials involving human subjects
Precursor: A forerunner or something that leads to the development of something else
Predictive modelling: Using data and algorithms to predict future outcomes
Predisposing: Making prone to a specific condition
Pre-fusion: Referring to a virus form before it binds to the host cell
Prejudice: Bias or preconceived opinion not based on reason or experience
Preservative: A substance that could prevent decay or spoilage
Presumed: Assumed or believed without a definite proof
Pretext: False reason or excuse
Prevail: Won or triumphed
Prevalence: A population that is affected by a condition at a given point in time
Preventives: Measures or actions taken to avoid a disease manifestation
Prioritising: Giving more importance to certain tasks or goals
prM: Pre-membrane
Proclamation: An official announcement or declaration
Pro-clotting: Promoting the formation of blood clots
Profuse: Excessive or abundant in quantity

Progenitor: An ancestor or source
Programmability: The ability to be programmed or controlled
Proinflammatory: Inducing or promoting inflammation
Projection: Estimate or prediction of future events or data
Prominent: Important, noticeable or well-known
Promulgated: Officially announced or publicly declared
Propel: Driven or pushed forward
Propensity: A natural tendency or inclination to do something
Prophylaxis: Prevention of disease or infection
Proprietary: Privately owned or controlled
Protamine: A protein that is used as a blood anticoagulant
Protease: An enzyme that breaks down proteins
Protein folding: The process by which proteins acquire their functional shape
Protein trafficking: The process by which proteins are transported within the cell
Proteomics: The study of proteins, including their functions and structures
Protocol: Established procedure or standard guidelines
Prototype: An initial or original model
PRP: Polysaccharide polyribosylribitol phosphate
Psychological: Relating to the mind or mental processes
Pulmonary: Related to the lungs or respiratory system
Pulmonologist: Doctor specialising in lung diseases
Pursued: Chased or followed with intent
Pus: A thick fluid (usually off-white) produced due to sepsis/infection

Q

QbD: Quality by design
QSAR: Quantitative structure activity relationship
Quadripartite: Something that involves four collaborative entities
Quantum: A large or significant amount
Quarantine: The act of isolating a population to prevent the further spread of disease

R

Rabies: A viral disease by a virus group (including Lyssa) affecting nervous system
Rabipur: A vaccine used to prevent rabies infection
Raccoons: Eutherian placental mammals often linked to rabies transmission
Race: Social group defined by physical characteristics
Radiology: A medical imaging system used for planned diagnosis and treatment
Raman spectroscopy: A technique to analyse molecular vibrations
Ramification: Consequence or outcome of a particular action
Ramping: Increasing or intensifying efforts or production
Rapid scaling: Quick increase in production or capacity
Rash: Skin eruption or irritation
RBD: Receptor-binding domain
RDIF: Russian direct investment fund
RDTech: Recombinant DNA technology
Reactogenicity: The ability to cause immune reaction
Readiness: The state of being prepared for action or an event
Realigning: Adjusting for better alignment or purpose

Realm: An area of expertise or activity
Reassortment: Genetic mixing, often in viruses
Recession: Usually a long period of economic decline
Reckless: Done without consideration for consequences or safety
Recombinant: Produced by genetic engineering
Recur: To happen again or reappear
Redefined: Given new or clearer definition
Redox potential: To measure the tendency of the oxidation-reduction reaction
Redundancy: Unnecessary repetition or excess of irrelevant components
Reemergence: Reappearance of previously controlled issues
Regenerate: To restore or grow again
Regenerative medicine: Treatments aimed at healing or replacing damaged tissues
Regimen: A planned course of treatment
Rehearsal: Practice or trial run of activity
Remedy: Curatives or treatments to treat an ailment
Remerging: Coming back into prominence
Renal: Related to the kidney
Render: Made or caused to become
Replicase polyproteins: Viral proteins involved in replication
Replication: The process of copying (usually a genetic material or cells)
Resource allocation: Distribution of resources for specific directed purpose
Respiratory distress: The difficulty in effective breathing
Respiratory droplet Tiny saliva/mucus drop containing pathogens during coughing or sneezing
Respite: A temporary relief from a difficult situation
Resurgence: Renewed increase or revival of activity
Revaccination: Repeat vaccination to enhance immunity
Revalidation: The process of confirming continued validity of a thing
Revamped: Improved or restructured effectively
Reverse vaccinology: The approach to develop a vaccine by analysing the pathogen's genome
Reverse zoonosis: The transmission of a disease from the humans to animals
Rhesus macaque: A type of monkey often used in biomedical research
Ribonucleoprotein: The RNA and protein complex found in the cell
Riboviria: A group of viruses that includes RNA viruses
Rigorous: Strict, thorough and demanding in approach
Rinderpest: A viral disease in cattle that is allegedly eradicated
RNA interference: The process of silencing the genes using small RNA molecules
RNN: Recurrent neural network
RNP: Ribonucleoprotein
Robust: Strong and resilient
Rodent: Small mammals, like rats and mice
ROHA: Radical one health approach
Rollout: The introduction or implementation of a plan or product
Rotavirus: A virus that causes severe diarrhoea
RPV: Recombinant protein vaccine
RSV: Respiratory syncytial virus
RTC: Replication-transcriptional complex
Rubella: A viral infection (known as German measles) that causes a rash and fever
RV: Reverse vaccinology

RVV: Replicating viral vectors

S

S: Spike
Safeguard: A measure to protect from a harm
SAGE: Strategic advisory group of experts
Salmonellosis: Bacterial infection through the consumption of contaminated food
Sane: Reasonable and rational
Sanitisation: The process of cleaning to reduce pathogens
SARS: Severe acute respiratory syndrome
Satiric: Containing or expressing satire
Scaffolding: Structural framework supporting growth or development
Scalability: The ability to be expanded or grown
Scale-down: Reduced in size or scope
Scale-up: Expanding production or capacity to larger levels
Scarifying: Scratching to stimulate growth
Schistosomiasis: Parasitic disease affecting the intestines
Scrub typhus: Bacterial disease spread by mites
Scrutinising: Examining or inspecting carefully
SDG: Sustainable development goal
Seamless: Smooth and uninterrupted
Sectoral integration: Cooperation across multiple societal sectors
Seemingly: Appearing to be true but uncertain
Self-adjuvant: Acting as its own immune enhancer
Self-amplification: The process where the effect increases over time
Sensitivity: The capacity to detect or respond to changes or a stimulus
Sensor: A device that detects a change or a stimulus
Septic shock: A severe infection causing widespread inflammation and organ failure
Serendipity: Finding something valuable by chance
Sero-conversion: Development of detectable antibodies
Serogroup: A group of microorganisms classified by shared antigens
Serology: The study of blood serum and immune responses
Seroprevalence: The level of a pathogen in a population, measured by antibodies
Serosurvey: A study assessing the presence of specific antibodies in a population
Serotype: Distinctive variation within a species
Serum: Clear liquid of blood after removing blood cells and clotting proteins
Sexually promiscuous: Engaging in multiple sexual partners and complicated sexual relationships
Shear stress management: Controlling forces that cause deformation in materials
Shield: Protection from harm
Shingles: A painful viral skin infection
Shortcomings: Deficiencies or weaknesses in something
Shrews: Small mammals that could potentially transmit diseases
SII: Serum Institute of India, Pune
Simulation: The imitation or modelling of real-world processes for a study
Single-shot: A vaccine that requires only one dose
SIRS: Systemic inflammatory respiratory syndrome
Size-exclusion chromatography: A technique to separate (protein) molecules based on size

Size-exclusion hydrophobic interaction: This technique combines the size and hydrophobicity properties
Skill-set A range of skills or abilities
Skunks: Wild mammals, carriers of rabies
Slated: Scheduled or planned for action
Smallpox: A deadly viral disease that causes skin lesions and scarring
SMS: Short messaging services
Sneak past: Move quietly or undetected
Socioeconomic: Relating to society and economy
SOFA: sequential organ failure assessment
Solid-formulated: Prepared in solid state form for administration
Sought: Attempted to find or obtain something
Spectroscopy: A technique to study matter through its interaction with light
Spectrum: The range or extent of something
Spike protein: The viral surface protein (like in SARS-CoV-2) that allows cellular entry
Spill: Unintentional release or overflow
Spillback: Human-to-animal disease transmission
Spillover: Disease transmission from animals to humans
ssDNA: Single-stranded DNA
SSHRC: Social sciences and humanities research council
ssRNA-RT: Single-stranded RNA with reverse transcriptase
Stack: Arranged or organised in a pile
Stalks: Supporting structures in cells or plants; may refer to viral attachment sites
Stark disparity: Sharp or stark difference or contrast
Starkly: In a clear and striking manner
State-of-art: Highly advanced or innovative
Static: Not moving or changing
Steadfast: Firm and unwavering commitment
Stem-loop: A structure formed in RNA or DNA when a strand folds back on itself
Sterilisation: The process of eliminating all the viable microorganisms in a system
Steroid A drug that reduces inflammation and suppresses the immune system
Stifling: Oppressively hot or restricting
Stipulated: Formally specified or required by a rule or agreement
Stockpile: A reserve of goods or resources for future use
Strangling angel: A metaphor for something deadly or suffocating
Strata: Layers or levels, often of society or material
Streamline: To make something more efficient or simple
Strides: Progress or significant advancements
Striking: Noticeable or remarkable in appearance
Stringent: Strict or severe in requirements or conditions
Strive: Make determined efforts toward goals
Stupendous: Extremely impressive or remarkable
Sturdy: Strong and wellbuilt in structure
Subcutaneous: Under the skin layer
Sublineages: Subdivisions within evolutionary lineages
Suboptimal: Less than the best possible condition
Subside: Become less intense or severe
Substantial: Significant or considerable in amount

Subtropics: Region just outside the tropics
Subunit vaccines: Vaccines made from specific protein components
Subvariants: Variants derived from another variant, often with slight differences
Succumbed: Yielded to force or disease
Supersite region: The area on a virus where mutations may occur that affect its properties
Surplus: An excess or amount beyond what is needed
Surveillance: Ongoing observation and monitoring of data or behaviour
Suspension: Particles dispersed in liquid but not dissolved
Swiftly: Moving or acting quickly
Swine: Domesticated pigs
Symptomatic: Showing signs or symptoms of a disease
Syndrome: Group of symptoms occurring together to characterise a clinical condition
Syphilis: A sexually transmitted bacterial infection
Systemic: Affecting the entire body or system

T

Tackling: Addressing or dealing with problem
Tailored: Customized to meet specific needs
Tangential flow filtration: Membrane filtration process for separation
Tangible interventions: Concrete measures with visible outcomes
TB: Tuberculosis
TBEV: Tickborne encephalitis virus
TCRdb: Comprehensive T-cell receptor database
Tecovirimat: Antiviral drug treating smallpox infections
Teleworking: Working remotely, often via digital tools
Temporal: Relating to time or duration
Tetanus: Bacterial infection causing muscle spasms and rigidity
Tetravalent: Having four components or effects
Therapeutic: Related to treatment of diseases or conditions
Thermostability: Resistance to changes under heat
Thriving: Flourishing or doing well
Thrombocytopenia: A condition of low platelet counts in the blood
Thrombosis: Formation of a blood clot in a vessel
Throttles: Regulates or limits flow or activity
Throughput: Amount of material processed in given time
THSTI: Translational Health Science and Technology Institute
Time lag: Delay between events or actions
Titre: The concentration or quantity of an antibody or antigen in a sample
TM: Transmembrane
TMPRSS 2: Transmembrane protease serine 2
Toll: The amount of damage or loss caused by an event or phenomenon
Toolkit: A set of tools or resources for a specific purpose
Topography: The arrangement of physical features in an area
Toxicants: Toxic substances or poisons
Toxicity: Degree to which substance can harm organisms
Toxoid: Inactivated toxin used in vaccines
Toxoplasmosis: Parasitic disease affecting humans and animals
Transcription: The synthesis of RNA from a DNA template

Transfer learning: A ML technique where the lessons learnt from a task is applied to another
Transfixed: Motionless due to shock or awe
Transformative: Causing significant change or improvement
Transfusion: Transfer of blood or fluids
Transgene: Gene introduced into an organism
Transgenic: Organism with genes from another species
Transient: Temporary or shortlived
Translation: The process of converting RNA into proteins
Transmembrane: Across or spanning a membrane, typically in biological contexts
Transmissive: Capable of spreading infections
Transnationally: Acrossmultiple countries
Treaties: Formal agreements between parties
Trimeric: Composed of three subunits or molecules
TRIPS: Trade-related aspects of intellectual property rights
Triumph: Great success or victory
Tropical: Relating to regions near equator
Tubercle: A small nodular lesion, especially in tuberculosis
Tubing: Flexible tubes used for conveying fluids or gases
Tumours: Abnormal growths of tissue, often cancerous
Typhus: Infectious disease caused by bacteria

U

UIP: Universal immunisation programme
Ultracentrifugation: Highspeed spinning used to separate particles
UN: United Nations
Underbelly: Weaker or vulnerable aspect
UNEP: UN environmental programme
Unforeseen: Unexpected or not predicted events
UNICEF: United Nations international children's emergency fund
Unprecedented: Never before experienced or done
Unravel: To disentangle or solve
UNSIC: United Nations system influenza coordination
Untoward: Unexpected or inappropriate
Untranslated regions: Noncoding parts of RNA sequences
Upfront: In advance or at beginning
Upstreaming: Moving processes closer to raw materials
Upsurge: Sudden increase or rise
US: The United States of America
USDA: United States department of agriculture
USFDA: United Statesfood and drug administration
Ushering: Guiding or introducing into a new phase
UTR: Untranslated region

V

Vacca: Likely referring to a genus or research term related to vaccines
Vaccinating: Administering vaccine to prevent disease
Vaccination: Administration of a vaccine to protect against disease
Vaccines: Biological preparation to induce immunity

Vaccinologists: Experts in vaccine development and research
Vaccinology: The study and science of vaccines
Variants: Different forms or strains
Varicella: Chickenpox viral infection
Variolae: The virus causing smallpox
Variolation: Early method of smallpox inoculation
Vector-borne: Transmitted by organisms like insects
Vectored Vaccines: Vaccines using a virus to deliver the vaccine genetic material
Venous thromboembolism: A condition where blood clots form in veins and travel to the lungs
Venturing: Daring or undertaking something risky
Vero cell-derived: Originating from a cell line used for growing viruses in vaccine production
Vero cell-line: Derived cells used in virology studies
Vesicular stomatitis: Viral disease affecting livestock
Viable: Capable of living or functioning
Vigilant: Watchful and alert for danger
ViPR: Virus pathogen resource
Virgin: Untouched or not previously affected
Virion: Complete, infectious form of a virus outside a host cell
Virtual screening: Computational technique for identifying potential drug candidates
Virulence: Degree of damage or harm caused by a pathogen
Virulent: Extremely infectious or harmful
Visceral: Related to internal organs, especially those in the abdomen
Vistas: Expansive views or prospects
VLP: Viruslike particle
VOC: Variants of concern
Void: Empty space
Voles: Small rodents similar to mice
Volunteers: Individuals who offer their services without compensation
Vowed: Promised solemnly or pledged
VPD: Vaccine preventable diseases
VUCA: Volatile, uncertain, complex and ambiguous
Vulnerable: Susceptible to harm or damage
VWF: Von Willebrand factor

W

Wake: Aftermath or trail left behind
Waned: Gradually decreased in strength
Waning immunity: Declining immune protection over time
War-footing: Emergency preparation for crisis situations
Wearable sensor: Devices worn on the body to monitor health or environmental data
Wet market: A marketplace to sell live animals, often linked to zoonotic diseases
Wet lab: Laboratory involving hands-on experiments with biological materials.
WFI: Water for injection
WHO: World health organisation
Whole genome sequencing: A process to determine the complete DNA sequence of an organism
Wildlife dynamics: Changes and interactions within wildlife populations
With ease: Accomplishing something without difficulty

WOAH: World organisation for animal health
Woodchuck: Type of rodent often used in biological studies
Worldviews: Comprehensive perspectives on life and society
Terminology Definition
Worrisome: Causing concern or anxiety
Wreaked: Caused destruction or damage
WTO: World trade organisation

X

Xenograft: Transplant from different species
Yellow fever: Viral disease transmitted by mosquitoes

Y

YNPRC: Yerkes national primate research centre

Z

Zaire ebolavirus: Strain of ebola virus causing severe outbreaks
Zoometric transition: Shift in patterns of zoonotic diseases
Zoonosis: Diseases that can be transmitted from animals to humans
Zoonotic diseases: Diseases spread from animals to humans

1

Historical Perspectives and Future Direction of Vaccine Development

Pratikhya Mohanty[1], Monali Kerketta[2] and Snehasish Mishra[1]

[1]School of Biotechnology, Kalinga Institute of Industrial Technology (KIIT) Deemed-to-be University, Bhubaneswar-751 024, Odisha, India
[2]Reseapro Scientific Services Pvt. Ltd., DCB-401, 4th floor, DLF Cyber City Chandaka Industrial Estate, Patia, Bhubaneswar-751024, Odisha, India

Abstract

This chapter attempts to travel the timeline and dissect historical perspectives of vaccination. Vaccine that protects and shields from numerous dangerous diseases (vaccine-preventable diseases; VPD) is an important area of research and development. Considering that vaccine has been very useful in successfully combating numerous infectious diseases in the past 200 years, they are considered as a historical turning point in the field of public health and medicines. Critical illnesses like the smallpox and wild polio (virus types 2 and 3) have mostly been eradicated as a result of mass immunisation programmes worldwide. Research, collaboration and widespread vaccination campaigns were necessary in vaccination efforts to control and ultimately eradicate infectious diseases. Biotechnological research has progressed to a level where producing recombinant vaccines is feasible. Research and development efforts on therapeutic vaccines are ongoing. Vaccine research in recombinant DNA/RNA technologies and therapeutic vaccinations for specific illnesses seem to be the future. This article offers a comprehensive history of vaccination since inception to its present forms, with future projections. Beginning with the variolation techniques in the early 17th century, it discusses the important turn of events from its discovery to the continued advancements and inventions till the covid-19 vaccine. Alongside the detailed core aspect, the chapter also describes the benefits of the one health approach with the zoonotic diseases in focus.

***Keywords*:** Infectious disease, Public health, Smallpox, Polio, Vaccination, Immunisation, One health approach.

1. Introduction

Profound research initiatives are perpetually thriving across the globe to address threats of the ever-evolving infectious diseases. Vaccines continue to shine as the most potent beacon of hope in the combat (Sah *et al.*, 2021; Mohapatra *et al.*, 2022). Over 20 vaccines are widely used at present to prevent various infectious viral diseases such as small pox, measles, mumps, etc. While vaccine discovery was noteworthy, the rapid increase in the numerous infectious diseases that inflict both humans and animals is worrisome (Mohapatra *et al.*, 2024a; Satapathy *et al.*, 2023). The increasing occurrences of the emerging and reemerging lethal infectious diseases have challenged human civilisation worldwide, threatening the very existence (Mohapatra *et al.*, 2020; Mohapatra *et al.*, 2021; Sarangi *et al.*, 2024). Due to constantly evolving mutated forms of the aetiological agents, a significant knowledge gap in understanding the intricate relationships between the host and the pathogen seems to exist (Conceição Silva *et al.*, 2023; Mohapatra *et al.*, 2023; Mohapatra *et al.*, 2024b).

In the wake of rapidly increasing deaths caused by the infectious disease smallpox in the 18th century, the basis of vaccination was laid by an English physician Edward Jenner along with his aide Benjamin Jesty. Their remarkable minute observations resulted in the development of vaccines that were adopted globally and contributed to critical advancements in medical sciences. Louis Pasteur further paved new ways that contradicted the traditional concept of spontaneous generations, while investigating into various manners of fermentations. Pasteur coined the term 'vaccination' honouring Edward Jenner's work (vacca means cow from which the vaccination term is adopted; Edward Jenner discovered smallpox vaccine from cowpox). Robert Koch, a German physician, is another great contributor to the advancements in vaccinology. Interested in microbial science, he successfully isolated *Bacillus anthracis* in its pure form and demonstrated the organismal interactions, manifestation of the disease and lifecycle of Anthrax.

The concept of booster vaccine arose later after the mechanism of the immune system in response to the vaccine was well-understood (Zakir *et al.*, 2019). Joseph Lister, a surgeon, attended the seventh International Medical Conference at London in 1881, and was inspired by Pasteur's findings that led to the origin of the principle of antisepsis in surgery. Koch demonstrated a technique to isolate and stain bacteria, and highlighted the significance. He refused to acknowledge Pasteur's discovery of attenuation techniques as he believed that the microbes possessed very specific biological and chemical properties. Contradictory to Koch's postulate, Pasteur believed that microbial constituents could be lost and regained. Later, he developed the rabies vaccine, a significant discovery in the history of medicines.

It was believed for a considerable duration that TB could be solely treated by antibiotics. Behring Kitasato prepared tubercle vaccine from human tubercle bacilli in 1902 adopting the process of attenuation. He termed it as 'Bovo vaccine', the ultimate significant vaccine made against tuberculosis bacilli. However, the vaccine posed an infection risk from the immunised animals (Montero *et al.*, 2024). Albert Calmette and Camille Guérin developed the 'Bacillus Calmette-Guérin' vaccine later using attenuated *Mycobacterium bovis* strain. With better safety profile, BCG remains the most globally used vaccines against tuberculosis till date. BCG brought reassurance for several decades (Zakir *et al.*, 2019). Vaccination lies on the principle of developing long-term immunity against one or more pathogen-specific antigens by fostering antibodies and development cytotoxic T-cells. The overall event is of three steps, i) Antigens Presenting Cells (APCs) take up antigens and adjuvants, ii) APCs maturation occurs, iii) Antibodies and cytotoxic T-cells are produced by the antigen-specific B- and T-cells (D'Amico *et al.*, 2021).

Several factors contribute to the increased human lifespan and decreased mortality rate, chief among which is controlling disease transmission, reducing host susceptibility, and adopting regular hygiene practices. Advances in public health have collectively played a major role in eradicating pathogenic diseases like polio (virus types 2, 3) and smallpox. Diseases like measles, mumps, diptheria, rubella and pertussis currently are widely under control. Despite the numerous progresses, there are still noticeable gaps in vaccine arsenal. One of the most prominent is HIV/AIDS, a global concern that has persisted for years and the vaccine is still under clinical trials. The challenge of emerging infectious diseases still remains a threat. It can be exemplified by recent COVID-19 global pandemic. Advancements in biotechnological techniques helped expedite vaccines development against COVID-19, although meant for 'emergency use' only (Montero *et al.*, 2024).

2. History of Vaccine Development

History is often regarded as ambivalence by some, but science can only be acknowledged as the evolution of ideas and inventions unlike other fields. Aeschylus quotes, "memory is the mother of all wisdom". Vaccine development has its origin in a discovery that is an oft-cited example of serendipity. The astounding rise in the occurrence of global pandemics had a huge impact on human civilisation which influenced the urgency to address these critical infectious diseases. Vaccination concept dates back to the 6th century wherein a Chinese classical text on medicines 'The Golden Mirror of Medicines' depicted the various inoculation techniques like variolation. The process involved inhaling the powder of the scabs obtained from human smallpox lesions or stuffing the smallpox vesicles filled cotton into the nose (Cleri *et al.*, 2006). Powdered scabs administration technique was tried in Turkey by scarifying the skin. Learning about viariolation in Constantinople, Mary Wortley Montagu is considered as the first person to practice it on her daughter, in 1721. Her practice gained public attention during the reign of King George I, and followed its mass inoculation on a gang of prisoners and orphans. Variolation resulted in positive outcomes, although the results were inconsistent in about 2–3% of the patients who succumbed to death. The deaths were however attributed to syphilis infection. Variolation technique was employed to counteract cattle plague and measles that had severely affected Europe during the time. Mentioning about measles, a British researcher Francis Home expressed his interest to alleviate the disease in 1758 in similar lines as the Turks had practiced it to combat smallpox.

Edward Jenner is credited for his initiatives to mitigate infectious disease smallpox by inoculating cowpox. After vigorous study for 25 years, Jenner published his work in 1798 on the relationship between cowpox and smallpox based on his 1796 path-breaking observations. He inoculated an eight-year old boy James Phipps with cowpox vesicles and later exposed him to smallpox virus with no visible health complications. The term 'Vaccination' was first coined by Paseur during the 19th century, as a tribute to Jenner. Modern day virus genome studies indicate that the cowpox virus was actually the 'poxvirus' in horses. Significance was attached to understanding infectious diseases thoroughly and developing relative pathology. It was soon realised that a contagious disease was caused by a living organism ('*contagium vivum*').

The fowl cholera by *Pasteurella multocida* remained static in microbiology field during the course of 82 years of Jenner's treaties on variolae vaccinae, vaccine development progenitor. Jacob Henle, a German pathologist and anatomist, demonstrated that living organisms were the cause of disease, and not miasmas. Henle emphasised that, it is necessary to culture the microbes outside of the hosts (*in vitro*) to decipher the interaction of the casual agent, infection and the disease manifestation mechanism. Robert Koch's postulate outlined the important characteristics of infection causing microbes. It involved isolating microbial pure culture and introducing it into a suitable host. It proved to be a remarkable breakthrough in the extensive investigation to develop prophylaxis (vaccine) and therapeutic serum treatments (Burke, 1993). Fig. 1 presents the timeline of vaccine discovery and development till date.

3. Earlier Scientific Endeavours

After Jenner's momentous discovery, Pasteur laid vaccine discovery platform and performed animal trials. He injected chicken with controlled dose of *Pasteurella multocida* pure culture that caused fowl cholera and observed no visible symptoms, a vital discovery in 1880.

Virulent culture subsequently injected in chickens showed no unfavourable development. His conclusions from his study were, a) the virulence property of pathogens can be attenuated if the culture is stored for some time, and b) immunity can be achieved artificially with the help of attenuated cultures. Poultry cholera vaccine was the chief experimentally produced vaccine that immediately followed the successes in anthrax (1881) and rabies (1885). Pasteur's immunisation studies were followed by many researchers, particularly by Von Behring and Kitasato who developed diphtheria antitoxin in 1890 (Kantha, 1991). This was the first therapy that demonstrated decrement in both mortality and morbidity rates.

Also called 'strangling angel of children', Diptheria was a deadly disease with almost 40% mortality (Galazka *et al.*, 1995). Investigations on diphtheria involved several processes including quality checking of immunobiologicals. Vaccine discovery and process fine-tuning during the late 19th century was a boon in combating infectious diseases like TB, typhus, typhoid and syphilis. There were numerous disease threats that prevailed and were difficult to manage due to limited knowledge on immunology. Even though vaccine development started earlier with smallpox and rabies, advanced techniques for mass vaccine development started during late 1950s with invent of tissue culture technology (Baker and Katz 2004).

The period 1900–1950 was the golden era of cell culture, pathology and immunology. Efforts focused to analyse disease mechanism that included transmission, use of adjuvants, immune response types; antibody-antigen interactions, specificity, and cellular and humoral immunity. Ramon succeeded in developing a cure for diphtheria and tetanus toxins in 1923 and 1927 respectively (Cavaillon, 2018). Roux developed *in vitro* cell culture in 1885 for the first time. A significant progress was also witnessed in 1928 when Fleming produced penicillin, which facilitated in fine-tuning the cell culture technique for vaccine production. Culturing the Lansing strain of poliovirus in non-nervous system human tissues gave a promising direction to mass production of polio vaccine, described in the published work of Enders, Weller and Robbin in 1949 (Eggers, 2002). Attenuated oral polio vaccine was successfully developed by Sabin in 1955, while Salk successfully used cell culture in 1960 and produced deactivated human polio vaccine in the early 1970s.

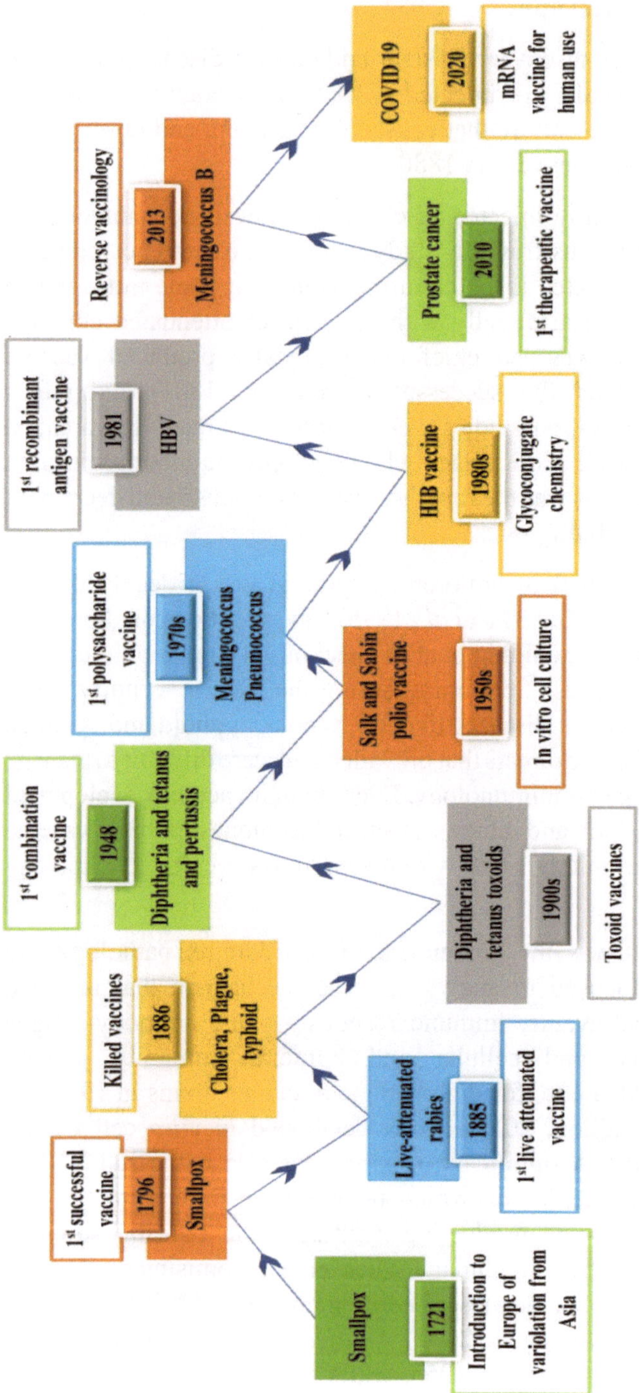

Fig. 1: A graphical presentation of the history and timeline of vaccine development

Emergence of combination (multivalent) vaccine offered prevention against multiple diseases (measles, mumps and rubella; MMR vaccine). It reduced the need for multiple inoculations and augmented traditional immunisation technique. Applying MMR vaccine considerably improved the global disease burden and wellbeing scenario. Measles recorded approximately 2.6 million annual deaths round the globe in the 1980s. The death rate has reduced to about 140,000 by 2018 and health standards have improved globally after vaccination campaigns. Michiaki Takahashi devised vaccines against varicella-zoster virus by primarily inoculating it in to human embryonic lung cells after its successful trial on guinea pig embryonic cells. It was approved in Korea and Japan in 1978 and in the US and other countries in 1995.

Hepatitis B vaccine discovery marked a breakthrough in immunology and its research helped understand the concept of the infection-induced cancers. The hepatitis B vaccine was first developed in 1982 by extracting and purifying the surface protein of the virus using molecular techniques. This technique proved to decrease the hepatocellular carcinoma risk and transmission of hepatotropic infections. The vaccine is currently employed in vaccinating children in many WHO member countries. *Neisseria meningitidis*, *Streptococcus pneumoniae* and *Haemophilus influenzae* type b (Hib) were considered in the 1980s as a common cause of child death. Several vaccines production strategies were simultaneously applied among which the capsular polysaccharides approach was popular. The polysaccharide-protein conjugation concept to enhance immunogenicity was laid in 1930s.

Implemented in 1981 to combat *N. meningitidis* serogroups A, C, W and Y, this strategy failed to show its potentials on serogroup B due to the hurdles that occurred in the biochemical interactions between the serogroup's pathogen capsule and the lipids in human nervous system. 23vPPV vaccine targeting *S. pneumoniae* was approved simultaneously with the polysaccharide vaccine against Hib in 1983. Hib Conjugated vaccine was also approved later. Conjugated polysaccharide (MenC) vaccine for *N. meningitidis* serogroup C in 1999 followed the approval of serogroups A, C, W and Y (MenACWY). *S. pneumoniae* conjugated vaccine (PCV) involving serotypes PCV7, PCV10 and PCV13, PCV15 and PCV20 was approved in early 2000s. Licensing of prime inactivated oral cholera vaccine (OCV) marked as a development in that year that was significant and influential during emergencies, natural disasters and military conflict regions with limited sanitary facilities. The vaccine effectively countered *Vibrio cholerae* that caused cholera. Whooping cough targeted recombinant acellular vaccine was first produced in 1992, considered as a good replacement to the existing whole-cell pertussis vaccine. Inactivated hepatitis A vaccine was approved the same year, followed by an array of other hepatitis A vaccines successively.

4. Emerging Technologies and Vaccinology in The 21st Century

The 21st century saw steady discoveries, including the vaccines against rotavirus and human papillomavirus (HPV). Rotavirus is the most common cause of acute diarrhoea worldwide among kids under five. Licenses for two rotavirus vaccines were granted in 2006, one based on the attenuation technique and the other based on a revolutionary molecular technique of virus reassortment that allowed expression of a particular gene in specific animal rotavirus strain as framework. Few others have been developed since then, embraced by more than 100 countries (O'Ryan *et al.*, 2015). Owing to the substantial impact of rotavirus disease in infants, the World Health Organisation (WHO) suggested including oral rotavirus vaccine in 2009 into regular childhood immunisation programmes. As a consequence, hospitalisations due to rotavirus decreased by 40% in children under the 5-years age in nations that embraced this vaccination programmes. The global annual rotavirus-induced diarrhoea-related fatalities declined by 25% during this period (Burnett *et al.*, 2020).

Introduction of first HPV vaccination approved in 2006 represented a significant advance in the fight against cervical cancer in women folks. This vaccine contained certain attenuated oncogenic forms and successfully prevented cervical and other HPV-linked malignancies (Gee *et al.*, 2016). Many nations have included HPV vaccine in their routine immunisation programmes, especially for women in their early teens. The vaccine is also suggested for men to avert penile cancer, anal cancer and other HPV-linked malignancies (Montero *et al.*, 2024). The vaccine provides protection against the most prevalent oncogenic HPV strains (Wang *et al.*, 2020). HPV vaccination is a preventive measure and does not guarantee safety against all HPV forms or act as therapeutics.

Development of *N. meningitidis* serogroup B (MenB) vaccine greatly changed our knowledge of and methods to conduct vaccine research, with invent of reverse vaccinology (RV). RV is a technique that uses powerful computer (*in silico*) analysis and examines the entire genetic makeup of a pathogen to predict the part (antigen) that triggered immune response, unlike the conventional 'isolate, inactivate, and inject' Pasteur's approach. Novel RV strategy is crucial for infections like MenB for which traditional strategies did not work (Adu-Bobie *et al.*, 2003). Antigenic resemblance of capsular polysaccharide of MenB with human glycoproteins caused weak immunogenic reactivity, posing autoimmunity concerns (Griffiss *et al.*, 1991).

Genome sequence of MenB MC58's was available online in 2000 (Montero *et al.*, 2024). After analysing this genome thoroughly, a total of 570 were shortlisted bioinformatically (*in silico*) as released or surface-exposed proteins. 350 of these were successfully cloned and expressed in *E. coli*. Many of the recombinant proteins had encouraging outcome when they were administered in mice: 91 of them showed immunogenicity and 28 elicited the creation of bactericidal antibodies, indicating at their suitability as candidates for vaccine production (Pizza *et al.*, 2000). Considering that the antigenicity of few of these were discovered even before the protein was identified, such unique approach to discover bactericidal antigens was breakthrough advancement in vaccine development (Masignani *et al.*, 2019). With more details about the MenB genome available, a thorough analysis of MenB strains in circulation was possible, providing valuable information about the variety and conserved sequences of the meningococcal antigens. Consequent to this assessment, three conserved bactericidal antigens were identified: factor H binding protein (fHbp), Neisseria heparin conjugated antigen (NHBA) and *N. meningitidis* adhesion A (NadA).

5. Recent Advancements in Vaccinology

Recent advancements in vaccine development have led to the numerous innovative strategies designed to improve immunogenicity, safety and efficacy of a discovered vaccine candidate. Some such path-breaking successful innovative interventions and their strategic beneficial outcomes are briefed below.

5.1. Adjuvants

Adjuvant is a compound that is added to a vaccine to enhance the functionality of the vaccine candidate by the virtue of which the vaccine recipient reveals greater immunological response against the target antigen. It was one of the history-defying discoveries with sustained benefits to vaccinological advancements. The modern-day adjuvants like aluminium salts, MF59 and AS01, not only enhance the immunogenicity of a vaccine but also modulate the immune system pathways, particularly by activating the innate immunity (Pulendran *et al.*, 2021). For instance, AS01 has demonstrated the ability to elicit humoral and cellular immunological responses, making it an essential component in the Mosquirix malaria vaccine (Stanisic and Good, 2023).

5.2. Monoclonal Antibodies (mAbs)

The discovery of monoclonal antibodies (mAbs) by Kohler and Milstein was a significant breakthrough and paved the way for vaccine development and immunotherapy. mAbs are bioengineered to recognise and bind to the specific target pathogen thereby either neutralising it directly or biomarking it to be destroyed by other specified immune cells. These antibodies could also serve as vaccine adjuncts, providing immediate and temporary but effective immunity while the body gets a buffer time to develop more robust and sustained immune response (Varadé *et al.*, 2021). The use of mAbs in COVID-19 vaccines during the recent pandemic demonstrated the protection that they offered even before the immune system of the subject produced its own protective antibodies (Chary *et al.*, 2023).

5.3. Molecular Vaccines

Molecular vaccines include DNA, RNA and protein subunit vaccines, and these have gained considerable attention owing to their precision and adaptability. DNA vaccine introduces a piece of DNA encoding the antigen of a subject pathogen into the host cells, leading to the production of the specified antigen and the immune response subsequently (Acosta-Coley *et al.*, 2022). RNA vaccines, such as the Pfizer-BioNTech and Moderna COVID-19 vaccines, used messenger RNA (mRNA) to instruct the host cell to produce the specified antigen qualitatively and quantitatively (Acosta-Coley *et al.*, 2022). RNA vaccine designing and production are faster, that make them a valuable tool in tackling a suddenly-emerging pandemic situation. Protein subunit vaccines deliver only the essential antigenic portion of a target pathogen to elicit immune responses. These vaccines do not need the introduction of the whole virus or bacterium, thus reducing the risk of side-effects and accidental manifestation of the disease. The Hepatitis B and human papillomavirus (HPV) vaccines exemplify such a vaccine development approach (Dadar *et al.*, 2018). Another molecular approach is seen in viral vector vaccines, like the COVID-19 vaccine of Johnson & Johnson, which used a modified virus (typically a harmless adenovirus) particle to deliver the genetic material from the target pathogen into the host body that elicited an immune response (Acosta-Coley *et al.*, 2022).

Likewise, the other advancements in vaccine development technology include the use of the virus-like particles (VLPs) and outer membrane vesicles (OMVs) that mimicked the structure of the virus while remaining non-infectious as they would lack the required pathogenic genetic material. VLPs and OMVs provide highly immunogenic platforms due to their ability to mimic natural infections. These are being explored in developing vaccines against diseases like influenza, HPV and malaria (Dadar *et al.*, 2018). The future of vaccine research and development lies in the advancements of such technological developments that would potentially offer more effective, expeditious and comprehensive protection against a range of diseases including the emerging ones.

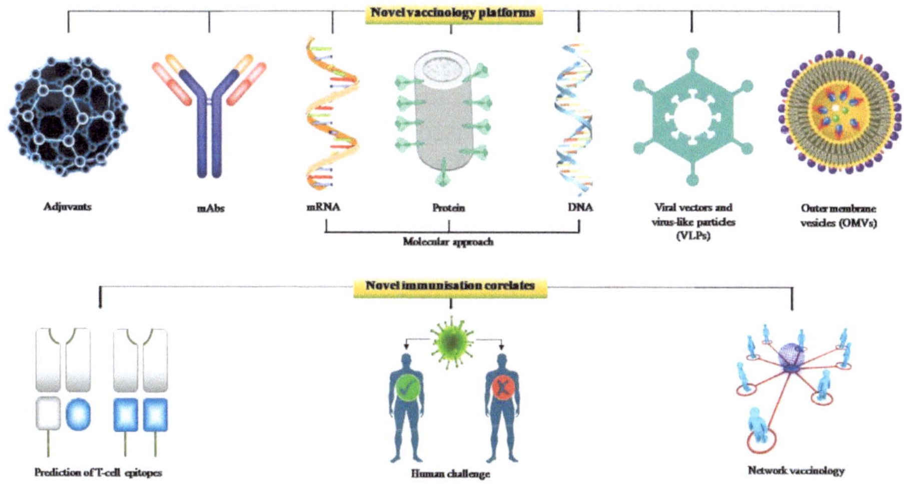

Fig. 2: Advancements in vaccine development platforms and immunity enhancement tools

The multi-component vaccine was approved in Europe and Canada (in 2013) and in the US (in 2015), and other nations followed suit (Masignani *et al.*, 2019). The US (in 2014) and Europe (in 2017) approved second MenB vaccine rLP2086 was concurrently produced. It comprised two fHbp protein versions (Villena *et al.*, 2018). Clinical trials to assess efficacy and safety of the combined vaccination of two licensed meningococcal ABCWY vaccines MenACWY and rLP2086 were started in 2017 (Peterson *et al.*, 2023). With the COVID-19 pandemic still round the corner, the pace of vaccine research and development need to be accelerated further. It is more critical with the emerging, reemerging and evolving infectious diseases, revealed through numerous recent literatures. COVID-19 pandemic has highlighted the benefits of the knowledge on vaccines and vaccinology, including integration of various related scientific fields to collaborate for the common good, the relevance of the 'One Health' strategy, and repositioning, repurposing and the potential usefulness of the less-practiced techniques and technologies.

Consequently, various SARS-CoV-2-targeted vaccines were developed at an unparalleled pace, although for 'emergency use' (complete safety, efficacy and human trials are pending) only. The efficient pace of the vaccines' development was possible owing to the on-site infrastructure already in place for novel vaccines (like vector-based delivery systems, mRNA and DNA-based vaccines) and substantial prior research data on SARS-CoV-1 and MERS (coronaviruses) with similar genetic make-up. Some top vaccine candidates could proceed rapidly from preclinical screening to Phase I clinical trials due to this (Chakraborty *et al.*, 2021). The mRNA-based vaccine synthesis technique (mRNA inserted into human cell using viral vector or delivered liposome-encapsulated) followed more rigorously during the pandemic was among the most inventive strategies. Such innovative vaccines successfully prevented SARS-CoV-2 from further damage caused by its wide spread around the world and sustenance for long which significantly helped to finally overcome the pandemic (Altmann and Boyton, 2022).

The formalin-inactivated RSV vaccine used in the 1960s during spontaneous RSV infections in children seemingly did not provide desired protection; rather it made lung inflammatory responses extremely worse. Consequently, the security issues significantly decelerated RSV vaccine development for decades (Venkatesan *et al.*, 2023). The fusion protein (F), known to be crucial to viral entrance and has a conserved sequence, is one of the proteins adorning the RSV surface. It is also an ideal target for vaccine manufacturing. The F protein existed in the pre-fusion and post-fusion phases with two intricate structural configurations. Significantly, formalin-inactivated RSV lacked the pre-fusion surface F protein while a contagious RSV possesses it (Killikelly *et al.*, 2016). Antigen diversity and the altered protein conformations were the obstacles that challenged the development of RSV vaccines. Table 1 lists the various vaccine types with their characteristics and limitations.

Table 1: A list of the various forms of vaccines, their characteristics and limitations

Type	Characteristics	Limitations/disadvantages
Live attenuated	Weakened form of pathogen offers long-lasting immunity, often with a single dose; multiple doses needed in certain cases	Not advised for people with weak immunity. Minimal chance that the infection may be seen as the attenuated form gains virulence
Inactivated	Incapable to replicate being inactivated; provides protection even to those with weak immunity	Protection is less persistent compared to live-attenuated vaccine; multiple doses needed
Subunit	Contains antigenic component of pathogen; safe for those with weak immune system	Protection is less persistent than live-attenuated vaccine; multiple doses needed
Toxoid	Benign toxin derivative; provokes immunity directed towards the toxin, not the infection	Multiple doses needed; could trigger allergic reactions in some
Vector-based	Microbes as vectors carrying gene sequences encoding for specific pathogenic antigen. Replicability of the vector is uncertain	Efficacy is less in people already immune to the vector. Immune-deficient populations are not advised to take these replicative vectors

Type	Characteristics	Limitations/disadvantages
Nucleic acid	Genetic material (mRNA or DNA) encoding specific virulence protein enclosed in a lipid vesicle or electroporation injected. It can be developed and manufactured rapidly	Requires very low storage temperature. The long-term consequences need assertion and are being investigated

Through many obstacles on way to the successful synthesis of Respiratory Syncytial Virus (RSV) vaccine, it was finally approved in 2023 by the US (USFDA) and Europe (EMA). The AS01 adjuvant and the pre-fusion F protein are present in this RSV vaccine (RSVpreF3OA) approved for the first time ever. This vaccination is approved in principle intended for individuals over the age of 60 (Papi *et al.*, 2023). The second vaccine (RSVPreF; a bivalent vaccine) contains equal levels of the pre-fusion F protein as it is prominent in the two (RSVA and RSVB) RSV subgroups. This second vaccination is licensed for the pregnant (between 32 and 36 gestation weeks) to protect the unborn till six months (Kampmann *et al.*, 2023) along with individuals over 60 years of age (Walsh *et al.*, 2023).

6. Immunity Enhancement Tools

In recent years, immunity enhancement tools have evolved that are capable of optimising the vaccine efficacy and providing enhanced protection against targeted infectious diseases. A critical area of advancements is the identification and application of T-cell epitopes in designing the vaccines. T-cell epitopes are short protein fragments that could be recognised by the T-cells, which play a pivotal role in cellular immunity. The objective to include these epitopes, especially from cytotoxic T-cells, into a vaccine candidate is to stimulate stronger and enduring immune responses which have the ability to eliminate the infected cells directly. T-cell epitope-based vaccines are particularly valuable against the diseases where the pathogen has been obligately internalised in the cells, such as viruses like the HIV or intracellular bacteria like *Mycobacterium tuberculosis* (Gong *et al.*, 2022). These epitopes could be combined with the adjuvants to further amplify the immune responses, providing a targeted approach to the development of a long-term immunity.

Yet another useful approach in enhancing immunity through vaccines involves the human challenge studies, where the human volunteers are deliberately exposed to the target pathogen after the vaccine is administered. However, such studies are often considered inhumane, being controversial and ethically compromising. Human challenge trials could nevertheless provide valuable information about the efficacy of a modified vaccine candidate, the immunological response it could elicit, and potential side-effects if any. Such studies have proven especially helpful in accelerating the development of vaccines against cholera, malaria, and the most recently, COVID-19 vaccines (Acosta-Coley *et al.*, 2022). Although the ethical considerations play a major deciding role in such studies, these seem to be important tools in modern vaccine research and development as they are capable of expediting vaccine development and optimising the dosing regimen.

With greater understandings of the need for equitable immunity and the role of herd immunity, vaccinology has undergone significant advancements. Herd immunity occurs when a sufficient portion of the population to a threshold level is vaccinated, that extend the provision of indirect protection to the unvaccinated individuals by reducing the overall transmission of the pathogen. The 'unvaccinated individuals' would include the human (or even animal) subjects that could not be vaccinated for health (immune-compromised), social (economic or population pressure), age (very old or very young age) or psychological (vaccine hesitancy) reasons. This concept has been central to the numerous vaccination campaigns for chronic diseases (like the measles, rubella and polio) wherein these disease outbreaks could be successfully prevented by the immunisation drives reaching to a significant level of the population. However, achieving herd immunity is only one part of addressing the immunisation challenge. Equitable vaccines distribution which ensures that the vaccines are accessible to all across the globe regardless of the socioeconomic status or geographical location has become crucial focus points. Disparities in equitable vaccine distribution, especially in poor and moderate income countries (LMICs) have highlighted the need for global initiatives to ensure that everyone benefits from the vaccines. Programmes like COVAX, which aim to distribute COVID-19 vaccines globally, emphasised the importance of equity in modern vaccine strategies to address the uneven burden of infectious diseases (Acosta-Coley *et al.*, 2022).

7. Vaccinology for Non-human Subjects: An Update

Infectious diseases could potentially spread from local (endemic) to global (pandemic) that threaten all the living species, and ultimately the ecology and the environment. Although advancements in public healthcare systems have enhanced the scale and speed of detection, prevention and management of infectious diseases, there is a large void in coordinated efforts to address the animal, human and environmental health that still remains primarily owing to the numerous emerging and remerging diseases (Zinsstag *et al.*, 2023). The interrelationships between the health of animals, humans, their habitats and the ecosystems, and the associated progressively denuding scenario were highlighted during the COVID-19 pandemic. To contain COVID-19, the

Chairs of the One Health Commission of Lancet recommended the formation of One Health research coalition (Amuasi *et al.*, 2020). The One Health initiative highlighted the interconnection between animals, humans and the environment to manage and prevent especially the zoonotic diseases at the origin thereby minimising the adverse impact of infectious diseases on public health (Adnyana *et al.*, 2023). The concerned committee recommended a holistic approach towards the health of humans, animals and the environment as an interconnected relationship within the ecosystem. It opined that the implementation of One Health approach was crucial to tackle COVID-19 pandemic and the preparedness for threats in the future to safeguard the global health and wellbeing.

The 2021-2030 roadmap of WHO for primarily the neglected tropical diseases (NTDs) emphasised on the One Health approach, detailed in a companion document released by it (World Health Organisation, 2022). This cross-disciplinary strategy unites humans, animals and the environmental health to achieve the ambitious NTD control and elimination goals, which outlined three pillars for action. The first pillar focuses on accelerating the programme-based action plans. It is achieved by developing One Health action plan for NTDs through technologically advanced evidence-based interventions and guidance, and fostering service and strategic delivery through joint risk assessments and surveillance. The second pillar prioritises the NTDs within the One Health framework (Forbes *et al.*, 2023). It involves strengthening the cross-sectoral coordination mechanisms and endeavouring NTD interventions in associated sectors. The third pillar focuses on facilitating the cultivation and sustenance of the nation-led One Health initiatives, aiming to transform the operation patterns and culture in line with the national mandates. A key intervention mechanism in this approach is promoting vaccination in animals. By breaking the transmission cycles by the animal reservoirs, these vaccines may significantly reduce the occurrence of zoonotic diseases in humans. The animal vaccine development strategies utilise the various technologies similar to the ones used in human vaccines. The inactivated (killed pathogen) and the live-attenuated vaccines (weakened pathogen) are common approaches. The potential of novel technologies like the recombinant subunit and DNA-based vaccines are also being explored. These novel approaches target the specific antigens of the target pathogen to potentially elicit more efficient immune responses.

The tripartite concept note by the WHO (World Health Organisation), WOAH (World Organisation for Animal Health) and FAO (Food and Agricultural Organisation of the United Nations) collectively agreed on focussing on the overall health and the risk complications at the animal-human interface, primarily focussed on rabies, antimicrobial resistance and avian influenza (Guarner and Jean, 2023). With the sharp rise of the severe COVID-19 pandemic and the possible environmental impact possibly attributed to the climate change, the UN Environmental Programme (UNEP) has also been involved as the fourth partner forming a quadripartite coalition duly supported by the independent high-level One Health expert panel (OHHLEP) comprising the specialised researchers. The quadripartite coalition collectively formed a One Health Joint plan of Action from the year 2022 till 2026 (Mettenleiter *et al.*, 2023). The alliance collectively works to devise the International Health Regulations (IHR) and disseminate public health awareness. Agencies like Natural Sciences and Engineering Research Council (NSERC), Canadian Institutes for Health Research (CIHR) and Social Sciences and Humanities Research Council (SSHRC) extended funds to study the potentially pandemic emerging diseases. The Institute of Infection and Immunity of the CIHR has formulated the study on zoonotic diseases. Rapid rise in the incidents of novel infectious diseases are being attributed to the increased human and animal interactions, resulting in the rapid transmission of diseases from animals to humans. It accelerated the spread of a disease further challenging the One Health efforts in mitigating infectious diseases (Mubareka *et al.*, 2023).

Thus, maintaining a scientifically and ecologically rational equilibrium among the various interdependent species is needed. Historically, majority of the pandemics, *viz.*, black-death, influenza, HIV, Rift Valley fever and most recently the SARS-CoV, SARS-CoV-2 and MERS-CoV, have originated from animal sources (zoonotic). The less-explored zoonotic pathogens (like the lesser-known *Salmonella*) that significantly impact public health are numerous. *Salmonella*, a food-borne infection from avian source, was estimated to cause 1.2 million illnesses in the US with 450 deaths. Nearly 14% of the salmonellosis cases in the early 1970s were by pet turtles. Approximately 11% of the various pathogen infections are zoonotic in nature (Abebe *et al.*, 2020). Control on the selling of such animal species could effectively decrease infections (Bosch *et al.*, 2016). Other zoonotic infections are influenza, bovine tuberculosis, west Nile fever etc. A joint study by the US Department of Agriculture (USDA) and Canada found the presence of SARS-CoV-2 in white-tailed deer (Vandegrift *et al.*, 2022). Mutated SARS-CoV-2 was found in minks in Denmark, identified through genome sequencing that posed infection threat in humans (Díaz *et al.*, 2021). Understanding the evolution of such infections plays a major role in finding a cure for the disease.

8. mRNA Vaccines to Prevent Infectious Diseases and Zoonoses in Animals

Only a handful of mRNA vaccines have been developed thus far, and the majority of these available mRNA vaccines are to safeguard humans against zoonotic illnesses like Zika virus sickness, rabies, influenza, Ebola and COVID-19. Foot-and-mouth disease (FMD) that affects animals through cloven hooves caused by the FMD virus is still one of the most contagious illnesses in the low- and medium-income countries. The virus has seven identified serotypes based on the antigenic and genetic characteristics, A, O, C, Asia1, SAT1, SAT2 and SAT3 (Wong *et al.*, 2020). The majority of the commercial FMD vaccines available are chemically inactivated virulent strains owing to one or many drawbacks with other approaches, like thermal instability, low immunogenicity, challenging serological analyses to differentiate between an infected and a vaccinated animal, and the high risk of the virulent virus spreading from the production facility (Belsham, 2020). As new and more sensitive techniques and approaches are needed, mRNA-based FMD vaccine development seemed promising. New lines of research have demonstrated the efficacy of the empty capsid-based vaccine against FMD in the natural host. The vaccine is produced by coexpressing FMDV P1-2A capsid precursor alongside 3Cpro in baculovirus or vaccinia virus (Newman *et al.*, 2021). Thus, a thermo-stable artificial RNA vaccine incorporating the FMDV P1-2A plus 3Cpro expressing genes could protect the livestock, especially in light of the advancements in mRNA vaccine technology during the COVID-19. mRNA vaccine could potentially overcome the drawbacks, including pathogenic virus or cell culture requirements, as in the conventional vaccines.

The Lyssavirus family that causes rabies is one of the deadliest forms of zoonotic viruses. Over 95% rabies infection cases, accounting for approximately 60,000 global human fatalities annually, are due to animal bites (especially dogs). Louis Pasteur made rabies vaccine from animal brain tissues to prevent rabies (Kaur *et al.*, 2015). The use of egg-culture or cell-culture based techniques were designed to address the significant adverse effects brought on by the myelin contaminant in inactivated viral vaccines and producing more efficient and safe vaccine. Temperature-stable mRNA encoding the rabies virus glycoprotein antigen and the cationic protein protamine as a stabiliser constituted the first rabies mRNA vaccine option CV7201 (Alberer *et al.*, 2017). By injecting mRNA intradermally, BALB/c mice were protected against rabies virus infection by producing antibodies that neutralised the virus (Stitz *et al.*, 2017). The rabies mRNA vaccine reportedly produced stronger cellular immunological response necessary for the protection than its other vaccine counterparts. The domesticated pigs had a shielding humoral immune response (Schnee *et al.*, 2016). To lower the dosage, the Phase I clinical research has been conducted on a new formulation that uses lipid nanoparticles encapsulated the same mRNA antigen (as CV7201). All the subject participants received two modest dosages of LNP-encapsulated mRNA (1 or 2 µg) to elicit the neutralising antibody responses that satisfied the WHO standards (Aldrich *et al.*, 2021). Apart from the non-amplifying mRNA rabies vaccine, many saRNA-based vaccines that targeted the glycoprotein G antigen have been designed. The primary objective is to work-out the possibilities to prevent rabies in canine population by injecting low LNP-encapsulated saRNAs dosages intramuscularly to elicit a protective immune response with minimal side-effect (Stokes *et al.*, 2020). Despite the encouraging advancements, the formulated mRNA vaccines have not yet been tested on cats or dogs. Consequently, to eradicate animal rabies especially in the wild, advancements in oral mRNA vaccines may be considered in future.

Various animal and bird species including pigs and dogs are infected by influenza virus that causes an exceptionally infectious respiratory disease. Influenza variants were responsible for four significant pandemics, H1N1 (1918), H2N2 (1957), H3N2 (1968) and H1N1 (repeated occurrence in 2009), in the past century apart from the periodic outbreaks (Jester *et al.*, 2020). As influenza virus is known to exhibit antigenic drift and shift, a compositionally altered influenza vaccine on regular bases is necessary to ensure protection through vaccination. The influenza vaccines that are administered to humans and birds presently are the inactivated and/or live-attenuated vaccine types, made in egg-based, cell-based and protein-based systems.

Usually, it takes 7-8 months for a vaccine from the conceptualisation of the designed vaccine to its field-scale trial which further undergoes complete clinical trial for a year or so. The rapid field-scale adoption of traditionally produced vaccines even for 'emergency use' after an outbreak is nearly impractical and scientifically irrational. Following the success of COVID-19 mRNA vaccines, the Phase I and II clinical trials to ascertain the efficacy and immunogenicity of the three-dose levels of Moderna's quadrivalent mRNA vaccine mRNA-1010 for seasonal influenza have been completed (Abbasi, 2021). An mRNA designed vaccine has two major advantages, one it could be rapidly designed and developed, and two it could be scaled-up fast to produce vaccines in large quantities. In this light, as swine or avian influenza viruses frequently spread to humans and cause serious illnesses, immunising these natural hosts (or carriers) with mRNA vaccines corresponding to the newly emerged viral strain/variant could help prevent fresh zoonotically transmitted outbreaks (from an endemic to pandemic).

Among the earliest mRNA vaccines against the infectious diseases, a RNA unit that encoded an attenuated strain of the tick-borne encephalitis virus (TBEV) was created in 1998. The RNA of the attenuated strain was encapsulated in gold particles, which showed the signs of antibody responses in the administered animal. In a comparative study, the mice inoculated with a full-length TBEV mRNA (that showed imunogenicity but lacked pathogenicity and the capability to multiply) could reportedly build protective immunity against the deadly viral infection (Aberle *et al.*, 2005). A SFV-based mRNA vaccine expressing the Louping-ill viral (LIV) envelope (ENV) and premembrane (prM) was designed in 2001. A zoonotic encephalitis flavivirus borne by ticks, LIV is primarily found in the Great Britain. When test mice were administered with a fatal dose of LIV (10 μg of naked mRNA administered intramuscularly) it could somehow protect the mice to certain extent. This suggested that the prM and ENV proteins could be the two potentially promising target molecules to develop vaccines (Pardi *et al.*, 2018).

9. Vaccine Development and Market Penetration

Driven by the advancements in technology and increased funding and the pressing need for the development of novel vaccines to contain the emerging diseases, vaccine development and the associated market demand has substantially grown in recent times. The advent in mRNA vaccines development platform during the COVID-19 marked a turning point in the rapid discovery and scaled-up production of vaccines, which has opened doors to apply the technology against an array of infectious diseases, cancers and even chronic health conditions. The success of Pfizer-BioNTech and Moderna's mRNA vaccines that were developed to counter COVID-19 showcased not only the effectiveness of this technology but also the potential to be rapidly scaled-up for mass production. This scalability has attracted investments from the private groups (like pharmaceutical companies) as well as the governments, opening up avenues to explore the mRNA vaccine development technology targeting diseases like HIV, Zika and influenza (Farlow *et al.*, 2023).

With the advent of vaccine innovations and technological breakthroughs, proactive public-private partnerships, increased government funding and global community healthcare collaborations, the global market for vaccines has opened up. The COVID-19 pandemic highlighted the importance of rapid vaccine development and its equitable distribution, prompting the governments to invest heavily in vaccine research and infrastructure. As a result, the capacity to innovate vaccines and foolproof supply chains has grown in recent times so that it could successfully and effectively combat the emerging infectious illnesses in the future too. Also, the success of vaccine development platforms (like the viral vectors and protein subunit vaccines, etc.) has encouraged the development of multivalent vaccines that could simultaneously target multiple strains of a target pathogen (Farlow *et al.*, 2023). Moreover, many such developed vaccines are age-defying thereby further facilitating the expansion of the vaccine market.

According to the sources working in close association with the COVID-19 vaccine research and development funding till March 2021, the US contributed \$2.23 billion leading the funding efforts with a notable portion of it coming from the various philanthropist sources. Germany followed after the US in public funding with \$1.51 billion, while the United Kingdom had a \$500 million contribution. Other notable contributors included the European Union with \$327 million, Canada with \$283 million, while Norway, Singapore and China provided significant amounts ranging from \$153 million to \$262 million (Wibawa, 2021). Fig. 3 highlights the global collaboration and investment that catalysed the accelerated vaccine development during the recent COVID-19 pandemic.

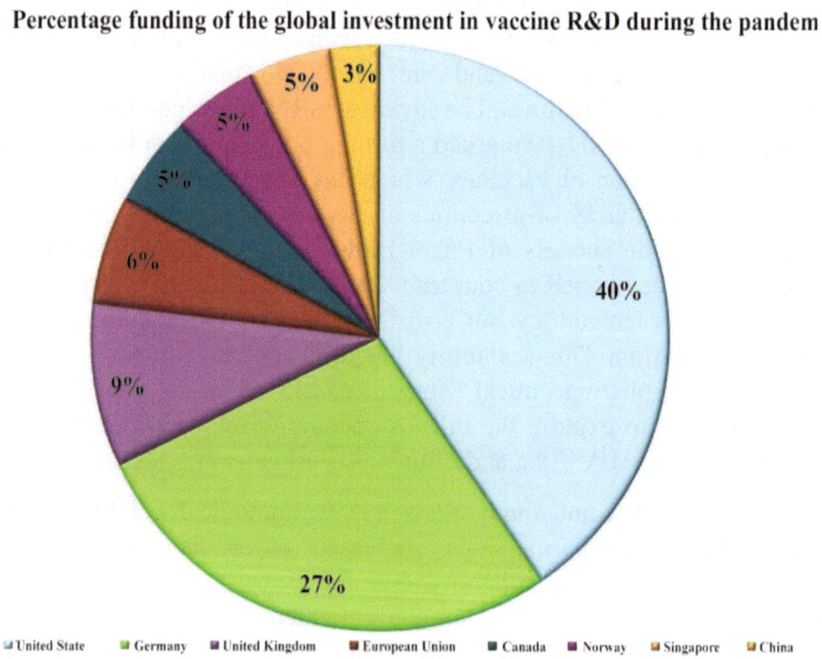

Fig. 3: The percent investment by various countries toward COVID-19 vaccine development

Another point of concern is the significantly varying cost of vaccines and types across different regions. The vaccine pricing was dependent on various factors like the cost of production, regulatory approval process, and the logistics requirements. Although, the rapid expansion of the vaccine development is driven through innovations in designing and production technologies (like the mRNA synthesis, viral vector production and protein subunit assembly) and by the market demand (Acosta-Coley *et al.*, 2022), but the vaccine cost is required to be rationalised, optimised and reduced to increase its affordability. Further advancements in innovations are undoubtedly expected to bring down the costs and improve the vaccine accessibility, primarily in the low-income regions (LMICs) where vaccine coverage remains perpetually suboptimal. Moreover to prevent future pandemics, market penetration also needs to focus on global distribution strategies, through well-prepared supply chains and equitable vaccine accessibility.

10. Future of Vaccinology

In the face of the rapidly evolving pathogens, traditional vaccines with poor targeting, low longevity, limited delivery methods, and possible side-effects seem underperforming to keep up with the pace and the needs. This is a critical challenge in ensuring community health worldwide. Vaccine development traditionally is known to trigger an immune response and provide protection against a targeted pathogen only irrespective of different people receiving the vaccine. Vaccines show effects beyond the target; it also elicits herd immunity. Age and gender factors play a vital role in determining the immunogenicity and efficacy of a vaccine. For instance, studies imply that the efficacy of Bacille Calmette-Guérin (BCG) vaccine could show varying effects based on its formulation and the age of the subject being vaccinated. Administrating BCG vaccine at an early age is beneficial. Usually BCG serves as a prototype to help in guiding future vaccine developments (Angelidou *et al.*, 2020).

Vaccines that are currently available over-the-counter are relatively poorly immunogenic, provided short-term protection, and might revert and again become the cause of the disease. Biomaterials and biotechniques advancements offer an array of opportunities to develop efficient next-generation vaccines. Global COVID-19 pandemic demonstrated the severity of infectious diseases and the detrimental effects on the physical health, mental health at individual level, and the local, regional and global economy. The COVID-19 pandemic saw the constantly emerging variants that challenged the efficacy of first-generation vaccines and also the vaccine side-effects supported by the ongoing discussion on Covishield causing heart attack (the vaccine by Moderna was also recalled from the market recently due to confirmed adverse health effects).

Learning a lesson from it, researchers could work collectively and collaboratively on the evidence-based vaccine delivery strategies to mitigate global pandemics in future. Discussion and awareness building among people to promote vaccine acceptance is important, especially in localities where hesitancy is high. The vaccine manufacturing sector has a critical role in effectively curbing infectious pandemics. The world community could potentially create a sustainable framework for production and distribution of vaccines. With a focus to address the limitations through innovative approaches of vaccine development and delivery, next-generation vaccines offer a ray of hope.

Vaccines, like those deployed against the COVID-19 pandemic, conventionally target single antigen (often the spike protein). While highly effective, even a small mutation in this target protein could reduce the efficacy of the vaccine as seen against Omicron variants (Shi *et al.*, 2022). Next-generation vaccines for broader and more foolproof antigen targeting strategies are being explored. One such approach involves targeting the conserved regions of viral genome that is least-prone to mutations that could potentially offer broader and reliable protection against even the variants (Hajnik *et al.*, 2022). Another strategy utilises multivalent vaccines that incorporate antigens from multiple strains to provide a wider immune responses and better assured protection (Kennedy *et al.*, 2020).

Durability or sustained effect of the protection shield by a vaccine is another area where the next-generation vaccines may be needed for enhanced benefits. Many conventional vaccines require booster shots to maintain the immunity for a longer duration. Next-generation vaccine approaches (like the self-amplifying mRNA vaccines) are being designed to generate stronger and more persistent immune responses that could potentially reduce the need for frequent booster dosing (Monet and Grandchamp, 2020). Investigations on suitable vectors or delivery vehicles like the liposome and nano-materials (like the nanoparticles and bacteriophages) are also being carried out that might enhance the sustainability (through sustained release for a long period of time) and targetability (through release at the desired location that would have maximal amplified result). Thus, the method of vaccine delivery is another innovation frontier.

Traditional injectable vaccines can have administration as well as logistical limitations, particularly in resource-limited settings. Next-generation vaccine development is exploring alternate delivery techniques like mucosal vaccine that is delivered orally or intranasally. Such techniques shall have the potential to induce mucosal immunity (potentially providing sterilising immunity) which could stifle the infection altogether and not just the severity of the disease (van Riel and de Wit 2020). Thermostable vaccine formulations could improve the stability and reduce the cold chain requirements. This shall facilitate transporting the vaccine and carry out vaccination campaigns more effectively in remote regions with limited access to refrigeration and cold storage. While the currently available vaccines underwent rigorous testing on safety parameters, next-generation vaccine platforms are still being investigated with regard to this aspect; safety is paramount in vaccinology. Careful evaluation of it through clinical trials is crucial to ensure the safety and efficacy of vaccines before they are approved for use.

With the advent of new-age vaccinology and novel approaches, three new terminologies have surfaced, biologics, biosimilars and biomimics. In essence, biologics are majorly natural, biomimics are purely artificial and biosimilars are somewhere in between. Biologics can be described as a broader term for all the products sourced from the living organisms, such as proteins, sugars or the DNA. Traditional vaccines, like those for influenza or hepatitis B, are considered as biologics in nature. The biological products that are highly similar to an existing FDA-approved biologics in terms of safety, purity and potency (as a reference product) are termed as biosimilars. Biosimilars offer a more affordable alternative to the reference product (biologics), thereby enhancing the scope of vaccine scalability and accessibility (Panda *et al.*, 2022). In vaccine development, biomimicry involves designing a vaccine that imitates the natural mechanisms through which a pathogen (virus or bacterium) interacts with the immune system. By mimicking these interactions, scientists can create vaccines that are more effective at stimulating a protective immune response. Biosimilars can help make biologics more affordable, and could potentially also increase the vaccination coverage. Biomimicry could inspire the designing of novel and more effective vaccines. Concerted efforts of the related fields hold great promise for vaccine development in the future, allowing for the creation of more accessible, effective and targeted vaccines.

11. Vaccination and Public Health Benefits

The primary effort of vaccination is to minimise the number of deaths due to a infectious disease that is considered lethal and is categorised under VPD (vaccine preventable disease). As hazardous infections are controlled, the humankind enjoys a longer and healthier life. A research conducted in the US by Roush *et al.* (2007) compared the revolutionary historical facts about the effect of immunisation on the occurrence of infectious diseases. They analysed the morbidity and mortality data linked to 13 VPDs comparing the rates prior to the establishment of vaccination programmes, and observed an almost 90%

decrement in occurrence. This incredible feat could be accomplished primarily due to the high vaccination rates for diseases like polio, diphtheria, tetanus and pertussis (DTaP), and MMR (Rodrigues and Plotkin, 2020). Significant obstacles to vaccine distribution are encountered in particularly the low- and middle-income countries (LMICs). In spite of this, the annual number of reported instances of VPDs has remarkably declined worldwide in the last 40 years with the rising immunisation rates.

Floods, varying temperature, a shift in disease vectors (like mosquitoes) due to climate change and global warming are the various contributing factors to the spread of infectious diseases (including the neglected tropical diseases) to other parts of the globe (Pecetta *et al.*, 2023). Diseases like dengue, yellow fever and cholera that are linked to climate change can be effectively prevented through the available vaccination measures. Vaccines combined with other community healthcare measures can contain outbreaks, epidemics and pandemics effectively. Ebola epidemic in the Democratic Republic of the Congo during 2018–2019 (Ilunga Kalenga *et al.*, 2019), cholera epidemic in Haiti during 2010–2019 (Rebaudet *et al.*, 2021) and the COVID-19 pandemic are a few such cases. Vaccines prevent diseases triggered by pathogenic germs that are currently prevalent in the public health domain. This preventive method reduces the selective pressure by minimising the use of antibiotics that promoted antibiotic resistance among the microbes. The increasing risk of multidrug-resistant bacteria could be the cause of future pandemics, which is crucial and must be addressed (Murray *et al.*, 2022).

Interestingly, vaccinations not only control the target virus but also are also effective against few other ailments. One (especially the convalescing, the immunocompromised, the elderly or a child) is predisposed to develop secondary microbial (bacterial, fungal and viral) infections and develop comorbidity. For instance, bacterial pneumonia and acute otitis media (AOM) frequently follow with influenza virus infection (Montero *et al.*, 2024). A small but considerable decrease in AOM instances could be achieved through influenza vaccination. Another instance is the influence of the measles vaccine introduced in the 1960s. It resulted in a notable decrease in child mortality and morbidity related to both measles and other associated infections (Mina *et al.*, 2015). Immunosuppression by measles increased the vulnerability to subsequent bacterial infections for a few weeks to months, especially those brought on by *S. pneumoniae* and Hib (Mina *et al.*, 2019). To guard against these secondary bacterial illnesses, measles vaccination was suggested.

Vaccination has a wider purpose in individuals than only prevention against infections. They also safeguard the community by establishing community resistance (herd immunity). The ability of a pathogen to spread is greatly reduced when a significant percentage of individuals develop immunity against the pathogen, either through vaccination or after having recovered from an infection. Even the individuals who are very old (elderly) or have health issues (like comorbidities) to receive the vaccine are protected through herd immunity. The benefits of this passive mode to protect the vulnerable, like the infants, the elderly and those with compromised immune systems, are in particular indispensible (Randolph and Barreiro 2020).

12. Conclusion

Vaccines are among the most crucial medical discoveries that protect the community against several infectious diseases. Even though several vaccines to cure infectious diseases have been developed, a significant disease burden still remains that vaccines can't control. However, modern techniques could significantly contribute to help prevent many other such diseases in future. In the era of vaccinology, the focus need to be broadened beyond the prophylactic vaccines, and therapeutic and personalised vaccine could be incorporate to combat both communicable (infectious) and non-communicable (non-infectious) diseases. Although it has greater potentials to target the emerging novel diseases, it has numerous issues and challenges to address first.

References

Abbasi J, 2021. Moderna's mRNA vaccine for seasonal flu enters clinical trials. Jama, 326(14): 1365–1365. doi: 10.1001/jama.2021.17499

Abebe E, Gugsa G and Ahmed M, 2020. Review on major food-borne zoonotic bacterial pathogens. J Trop. Med., 2020(1): 4674235. doi: 10.1155/2020/4674235

Aberle JH, Aberle SW, Kofler RM and Mandl CW, 2005. Humoral and cellular immune response to RNA immunization with flavivirus replicons derived from tick-borne encephalitis virus. J. Virol., 79(24): 15107–15113. doi: 10.1128/jvi.79.24.15107-15113.2005

Acosta-Coley I, Cervantes-Ceballos L, Tejeda-Benítez L, Sierra-Márquez L, Cabarcas-Montalvo M, García-Espiñeira M, Coronell-Rodríguez W and Arroyo-Salgado B, 2022. Vaccines platforms and COVID-19: what you need to know. Trop. Dis. Travel Med. Vaccines, 8(1): 20. doi: 10.1186/s40794-022-00176-4

Adnyana IM, Utomo B, Eljatin DS and Sudaryati NL, 2023. One Health approach and zoonotic diseases in Indonesia: Urgency of implementation and challenges. Narra. J., 3(3): e257. doi: 10.52225/narra.v3i3.257

Adu-Bobie J, Capecchi B, Serruto D, Rappuoli R and Pizza M, 2003. Two years into reverse vaccinology. Vaccine, 21(7–8): 605–610. doi: 10.1016/S0264-410X(02)00566-2

Alberer M, Gnad-Vogt U, Hong HS, Mehr KT, Backert L, Finak G, Gottardo R, Bica MA, Garofano A, Koch SD and Fotin-Mleczek M, 2017. Safety and immunogenicity of a mRNA rabies vaccine in healthy adults: an open-label, non-randomised, prospective, first in human phase 1 clinical trial. Lancet, 390(10101): 1511–1520. doi: 10.1016/S0140-6736(17)31665-3

Aldrich C, Leroux–Roels I, Huang KB, Bica MA, Loeliger E, Schoenborn-Kellenberger O, Walz L, Leroux-Roels G, von Sonnenburg F and Oostvogels L, 2021. Proof-of-concept of a low-dose unmodified mRNA-based rabies vaccine formulated with lipid nanoparticles in human volunteers: A phase 1 trial. Vaccine, 39(8): 1310–1318. doi: 10.1016/j.vaccine.2020.12.070

Altmann DM and Boyton RJ, 2022. COVID-19 vaccination: The road ahead. Science, 375(6585): 1127–1132. doi: 10.1126/science.abn1755

Amuasi JH, Walzer C, Heymann D, Carabin H, Haines A and Winkler AS, 2020. Calling for a COVID-19 one health research coalition. The Lancet, 395(10236): 1543–1544. doi: 10.1016/S0140-6736(20)31028-X

Angelidou A, Diray-Arce J, Conti MG, Smolen KK, van Haren SD, Dowling DJ, Husson RN and Levy O, 2020. BCG as a case study for precision vaccine development: lessons from vaccine heterogeneity, trained immunity, and immune ontogeny. Front. Microbiol., 11: 481431. doi: 10.3389/fmicb.2020.00332

Baker JP and Katz SL, 2004. Childhood vaccine development: an overview. Pediatr. Res., 55(2): 347–356. doi: 10.1203/01.PDR.0000106317.36875.6A

Belsham GJ, 2020. Towards improvements in foot-and-mouth disease vaccine performance. Acta Vet. Scand., 62(1): 20. doi: 10.1186/s13028-020-00519-1

Bosch S, Tauxe RV and Behravesh CB, 2016. Turtle-associated salmonellosis, United States, 2006–2014. Emerg. Infect. Dis., 22(7): 1149–1155. doi: 10.3201/eid2207.150685

Burke DS, 1993. Of postulates and peccadilloes: Robert Koch and vaccine (tuberculin) therapy for tuberculosis. Vaccine, 11(8): 795–804. doi: 10.1016/0264-410X(93)90354-Z

Burnett E, Parashar UD and Tate JE, 2020. Real-world effectiveness of rotavirus vaccines, 2006–19: a literature review and meta-analysis. Lancet Glob. Health., 8(9): e1195–e1202. doi: 10.1016/S2214-109X(20)30262-X

Cavaillon JM, 2018. Historical links between toxinology and immunology. Pathog. Dis., 76(3): fty019. doi: 10.1093/femspd/fty019

Chakraborty S, Mallajosyula V, Tato CM, Tan GS and Wang TT, 2021. SARS-CoV-2 vaccines in advanced clinical trials: Where do we stand?. Adv. Drug Deliv. Rev., 172: 314–338. doi: 10.1016/j.addr.2021.01.014

Chary M, Barbuto AF, Izadmehr S, Tarsillo M, Fleischer E and Burns MM, 2023. COVID-19 therapeutics: use, mechanism of action, and toxicity (vaccines, monoclonal antibodies, and immunotherapeutics). J. Med. Toxicol., 19(2): 205–218. doi: 10.1007/s13181-023-00931-9

Cleri DJ, Porwancher RB, Ricketti AJ, Ramos-Bonner LS and Vernaleo JR, 2006. Smallpox as a bioterrorist weapon: myth or menace?. Infect. Dis. Clin., 20(2): 329–357. doi: 10.1016/j.idc.2006.03.005

Conceição Silva F, De Luca PM and Lima-Junior JDC, 2023. Vaccine Development against Infectious Diseases: State of the Art, New Insights, and Future Directions. Vaccines, 11(11): 1632. doi: 10.3390/vaccines11111632

Dadar M, Chakraborty S, Dhama K, Prasad M, Khandia R, Hassan S, Munjal A, Tiwari R, Karthik K, Kumar D and Iqbal HM, 2018. Advances in designing and developing vaccines, drugs and therapeutic approaches to counter human papilloma virus. Front. Immunol., 9: 2478. doi: 10.3389/fimmu.2018.02478

Díaz AV, Walker M and Webster JP, 2021. Surveillance and control of SARS-CoV-2 in mustelids: An evolutionary perspective. Evol. Appl., 14(12): 2715–2725. doi: 10.1111/eva.13310

D'Amico C, Fontana F, Cheng R and Santos HA, 2021. Development of vaccine formulations: past, present, and future. Drug Deliv. Transl. Res., 11: 353–372. doi: 10.1007/s13346-021-00924-7

Eggers HJ, 2002. History of poliomyelitis and poliomyelitis research. Mol. Biol. Picornavirus., 1–14. doi: 10.1128/9781555817916.ch1

Farlow A, Torreele E, Gray G, Ruxrungtham K, Rees H, Prasad S, Gomez C, Sall A, Magalhães J, Olliaro P and Terblanche P, 2023. The future of epidemic and pandemic vaccines to serve global public health needs. Vaccines, 11(3): 690. doi: 10.3390/vaccines11030690

Forbes K, Basáñez MG, Hollingsworth TD and Anderson RM, 2023. Introduction to the special issue: challenges and opportunities in the fight against neglected tropical diseases: a decade from the London Declaration on NTDs. Phil. Trans. R. Soc. B, 378(1887): 20220272. doi: 10.1098/rstb.2022.0272

Galazka AM, Robertson SE and Oblapenko GP, 1995. Resurgence of diphtheria. Euro. J Epidemiol., 11: 95–105. doi: 10.1007/BF01719954

Gee J, Weinbaum C, Sukumaran L and Markowitz LE, 2016. Quadrivalent HPV vaccine safety review and safety monitoring plans for nine-valent HPV vaccine in the United States. Hum Vaccin. Immunother., 12(6): 1406–1417. doi: 10.1080/21645515.2016.1168952

Gong W, Pan C, Cheng P, Wang J, Zhao G and Wu X, 2022. Peptide-based vaccines for tuberculosis. Front. Immunol., 13: 830497. doi: 10.3389/fimmu.2022.830497

Griffiss JM, Yamasaki R, Estabrook M and Kim JJ, 1991. Meningococcal molecular mimicry and the search for an ideal vaccine. Trans. R. Soc. Trop. Med. Hyg., 85: 32–36. doi: 10.1016/0035-9203(91)90338-Y

Guarner J and Jean S, 2023. One Health: The Role of Pathology as it pertains to Diagnosis of Zoonoses and Discovery of Emerging Infections. Mod. Pathol., 36(8): 100236. doi: 10.1016/j.modpat.2023.100236

Hajnik RL, Plante JA, Liang Y, Alameh MG, Tang J, Bonam SR, Zhong C, Adam A, Scharton D, Rafael GH and Liu Y, 2022. Dual spike and nucleocapsid mRNA vaccination confer protection against SARS-CoV-2 Omicron and Delta variants in preclinical models. Sci. Transl. Med., 14(662): eabq1945. doi: 10.1126/scitranslmed.abq1945

Ilunga Kalenga O, Moeti M, Sparrow A, Nguyen VK, Lucey D and Ghebreyesus TA, 2019. The ongoing Ebola epidemic in the Democratic Republic of Congo, 2018–2019. N. Eng. J. Med., 381(4): 373–383. doi: 10.1056/NEJMsr1904253

Jester BJ, Uyeki TM and Jernigan DB, 2020. Fifty years of influenza A (H3N2) following the pandemic of 1968. Am J Public Health, 110(5): 669–676. doi: 10.2105/AJPH.2019.305557

Kampmann B, Madhi SA, Munjal I, Simões EA, Pahud BA, Llapur C, Baker J, Pérez Marc G, Radley D, Shittu E and Glanternik J, 2023. Bivalent prefusion F vaccine in pregnancy to prevent RSV illness in infants. N. Eng. J. Med., 388(16): 1451–1464. doi: 10.1056/NEJMoa2216480

Kantha SS, 1991. A centennial review; the 1890 tetanus antitoxin paper of von Behring and Kitasato and the related developments. Keio J Med., 40(1), 35–39. doi: 10.2302/kjm.40.35

Kaur M, Garg R, Singh S and Bhatnagar R, 2015. Rabies vaccines: where do we stand, where are we heading?. Expert Rev. Vaccines, 14(3): 369–381. doi: 10.1586/14760584.2015.973403

Kennedy RB, Ovsyannikova IG, Palese P and Poland GA, 2020. Current challenges in vaccinology. Front. Immunol., 11: 1181. doi: 10.3389/fimmu.2020.01181

Killikelly AM, Kanekiyo M and Graham BS, 2016. Pre-fusion F is absent on the surface of formalin inactivated respiratory syncytial virus. Sci. Rep., 6(1): 34108. doi: 10.1038/srep34108

Masignani V, Pizza M and Moxon ER, 2019. The development of a vaccine against meningococcus B using reverse vaccinology. Front. Immunol., 10: 441439. doi: 10.3389/fimmu.2019.00751

Mettenleiter TC, Markotter W, Charron DF, Adisasmito WB, Almuhairi S, Behravesh CB, Bilivogui P, Bukachi SA, Casas N, Becerra NC and Chaudhary A, 2023. The one health high-level expert panel (OHHLEP). One Health Outlook, 5(1): 18. doi: 10.1186/s42522-023-00085-2

Mina MJ, Kula T, Leng Y, Li M, De Vries RD, Knip M, Siljander H, Rewers M, Choy DF, Wilson MS and Larman HB, 2019. Measles virus infection diminishes preexisting antibodies that offer protection from other pathogens. Science, 366(6465): 599–606. doi: 10.1126/science.aay6485

Mina MJ, Metcalf CJE, De Swart RL, Osterhaus ADME and Grenfell BT, 2015. Long-term measles-induced immunomodulation increases overall childhood infectious disease mortality. Science, 348(6235): 694–699. doi: 10.1126/science.aaa3662

Mohapatra RK, Das PK and Kandi V, 2020. Challenges in controlling COVID-19 in migrants in Odisha, India. Diabetes Metab. Syndr., 14(6):1593-9. doi: 10.1016/j.dsx.2020.08.024

Mohapatra RK, El-Shall NA, Tiwari R, Nainu F, Kandi V, Sarangi AK, Mohammed TA, Desingu PA, Chakraborty C and Dhama K, 2022. Need of booster vaccine doses to counteract the emergence of SARS-CoV-2 variants in the context of the Omicron variant and increasing COVID-19 cases: An update. Hum. Vaccin. Immunother., 18(5):2065824. https://doi.org /10.1080/21645515.2022.2065824

Mohapatra RK, Kandi V, Gaidhane AM, Zahiruddin QS, Rustagi S, Satapathy P, Mishra S and Tuglo LS, 2024b. Global domination of the recently VoI-classified'JN. 1′ outcompeting other variants–Comparing the vaccines' efficacy. Clinical Infection in Practice, 22:100358. https://doi.org/10.1016/j.clinpr.2024.100358

Mohapatra RK, Mishra S, Azam M and Dhama K, 2021. COVID-19, WHO guidelines, pedagogy, and respite. Open Med., 16(1):491-3. doi: 10.1515/med-2021-0266

Mohapatra RK, Mishra S, Kandi V, Branda F, Ansari A, Rabaan AA and Kudrat-E-Zahan M, 2023a. Analyzing the emerging patterns of SARS-CoV-2 Omicron subvariants for the development of next-gen vaccine: An observational study. Health Sci. Rep., 6(10):e1596. doi: 10.1002/hsr2.1596

Mohapatra RK, Mishra S, Tuglo LS, Kutikuppala LV, Mohapatra PK, Kandi V, Panda SK and Desai DN, 2024a. Need of Monkeypox animal vaccine and its global distribution: right time to address?. Int. J. Surg., 110(12):8164-6. doi: 10.1097/JS9.0000000000000100

Mohapatra RK, Verma S, Kandi V, Sarangi AK, Seidel V, Das SN, Behera A, Tuli HS, Sharma AK and Dhama K, 2023b. The SARS-CoV-2 Omicron variant and its multiple sub-lineages: transmissibility, vaccine development, antiviral drugs, monoclonal antibodies, and strategies for infection control–a review. ChemistrySelect., 8(9):e202201380. https://doi.org/10.1002/slct.202201380

Monet L and Grandchamp N, 2020. The Emergence of the Next-Generation Vaccines. Arch. Clin. Biomed. Res., 4(4): 325–348. doi: 10.26502/acbr.50170107

Montero DA, Vidal RM, Velasco J, Carreño LJ, Torres JP, Benachi O MA, Tovar-Rosero YY, Oñate AA and O'Ryan M, 2024. Two centuries of vaccination: historical and conceptual approach and future perspectives. Front. Public Health, 11: 1326154. doi: 10.3389/fpubh.2023.1326154

Mubareka S, Amuasi J, Banerjee A, Carabin H, Copper Jack J, Jardine C, Jaroszewicz B, Keefe G, Kotwa J, Kutz S and McGregor D, 2023. Strengthening a One Health approach to emerging zoonoses. Facets, 8(1): 1–64. doi: 10.1139/facets-2021-0190

Murray CJ, Ikuta KS, Sharara F, Swetschinski L, Aguilar GR, Gray A, Han C, Bisignano C, Rao P, Wool E and Johnson SC, 2022. Global burden of bacterial antimicrobial resistance in 2019: a systematic analysis. Lancet, 399(10325): 629–655. doi: 10.1016/S0140-6736(21)02724-0

Newman J, Rowlands DJ and Tuthill TJ, 2021. An engineered maturation cleavage provides a recombinant mimic of foot-and-mouth disease virus capsid assembly-disassembly. Life, 11(6): 500. doi: 10.3390/life11060500

O'Ryan M, Vidal R, del Canto F, Salazar JC and Montero D, 2015. Vaccines for viral and bacterial pathogens causing acute gastroenteritis: Part I: Overview, vaccines for enteric viruses and Vibrio cholerae. Hum Vaccin. Immunother., 11(3): 584–600. Doi: 10.1080/21645515.2015.1011019

Panda S, Singh PK, Mishra S, Mitra S, Pattnaik P, Adhikary SD and Mohapatra RK, 2022. Indian biosimilars and vaccines at crossroads–replicating the success of pharmagenerics. Vaccines, 11(1): 110. doi: 10.3390/vaccines11010110

Papi A, Ison MG, Langley JM, Lee DG, Leroux-Roels I, Martinon-Torres F, Schwarz TF, van Zyl-Smit RN, Campora L, Dezutter N and De Schrevel N, 2023. Respiratory syncytial virus prefusion F protein vaccine in older adults. N. Engl. J. Med., 388:595–608. doi: 10.1056/NEJMoa2209604

Pardi N, Hogan MJ, Porter FW and Weissman D, 2018. mRNA vaccines—a new era in vaccinology. Nat. Rev. Drug Discov., 17(4): 261–279. doi: 10.1038/nrd.2017.243

Pecetta S, Nandi A, Weller C, Harris V, Fletcher H, Berlanda Scorza F, Pizza M, Salisbury D, Moxon R, Black S and Bloom DE, 2023. Vaccines for a sustainable planet. Sci. Transl. Med., 15(685): eadf1093. doi: 10.1126/scitranslmed.adf1093

Peterson J, Drazan D, Czajka H, Maguire J, Pregaldien JL, Seppa I, Maansson R, O'Neill R, Balmer P, Jodar L and Jansen KU, 2023. Immunogenicity and safety of a pentavalent meningococcal ABCWY vaccine in adolescents and young adults: an observer-blind, active-controlled, randomised trial. Lancet Infect. Dis., 23(12): 1370–1382. doi: 10.1016/S1473-3099(23)00191-3

Pizza M, Scarlato V, Masignani V, Giuliani MM, Arico B, Comanducci M, Jennings GT, Baldi L, Bartolini E, Capecchi B and Galeotti CL, 2000. Identification of vaccine candidates against serogroup B meningococcus by whole-genome sequencing. Science, 287(5459): 1816–1820. doi: 10.1126/science.287.5459.1816

Pulendran B, SArunachalam P and O'Hagan DT, 2021. Emerging concepts in the science of vaccine adjuvants. Nat. Rev. Drug Discov., 20(6): 454–475. doi: 10.1038/s41573-021-00163-y

Randolph HE and Barreiro LB, 2020. Herd immunity: understanding COVID-19. Immunity, 52(5): 737–741. doi: 10.1016/j.immuni.2020.04.012

Rebaudet S, Dély P, Boncy J, Henrys JH and Piarroux R, 2021. Toward cholera elimination, Haiti. Emerg. Infect. Dis., 27(11): 2932–2936. doi: 10.3201/eid2711.203372

Rodrigues CM and Plotkin SA, 2020. Impact of vaccines; health, economic and social perspectives. Front. Microbiol., 11: 1526. doi: 10.3389/fmicb.2020.01526

Roush SW, Murphy TV and Vaccine-Preventable Disease Table Working Group, 2007. Historical comparisons of morbidity and mortality for vaccine-preventable diseases in the United States. Jama, 298(18): 2155–2163. doi: 10.1001/jama.298.18.2155

Sah R, Khatiwada AP, Shrestha S, Bhuvan KC, Tiwari R, Mohapatra RK, Dhama K and Rodriguez-Morales AJ, 2021. COVID-19 vaccination campaign in Nepal, emerging UK variant and futuristic vaccination strategies to combat the ongoing pandemic. Travel Med. Infect. Dis., 41:102037. doi: 10.1016/j.tmaid.2021.102037

Sarangi AK, Salem MA, Younus MD, El-Haroun H, Mahal A, Tripathy L, Mishra R, Shabil M, Alhumaydhi FA, Khatib MN and Bushi G, 2024. Advanced biomaterials for regenerative medicine and their possible therapeutic significance in treating COVID-19: a critical overview. Int. J. Surg., 110(12):7508-27. doi: 10.1097/JS9.0000000000002110

Satapathy BS, Pattnaik G, Sahoo RN, Pattanaik S, Sarangi AK, Kandi V, Mishra S, Rabaan AA, Mohanty A, Sah R and Mohapatra RK, 2023. COVID-19 vaccines and their underbelly: Are we going the right way?. Health Sci. Rep., 6(9):e1540. doi: 10.1002/hsr2.1540

Schnee M, Vogel AB, Voss D, Petsch B, Baumhof P, Kramps T and Stitz L, 2016. An mRNA vaccine encoding rabies virus glycoprotein induces protection against lethal infection in mice and correlates of protection in adult and newborn pigs. PLoS Negl. Trop. Dis., 10(6): e0004746. doi: 10.1371/journal.pntd.0004746

Shi J, Wang G, Zheng J, Verma AK, Guan X, Malisheni MM, Geng Q, Li F, Perlman S and Du L, 2022. Effective vaccination strategy using SARS-CoV-2 spike cocktail against Omicron and other variants of concern. npj Vaccines, 7(1): 169. doi: 10.1038/s41541-022-00580-z

Stanisic DI and Good MF, 2023. Malaria vaccines: progress to date. BioDrugs, 37(6): 737–756. doi: 10.1007/s40259-023-00623-4

Stitz L, Vogel A, Schnee M, Voss D, Rauch S, Mutzke T, Ketterer T, Kramps T and Petsch B, 2017. A thermostable messenger RNA based vaccine against rabies. PLoS Negl. Trop. Dis., 11(12): e0006108. doi: 10.1371/journal.pntd.0006108

Stokes A, Pion J, Binazon O, Laffont B, Bigras M, Dubois G, Blouin K, Young JK, Ringenberg MA, Abdeljelil NB and Haruna J, 2020. Nonclinical safety assessment of repeated administration and biodistribution of a novel rabies self-amplifying mRNA vaccine in rats. Regul. Toxicol. Pharmacol., 113: 104648. doi: 10.1016/j.yrtph.2020.104648

Vandegrift KJ, Yon M, Surendran Nair M, Gontu A, Ramasamy S, Amirthalingam S, Neerukonda S, Nissly RH, Chothe SK, Jakka P and LaBella L, 2022. SARS-CoV-2 Omicron (B. 1.1. 529) infection of wild white-tailed deer in New York City. Viruses, 14(12): 2770. doi: 10.3390/v14122770

van Riel D and de Wit E, 2020. Next-generation vaccine platforms for COVID-19. Nat. Mater., 19(8): 810–812. doi: 10.1038/s41563-020-0746-0

Varadé J, Magadán S and González-Fernández Á, 2021. Human immunology and immunotherapy: main achievements and challenges. Cell Mol. Immunol., 18(4): 805–828. doi: 10.1038/s41423-020-00530-6

Venkatesan P, 2023. First RSV vaccine approvals. Lancet Microbe, 4(8): e577. doi: 10.1016/S2666-5247(23)00195-7

Villena R, Safadi MAP, Valenzuela MT, Torres JP, Finn A and O'Ryan M, 2018. Global epidemiology of serogroup B meningococcal disease and opportunities for prevention with novel recombinant protein vaccines. Hum Vaccin. Immunother., 14(5): 1042–1057. doi: 10.1080/21645515.2018.1458175

Walsh EE, Pérez Marc G, Zareba AM, Falsey AR, Jiang Q, Patton M, Polack FP, Llapur C, Doreski PA, Ilangovan K and Rämet M, 2023. Efficacy and safety of a bivalent RSV prefusion F vaccine in older adults. N. Eng. J. Med., 388(16): 1465–1477. doi: 10.1056/NEJMoa2213836

Wang R, Pan W, Jin L, Huang W, Li Y, Wu D, Gao C, Ma D and Liao S, 2020. Human papillomavirus vaccine against cervical cancer: Opportunity and challenge. Cancer Lett., 471: 88–102. doi: 10.1016/j.canlet.2019.11.039

Wibawa T, 2021. COVID-19 vaccine research and development: ethical issues. Trop. Med. Int. Health, 26(1): 14-19. doi: 10.1111/tmi.13503

Wong CL, Yong CY, Ong HK, Ho KL and Tan WS, 2020. Advances in the diagnosis of foot-and-mouth disease. Front. Vet. Sci., 7: 477. doi: 10.3389/fvets.2020.00477

World Health Organization, 2022. Ending the neglect to attain the sustainable development goals: One health: approach for action against neglected tropical diseases 2021-2030.

Zakir F, Islam F, Jabeen A and Moni SS, 2019. Vaccine development: a historical perspective. Biomed. Res., 30(3): 452–455.

Zinsstag J, Kaiser-Grolimund A, Heitz-Tokpa K, Sreedharan R, Lubroth J, Caya F, Stone M, Brown H, Bonfoh B, Dobell E and Morgan D, 2023. Advancing One human–animal–environment Health for global health security: what does the evidence say? The Lancet, 401(10376): 591–604. doi: 10.1016/S0140-6736(22)01595-1

2

Vaccine Development to Counter Infectious Diseases: The COVID-19 Saga

Lizaranee Tripathy[1], Ashish K. Sarangi[1,*], Sanjib Kumar Naik[2]
Ajit Behera[3], Ranjan K. Mohapatra[4,*]

[1]Department of Chemistry, Centurion University of Technology and Management, Balangir-767 001, Odisha, India
[2]Department of Information Technology, Centurion University of Technology and Management, Balangir-767 001, Odisha, India
[3]Department of Metallurgical & Materials Engineering, National Institute of Technology, Rourkela-769 008, Odisha, India
[4]Department of Chemistry, Government College of Engineering, Keonjhar – 758 002, Odisha, India

Abstract

The process of vaccine development involves numerous stages from research, discovery, innovation, formulation, testing, mass production, logistics, deployment and administering the vaccine to the target population. The COVID-19 pandemic expedited the endeavour to develop vaccine worldwide that is unparalleled in history. In addition to the steps that were similar during the usual vaccine development process, it called for stronger collaborative teamwork with stricter deadlines during the pandemic due to the emergency situation that built up everywhere (in its spread as well as severity). Research was expedited, potential candidate vaccines were discovered and the proofs of concept were designed that paved the way for pre-clinical efficacy testing. Multiple-step clinical trials to ascertain that the vaccines were effective and safe at least for 'emergency use' in human subjects were carried out swiftly. The emergency usage regulatory approval and recommending the usage pattern involved accelerated review procedures. It immediately followed rapid scaling-up for increased production in order to meet the need to save as many human lives as possible across the globe. The approved vaccines were simultaneously evaluated for safety through dedicated pharmacovigilance systems. The future of vaccine development shall also focus on improving the worldwide access to vaccines, managing the virus variants and streamlining mass vaccination campaigns. Comprehending the research, development and administration phases to create and implement life-saving vaccinations within the regulatory framework amid international health emergencies as encountered during the COVID-19 pandemic and the enormous collective endeavours are highlighted in this chapter.

***Keywords*:** COVID-19, vaccine, clinical trial, vaccination, community health, infectious disease

1. Research and Discovery of COVID-19 Vaccines

The virus SARS-CoV-2 known to cause pneumonia reportedly first appeared in December 2019 from China's Hubei Province, which could have appeared prior to that as well that had gone unrecognised, unnoticed or undocumented (Andersen *et al.*, 2020). Prior to zoometric transition, natural selection for animal hosts like bats and pangolins most likely led to its current evolution (Wu *et al.*, 2020). Seven virus members of Coronaviridae Family and Coronavirinae Subfamily have been identified as human pathogens as of now, three of which could potentially induce harmful respiratory clinical conditions (Zhou *et al.*, 2020). These are collectively referred as corona viruses (CoVs). Infecting an array of hosts, these could cause illnesses that ranged from a usual flu to a serious and often lethal condition (Zhu *et al.*, 2020). The ICVT initially designated the novel COVID-19 virus as 2019-nCoV. Afterwards, it was renamed as SARS-CoV-2 as its genomic make-up was very similar to it sister virus SARS-CoV-1 (Gorbalenya *et al.*, 2020). It is a beta corona virus that is a close cousin of the SARS virus, as per gene sequence of the virus (Silva *et al.*, 2023). The WHO (World Health Organisation) classified the ongoing threat posed by this virus as a global health emergency due to its rapid spread from its origin in China to other regions (Dhama *et al.*, 2020).

Vaccination was a breakthrough life-shaping development in medical microbiology to reduce the spread and consequences of infectious diseases (Funk *et al.*, 2020; Satapathy *et al.*, 2023; Sarangi *et al.*, 2024). Vaccination is the most effective strategy to prevent an infectious disease as it is more affordable than therapeutics with a shorter half-life (André *et al.*, 2001). Immunisation prevents 2-3 million deaths from over 20 deadly infectious illnesses presently and tremendous efforts were made to counter COVID-19 too. Like any other viral disease, the corona virus diseases could be prevented through vaccination (Velásquez *et al.*, 2022). WHO brings together public health practitioners and scientists from around the world to expedite research and development create new guidelines stop the corona virus pandemic from spreading, and treat those who are affected.

Curative as well as preventive vaccinations would be essential as obvious means to guarantee public healthcare (Pronker *et al.*, 2013). Safe and effective vaccines were required develop to counter the highly transmitting and lethally infectious COVID-19 pandemic to occur and recur (Liu *et al.*, 2020). Vaccine discovery against SARS-CoV-2 was aided by the significant sequence homology of this coronavirus with two other deadly CoVs (MERS-CoV and SARS-CoV-1). Vaccine provided sustained immunity by exposing an individual to antigens that triggered the development of immunological memory prior to an incidental contact with the viable infective virus. Humoral antibody activation and the effectors role of cellular T-cells mediate the process (Sharpe *et al.*, 2020). The industry, government and academia needed to work together on novel techniques to produce an effective vaccine against SARS-CoV-2 with each group showcasing unique capabilities (Corey *et al.*, 2020). The antigens that are preferred in vaccine development to successfully elicit antigen-specific immune response are, the S proteins or its fragments (S1), nucleocapsid proteins (N), membrane protein (M) or envelope protein (E).

As the COVID-19 viral infection was encountered by the humanity for the first time ever, knowledge about its biological characteristics, epidemiology, individualised immune responses and other traits was lacking. It made designing of the vaccines to counter its spread among human population is challenging (Ahmed *et al.*, 2020). The S (spike) protein seemed to be a promising target for vaccine development as it contained both antigenicity and receptor-binding domain (RBD). It was imperative to verify the clinical significance of SARS-CoV-2 binding, the neutralising antibody titre and predicting the efficacy (Yu *et al.*, 2020). The only feasibility test to validate the relationship between antibody titre and the efficacy (protecting against COVID-19) is a well-designed large-scale clinical trial (Heaton *et al.*, 2020). The potential of a regularly administered approved vaccine to make a subsequent SARS-CoV-2 illness worse is also high as evidenced in several SARS-CoV-1 animal vaccine (against feline coronaviruses) challenge models and verified (Bolles *et al.*, 2011).

The ability to create vaccines using only the sequencing data is the major advantage in developing next-generation vaccines (Van *et al.*, 2020). The available coding sequences of the viral protein necessary to counter the infection or sickness is taken and included in the discovered vaccine ensuring that the amount of viral proteins is sufficiently high to initiate immunity activation rather than depending on the ability of the virus to develop it

(Craven *et al*., 2021). The fact that most COVID-19 vaccines under clinical trials contained the next-generation platform indicated the high adaptability of these platforms for rapid vaccine development. Once a potential vaccine candidate is identified, it is applied for reviewing as a novel vaccine to the Food and Drug Administration (USFDA) or other regulatory agencies (Shang *et al*., 2020).

After the declaration of COVID-19 pandemic by the WHO on 11 March 2020, there was an increasing demand for its immediate therapy and potential prevention owing to the severity of the infection (especially the lower respiratory tract), widespread distribution, the lack of prophylaxis and therapies, and the rapidly growing afflicted population (Casadevall *et al*., 2020; Begum *et al*., 2021). Efforts to develop safe and effective preventive measures were immediately initiated (Pang *et al*., 2020). As the prevailing situation lacked a time-tested prophylaxis, numerous vaccines were developed that were subjected to clinical trial (Dhama *et al*., 2020). Numerous efforts were attempted to produce vaccines to contain COVID-19, with the majority of these attempts utilising the spike(S)-protein of SARS-CoV-2 virus as the antigen. Fig. 1 summarises the numerous vaccine candidates in various trial stages, with the major proportion of the candidates at Phases I and II clinical trial and the percentage. The available worldwide data on the vaccine candidates registered for clinical trial evaluation till 15 October 2020 was compiled to construct the figure.

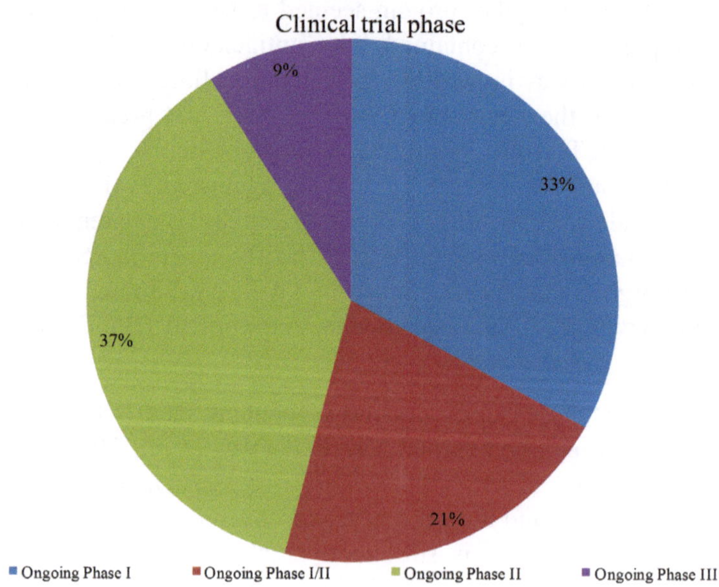

Fig. 1: A summary of COVID-19 vaccine candidates under clinical trial as by 15 October 2020

Fig. 2 depicts a summary of the clinical development landscape of COVID-19 vaccines at the global scale. Viral particles that resemble the virus (virus-like particle; VLP), protein subunit, nucleic acid-based, replicating and non-replicating viral vectors are the seven main types of the COVID-19 vaccine development platforms employed for the purpose. Fig. 2 also displays the proportionate potential vaccines presently under clinical trial. Protein subunit-based vaccines make up to the third highest of the seven categories under clinical trial, while VLP-based vaccines and replicating viral vectors constitute only 5%. Nucleic acid platform based vaccine development included both DNA and RNA vaccines.

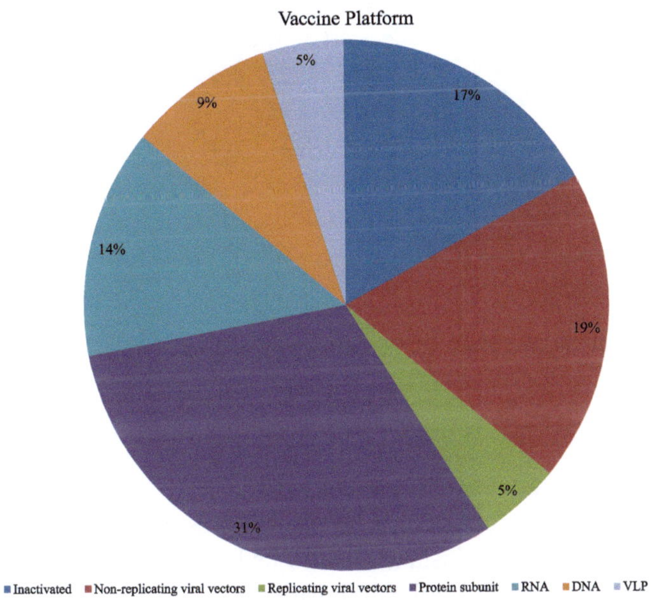

Fig. 2: A summary of worldwide vaccines against COVID-19 under clinical trial across the various platforms

Fig. 3 summarises the developed COVID-19 vaccines around the globe at preclinical stages. It lists ten main categories of COVID-19 vaccine types, based on the inactivated replicating bacterial vector, T-cells based protein subunits replicating viral vectors, non-replicating viral vector, DNA, RNA, VLP and live attenuated virus. It shows proportion of the prospective vaccines that are at preclinical stage. T-cell-based and replicating bacterial vector vaccines are the least advanced vaccine types among the ten, and protein subunit-based vaccine has the major share. While 36% of these are under preclinical stage, only 1% of the RNA-based ones are at the preclinical stage worldwide.

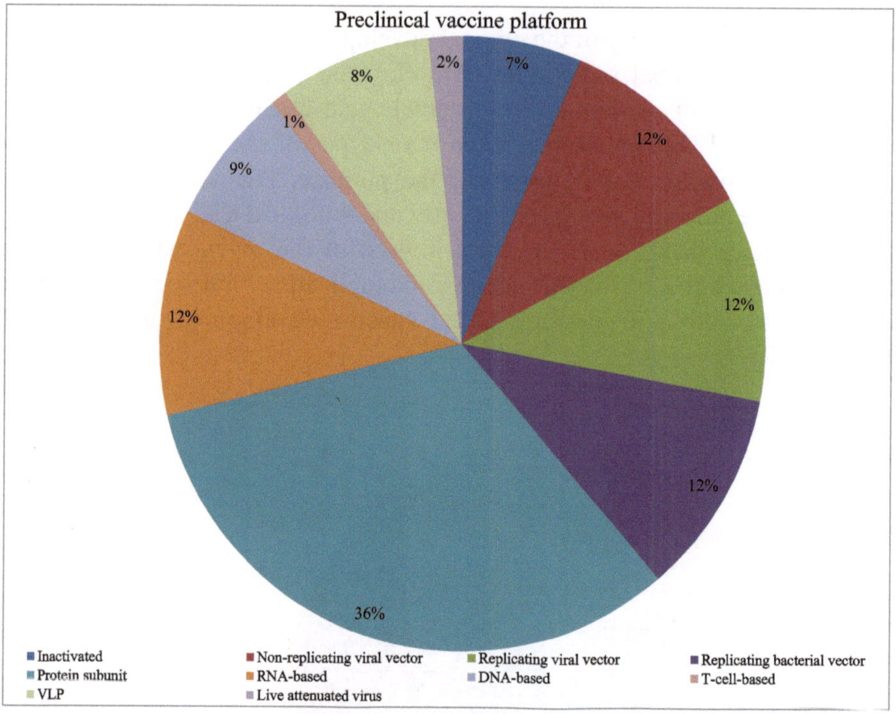

Fig. 3. A summarised worldwide state of vaccine development at preclinical stage till 2019

1.1. RNA-based vaccine

Significant biotechnological advancements seemingly have significantly developed over conventional vaccine development strategies in recent times, and mRNA vaccine is one such case instance due to its higher efficacy, rapid development cycles, affordability and safe administration (Pardi *et al*., 2018). The mRNA vaccine development platform is dynamic with a minimal risk of inspectional mutagenesis, non-integration and infectiousness. mRNA vaccine development and production involves numerous steps: identifying antigen sequence, examining and improving nucleotide screening, identifying delivery mechanisms and evaluating their safety and immunological response (Jahanafrooz *et al*., 2020). The two main RNA-based vaccine types are virally-generated RNA (self-replicating) and mRNA (non-replicating) type. While mRNA-based vaccine typically has 50–30 untranslated regions (UTRs) that solely encode the target antigen, a self-replicating RNA vaccine usually has both the antigen and the essential viral replication apparatus. Improving stability and reducing the immunogenicity of mRNA vaccine is possible (Kaur *et al.*, 2020). Being a less immunogenic genetic vector, anti-vector immunity of mRNA vaccine is also resisted thereby permitting for repeated vaccination (Zhang *et al.*, 2019). Also, rapid vaccine development programme could be strengthened as the adaptability and capacity of this platform to structurally mimic the antigen and express it similar to a natural infection are quite high (Patel *et al.*, 2021). Another potential advantage of mRNA vaccines is the accessible and portable 'printing' device to manufacture mRNA (Saif *et al.*, 2020). Below are discussed the two most successful case discoveries of mRNA vaccines during the COVID-19 pandemic.

1.1.1. The mRNA-1273 – Moderns TX Inc.

Moderna mRNA vaccine is an artificial mRNA encoding the complete prefusion stabilised spike protein (S) for SARS-CoV-2 encapsulated in LNP. It potentially triggers a very specific antiviral S-protein response. It is recognised as relatively safe as it does not include any active or inactivated pathogen subunit (Tu *et al.*, 2020). The USFDA approved the vaccine with fast-track status to conduct Phase II clinical trial, after the interim antibody data of Phase I for eight subjects at varying dose levels was released. The levels of the neutralising antibody were substantially high in subjects who received 100 μg dosage compared to the sera in convalescing patients. Cohorts that received 25 μg and 100 Pl doses demonstrated that the vaccine was mostly safe and well-tolerated. However, three subjects experienced grade 3 systemic symptoms after the administration of 250 μg second dose.

A major advantage of prophylactic mRNA vaccine approach is that while mimicking natural infection it integrates many mRNAs in single vaccine and elicits immune response better. On 24 February 2020, Moderna announced that it had produced 'mRNA-1273' using techniques and approaches as detailed in its earlier patents, and that the initial batch was available for human use against SARS-CoV-2. Its patent application WO2018115527 details the mRNA-expressing vaccine using at least one MERS coronavirus antigen. Humoral immune response activation and *in vivo* translation were observed in mice when LNP encapsulated MERS-CoV S protein-expressing mRNA was intradermally administered (Safety *et al.*, 2020). Moderna developed the mRNA-1273 (mRNA) vaccine that targeted stable state SARS-CoV-2-linked perfusion S protein in collaboration with NIAID Vaccine Research Centre. The NIAID, a division of NIH, US received mRNA-1273 vials for Phase 1 trial.

1.1.2. BNT162b1 – Pfizer and BioNTech

BNT162b1 is a codon-optimised mRNA vaccine encoding for the trimerised spike glycoprotein neutralising antibody RBD of SARS-CoV-2 as principal antigen target. The immunogenicity of RBD antigen is enhanced in the vaccine by including the T-4 fibrin-derived fold on the trimerisation domain. The mRNA was encased in the ionisable cationic LNPs of 80 nm size to ensure efficient dispersion of the vaccine. An elevated level of IgG (immunoglobulin G) that was specific to RBD was found in the Phase I/II clinical trials with the geometric mean concentration being 8–46.3 times higher than the serum titre levels found in a convalescing patient. On the other hand, the geometric mean titre of the neutralising antibody against SARS-CoV-2 was 1.8–2.8 times higher than the convalescence serum panel. The study detailed the immunogenicity, safety and efficacy of BNT162b1 (nucleoside-modified LNP-encased mRNA vaccine). Two dosages of BNT162b1 were administered with 21-day gap in the trial to 18 to 55 years age independent adults with good health conditions. They were randomly assigned to receive 10 μg, 30 μg and 100 μg in cohorts. The usually mild to moderate and transient effects of the vaccine, including the local reactions and systemic events, were found to be dose-dependent. The BNT162b1 vaccine candidate in point that underwent clinical trial incorporated a nucleoside-modified mRNA. The mRNA-encoded protein in the vaccine is the antibody that neutralised SARS-CoV-2 by targeting the RBD on the spike protein. The RBD-binding IgG and SARS-CoV-2 neutralising titre in the sera increased proportionately with the vaccine dosage level, especially after the second shot being administered. The serum profile in the convalescent human patients was estimated as containing the neutralising antibody titre in geometric mean, which was 1.8–2.8 times higher in COVID-19 cases.

These results are certainly encouraging and prompt for extended research to unravel the potentials of mRNA-based vaccines. The multivalent presentation and immunogenicity of the RBD antigen which is expressed in BNT162b1 could be further enhanced with the addition of 'fold on' trimerisation domain obtained from T-4 fibroin. This mRNA vaccine was packaged in lipid nanoparticles (LNPs) so that the intramuscularly administered vaccine transports through the cells more efficiently. Although only minor notable local fleeting reactions and systemic events without critical negative effects were observed, however the assessed data did not measure the immune response, neither the protection level even after administration of the second dosage after the two-week gap (Chalkias *et al.*, 2020). Prospective RNA-based vaccine candidates to combat the COVID-19 that were registered worldwide, and were at the various clinical trial stages are detailed in Table 1 (Rego *et al.*, 2020; Zhang *et al.*, 2021).

Table 1: A list of the various mRNA-based COVID-19 vaccine candidates registered for clinical trials worldwide

Sl. No.	Title of the work	Description	Formulated vaccine form	Clinical trial stage	Sponsor and collaborator	Source
1.	Safety and immunogenicity study of mRNA-1273 vaccine for prophylaxis of SARS-CoV-2 infection	Encodes for a full-length, perfusion stabilised SARS-CoV-2S protein; safety, reactogenicity and immunogenicity was assessed	LNP-encapsulated mRNA	Phase I	NIAID	Le *et al.*, 2020
2.	mRNA-1273 COVID-19 vaccine safety, reactogenicity, and immunogenicity in 18 years and older individuals: a dose-confirmation study	The safety, immunogenicity and reactogenicity of two dose levels of the mRNA-1273 vaccine evaluated in this clinical investigation	LNP-encapsulated mRNA	Phase II	Moderna TX Inc. in collaboration with Advanced Biomedical Research & Dev. Authority	Iqbal *et al.*, 2020
3.	An investigation to assess the mRNA-1273 vaccine's immunogenicity, safety and efficacy in preventing COVID-19 in 18 years and above adults	The trial assessed the immunogenicity, tolerability and ability of the vaccine (mRNA-1273) to prevent COVID-19 infection	LNP-encapsulated mRNA	Phase III	Moderna TX Inc. in collaboration with Advanced Biomedical Research & Dev. Authority and NIAID	Ura *et al.*, 2014
4.	Phase I clinical trial of COVID-19 mRNA vaccine BNT162b1 in China	Evaluated safety and tolerability profiles of BNT162b1 P/B immunisation given 21 days apart on healthy Chinese subjects through 28 days after vaccination booster	Three LNP-mRNAs	Phase I	Jiangsu Provincial in collaboration with CDC	Henao *et al.*, 2017
5.	A study to examine the safety and efficacy of a single BNT162 vaccination against COVID-19	BNT162b3 was administered using a P/B regimen. The trial was divided into two parts for dose-escalation cohorts in older subjects	Three LNP-mRNAs	Phase I/II	Biotech RNA Pharmaceuticals GmbH	Van *et al.*, 2020

Sl. No.	Title of the work	Description	Formulated vaccine form	Clinical trial stage	Sponsor and collaborator	Source
6.	Investigation to characterise the immunogenicity, safety, efficacy and tolerability of RNA vaccines against COVID-19 in healthy individuals	Phase I/II/III randomised trial; placebo-controlled, dose-finding, observer-blind, vaccine candidate-selection, and efficacy in healthy individuals	Three LNP-mRNAs	Phase III	BioNTech collaborating with Pfizer	Zhu *et al.*, 2020
7.	An investigation on the immunogenicity, reactogenicity and safety of the CVnCoV vaccine in healthy adults	The investigation assessed the reactogenicity and safety profile following CVnCoV administrations at various dose levels	mRNA	Phase I	CureVacAG with the CEPI	-
8.	Investigational SARS-CoV-2 vaccine ARCT-021 ascending dosage study in healthy adults	Evaluated the safety, acceptability and immunogenicity of ARCT-021 experimental vaccination in volunteers	mRNA	Phase I/II	Arcturus Therapeutics Inc.	Ou *et al.*, 2020
9.	A study evaluating the safety of CoV vaccine in healthy men and women individuals	Evaluated the vaccine's safety and immune-system effects as the primary goal	LNP-nCoVsaRNA	Phase I	Imperial College, London	-
10.	A phase I clinical research to assess safety, tolerability and initial immunogenicity of varying SARS-CoV-2 mRNA vaccine doses in 18–59, and 60 and older individuals	Investigated the cellular immunological response to the RBD of S protein and the immune persistence of the investigated vaccine at the suggested dose	mRNA	Phase I	PLA Academy of Military Sciences, Walvax Biotech, China	Chen *et al.*, 2020

2. Proof of Concept (pre-clinical stage)

The repurposing and repositioning of potential heterogonous SARS RBD219-N1 as the vaccination antigen to guard against SARS-CoV-2 infection was considered, once the SARS-CoV-2 sequence was available in 2020 after the COVID-19 appeared (Hotez *et al.*, 2020). It was seen that SARS RBD219-N1 and the matching SARS-CoV-2 antigen had 75% identity and 83% similarity. Certain monoclonal antibodies (Mabs) produced against SARS-CoV-2 antigens and SARS-CoV RBD cross-reacted. Due to concerns about likelihoods of enhancing immunity using this especially when the antigen was formed atop an adjuvant like aluminium hydroxide (alum) that induced Th2 production, scientific community and the policymakers lost enthusiasm on the idea of heterogonous antigen immunisation. However, it disregarded the experimental findings that aluminium hydroxide adjuvant reduced the immunological performance in the virus-challenged mouse models and that the Th-17 host responses and the eosinophilic enhancement linked to coronavirus vaccinations were strongly correlated (David *et al.*, 2020; Ulrich *et al.*, 2020). Although an independent NIH study panel confirmed the latter observations too (Haynes *et al.*, 2020), the human clinical trials of SARS RBD219-N1 antigen as a possible COVID-19 vaccine antigen was yet to be evaluated. Texas Children's CVD created a novel RBD that was unique to COVID-19 and SARS-CoV-2, instead of using SARS RBD219-N1 as the foundation for a COVID-19 vaccine. Preferring it sparks from the success of yeast-derived RBD in experimental SARS infections earlier (Jiang *et al.*, 2020), and that yeast microbial fermentation is a typical technique to generate antigens used to make recombinant protein hepatitis B vaccines for the low- and medium-income countries (LMICs) (Hotez *et al.*, 2020). The reasoning was that successfully created SARS-CoV-2 RBD vaccine antigen could hasten the manufacturing of vaccines in numerous LMICs locally and support international initiatives aimed at achieving equity in COVID-19 vaccination.

Genetic engineering was used for the first time to create three distinct constructs resembling the original (Wuhan strain) SARS-CoV-2 sequence based on the native SARS-CoV RBD219 (Fig. 4). They contained both a N1 deleted variant and a wild-type molecule (Wen-Hsiang *et al.*, 2021). The N-terminal asparagine (N331) of S-protein was deleted to prevent hyper-glycosylation that could affect both immunogenicity and consistency of production, similar to what happened with primordial SARS antigen. Oligomerisation and aggregation via intermolecular disulphide bonds were brought about by a cytokine residue at position 538, which was resolved by replacing the cytokine with an alanine residue. Compared to the wild-type molecule a novel antigen known as SARS-CoV-2 RBD219-N1C1 consequently had several benefits, like increased fermentation yield, lack of hyper-glycosylation and oligomer formation, and decreased aggregation. Also, high yield and purification of the novel molecule could be achieved. Further, it was discovered later that the protein antigen binds to ACE-2 receptor that was thought to be the primary host receptor for the coronavirus in humans. The antibodies against the mouse protein showed strong neutralisation of the virus in a mock viral assay, with IC_{50} values ranging between 1:1000 and 1:10000 (Pollet *et al.*, 2021). A balanced Th1/Th2 cellular immune response was indicated by the high levels of cross-neutralising antibodies against alpha, beta, delta and Omicron (BA.1) pseudoviral variants. These responses were induced when alum or alum-mixed with a second immunostimulant like a CpG1826 oligonucleotide (Invivogen, San Diego, USA) was used alongside the SARS-CoV-2 RBD219-N1C1 antigen (Pollet *et al.*, 2022). These include lentiviral particles contained in the surging SARS-CoV-2. A comparable medication generated protective antibodies in a CpG formulation in adult animals. *P. pastoris* was used to create and scale-up the SARS-CoV-2 RBD219-N1C1 antigen process to 1-L and 5-L levels.

It was demonstrated that the method produced notably high yield (>400 mg/L of fermentation supernatant) that could be purified using a combined size-exclusion hydrophobic interaction and ion-exchange chromatography (Lee *et al.*, 2021). The purified molecule was evaluated and described through ACE-2 affinity dynamic light scattering, HPLC and other biophysical techniques at the YNPRC at Emory University. RBD219-WT antigen (same as RBD219-N1C1 but lacked the two mutations of the construct) was tested for protective immunity against SARS-CoV-2 challenge paradigm in non-human primates (Pino *et al.*, 2021). Being the first one accessible for animal testing, WT antigen was selected for non-human primate testing after combining it with aluminium hydroxide before the test. Inducing Th1-biased $CD4^+$ and cytotoxic $CD8^+$ T cell responses and high virus-neutralising antibody levels, the vaccination produced a strong protective effect as demonstrated by decreased virus titre in both nasal secretions and bronchoalveolar ravage (BAL) samples. Further, a decrease in lung pathology in comparison to the control group was noted. Anti-RBD antibodies level was inversely correlated with BAL fluid viral nucleic acid levels. In addition to the quantity of viral mRNA in secretions from nose, RBD-specific plasma cells in draining lymph nodes and other related immune observations further linked to protective immunity (Thuluva *et al.*, 2020).

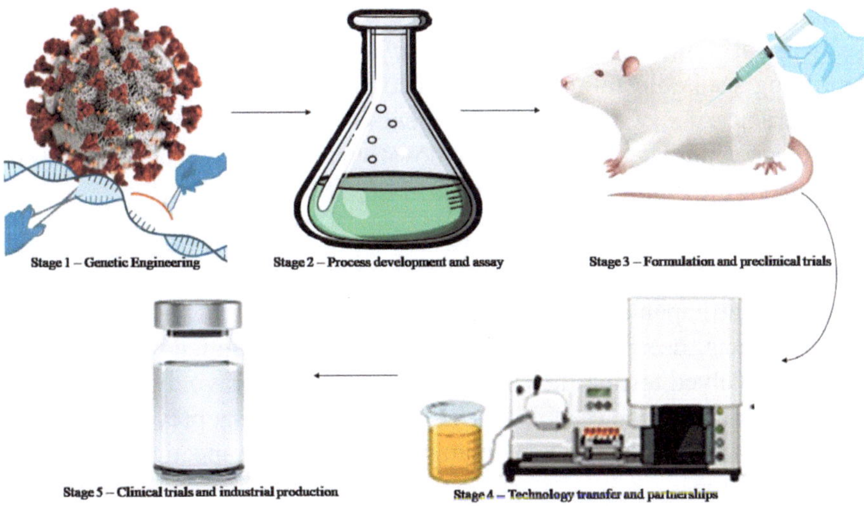

Fig. 4: The COVID-19 vaccine strategy: Stages in research, development and translation

3. Clinical (human subject testing) evaluation

At present, no approved therapeutics for COVID-19 illness by SARS-CoV-2 coronavirus and no vaccine to protect from the virus are there (Docea *et al.*, 2020), although numerous vaccine are available for 'emergency use' only. Medical professionals from around the world repositioned many currently available medications to treat COVID-19 patients albeit with varying results and challenges in determining the efficacies (Nitulescu *et al.*, 2020). Global spread of COVID-19 pandemic made it imperative for researchers and medical professionals to expedite the development of an optimal vaccine against SARS-CoV-2, even if it meant taking a more 'relaxed' approach to accepted protocols (Tsatsakis *et al.*, 2020). About 105 vaccine development projects were initiated as of early April 2020, which was still counting.

Novel COVID-19 vaccine discovery process starts with the basic ideation to its distribution. Intended to provide efficient prevention, vaccine development could take several years (up to decades). Usually the average duration is 10.7 years (Torequl *et al.*, 2020). This is due to the systematic processes behind ascertaining the mechanisms of action of the newly developed molecule and evaluating the toxicity and immunogenicity characteristics of the preparation (Busquet *et al.*, 2020). Preclinical studies typically test the newly discovered bioactive compound on animal models, and clinical trials later test the same on humans. However, due to the desperate situation that emerged during the pandemic, the goal to acquire COVID-19 vaccine had to be accelerated. As a result, the vaccines developed then were released for 'emergency human use' without animal testing (Docea *et al.*, 2016). The challenges included identifying a suitable animal model that comparably exhibited both important characteristics, *i.e.*, COVID-19 pathogenesis and immune response toward the vaccine candidate. Due to this, innovative approaches like animal testing substitutes were employed (Lakdawala *et al.*, 2020).

Human clinical trials for vaccines use the approaches that were similar to the testing of other medications: Phase I involved testing the vaccine's safety profile on healthy participants, Phase II focused on examining the immune responses, adverse effects, determining the right dosage and treatment frequency, and Phase III involved testing the efficiency of a vaccine in avoiding the intended viral/bacterial infection (Calina *et al.*, 2020). Vaccine as a preventive measure is of great significance from the community health perspectives (Rostami *et al.*, 2020). It means, a large population of healthy individuals are immunised to estimate the impact and effects of vaccination on the likelihood of getting infected by the virus and the severity of the course of infection. The test cohort of the individuals to be immunised under the trial typically comprise a group of high-risk subjects of infection (Stokes *et al.*, 2020). Vaccination against the novel CoV was otherwise time-consuming mostly attributed to the requirements of a lot of testing in the conventional third stage of the trial; it is the phase where tens of thousands human subjects volunteer to participate in the test. Ascertaining if those who received the test vaccine developed immunity against the coronavirus was the process outcome wherein some received the vaccine (test cohort) and others did not (placebo cohort). As this trial process consumes lot of time, researchers debated whether to replace this test with an expeditious one due to the prevailing pandemic's pressure. The agreed upon alternate Phase III approach in humans was to vaccinate a small number of volunteers after being exposed to coronavirus and examine whether they developed the immunity.

About 40 out of every 10,000 Americans were infected with COVID-19 by 30 May 2020, as reported by the US CDC. It meant that whether the vaccination reduced the infection to less than 40 typically in every 10,000 cases needed to be confirmed. Given the low number of new infections occurring in Europe then and no prior scientific knowledge about the novel virus, undertaking such research was difficult. Also, the peak infection around April 9 fell by 80% two months later (with a frequency of 2.8 in every 10,000 people). The statistical odds were considerably improved by categorising high-risk people like the healthcare workers, but these straightforward number plays highlighted other difficulties to address. It is increasingly harder considering that no vaccination would work 100% satisfactorily. The CDC found that the vaccine's efficiency ranged between 19 and 60%, using influenza vaccine as an example through the previous decade. It poses significant statistical challenges over and above the significant limitations in COVID-19 test accuracies.

In a quest to perfect COVID-19 vaccine, researchers suggested expediting the conventional idea of vaccine assessment by exposing willing healthy individuals to COVID-19 (Pronker *et al.*, 2013). Given the lack of a licensed medication or antibody treatment for COVID-19, deliberately infecting an individual presented an ethical hurdle too. Medical experts endorsed the advantages of vaccine trials especially against SARS-CoV-2 infection highlighting a major benefit of expedited investigation and approval. Nonetheless, the ethical aspects of the voluntary infection of COVID-19 were necessary to address (Plotkin *et al.*, 2020). Assuming the efficacy of influenza vaccine would require a significant number of volunteers to contract the complete illness maybe at an even higher rate given that they are merely experimental vaccinations. Subjects between 20 and 30 years are most likely considered for such risky trials and considering that the influenza vaccination mortality rate in the group is roughly 0.2% (Bullen *et al.*, 2020). It suggests that two out of every 1,000 volunteers would probably pass away with time even in the absence of vaccination, and one of every 1,000 volunteers are likely do so in the event of vaccine efficacy. Recent research indicated that SARS-CoV-2 infects human brain cells and is consistent with neurological symptoms. As a human brain is extremely sensitive and immune cell invasion and inflammation are rare, it is unclear if such infection could be totally eradicated. It shows that concerns for volunteers are not just whether to take a chance on life, but also whether to get a persistent infection that could have long-term health effects with accelerated neurodegenerative disorders (Delany *et al.*, 2014).

In addition to understand the safety and efficacy of COVID-19 vaccines, the clinical trials could obviously have additionally beneficial to infection studies for various reasons. These include, i) learning more about how a immune system would develop in response to the infection; ii) verifying the results of diagnostic test; iii) offering added information regarding the dynamics of the infection process; and iv) determining if the infected person is still able to disseminate the virus even after the symptoms subside (Bompart *et al.*, 2019). Human challenge studies have been effective in the past to treat malaria, yellow fever and smallpox. Typhoid fever, cholera and influenza are more recent such instances for which expeditious approaches for an accelerated vaccine development as detailed in Fig. 5 became imminent (He *et al.*, 2004).

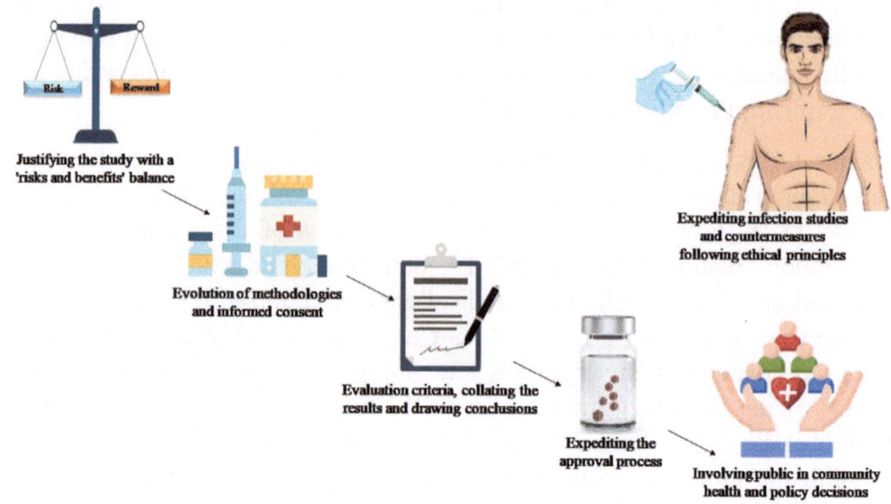

Fig. 5: Flow-chart detailing the expeditious approaches in vaccine development and approval

4. Vaccine manufacturing process

4.1. Recombinant Protein Vaccines (RPV)

The antigen employed in RPV is a partial fragment (like the RBD) alone or in combination with a carrier protein instead of the entire viral entity (Du *et al.*, 2007). The protein antigen is taken up by the antigen-presenting cells (APC) where endosome breaks it down. As the protein fragments break down, the slices are delivered to the major histocompatibility complex II molecules to trigger the subsequent immune responses. It was demonstrated that the animal models vaccinated with candidate recombinant protein vaccine developed neutralising antibodies against SARS-CoV-2 (Fang *et al.*, 2006). A major drawback of recombinant protein vaccine is that it often offered protection against the viral infection only partially, and typically elicited humoral immune responses only (Galmiche *et al.*, 1999; Wang *et al.*, 2020). Thus, recombinant protein vaccines would need an adjuvant to boost immunogenicity while formulating. Matrix-M adjuvant was used in NVX-CoV2373, a COVID-19 vaccine candidate (Du *et al.*, 2008).

4.2. Viral Vector-Based Vaccines

Viral vector vaccine clones the antigen in the vector that could not proliferate. Lentivirus, adenovirus and AAV are examples of some common vectors. Viral vector vaccine elicits greater cellular immune responses compared to a RPV as it mimics the disease state of the original viral infection. An AAV vector was used to create a potential SARS-CoV vaccine.

4.3. Bacterial Vector-Based Vaccines

An additional choice for vector-based vaccine development is the bacterial vector. The most promising among them is LAB, the harmless lactic acid bacteria (Detmer *et al.*, 2006). LAB was used as the vector in the COVID-19 vaccine candidate bacTRL-Spike from Symvivo, currently undergoing clinical studies. The LAB vector has few benefits that included, i) it could be lyophilised to improve stability profile, ii) it is regarded as safe (GRAS) in food and feed, and iii) its manufacturing cost was low (Montel *et al.*, 2014; Thi *et al.*, 2015).

4.4. Plasmid DNA Vaccines

DNA vaccine has higher safety rating as live virus is not required. Producing a plasmid DNA is somewhat simple, and the DNA strand could be freeze-dried and stored for long term. A preserved DNA strand is more stable than viruses, proteins and mRNA. However a primary deterrent in this approach is the low transfection efficacy of the plasmid DNA vaccine. The COVID-19 vaccine candidate from Invivo INO-4800 employed CELLECTRA handheld electroporation tool to achieve it. Electrodes and the vaccine are intradermally injected, by cracking apart the cell membrane by an electric pulse, enabling the plasmid to enter the cell. While biotechniques expedite the clinical study initiation, it throttles mass immunisation.

4.5. mRNA Vaccines

The mRNA vaccine generated entirely *in vitro* is the trending novel vaccine generation that seems to be highly promising in terms of flexibility of development (the RNA fragment engineering) and scaled up production. As mRNA-based antigen expression is a transient process, the risk of it integrating with the host DNA is very little and thus the safety aspect is high. Therefore, the approach benefits from non-requirement of a removal process for the live material (from quality perspective) and an enabled rapid swapping between products during manufacturing. This is due to the fact that the desired protein could be generated through translation by altering only the RNA molecules' sequence, which is easy to acquire during the manufacturing process. By being totally synthetically generated *in vitro*, disease transmission risk within the production facility is also negligible, particularly while synthesising vaccines for high-risk infectious diseases like Ebola.

The natural mRNA molecule has inherent poor transfection efficiency. Thus, these molecules are frequently incorporated within a lipid nanoparticle (LNP) as a carrier for transfection (Kowalski *et al.*, 2019). A typical LNP for formulation is a structurally stiff helper lipid that contains an mRNA condensed in to the lipid. The lipidised polymer cover alters the particle surface characteristics. As the LNP is phagocytised by the cell and is exposed to a low pH environment of the endosome, the lipid containing the condensed mRNA penetrates the endosome and release the mRNA molecule into the cytoplasm. The condensed mRNA lipid milieu serves as the central component of the mRNA-based vaccine development platform. The two frequently employed commercially available lipids (positively charged) are DLin-MC3-DMA and DOTAP. Developed by Moderna, LNP-encapsulated mRNA vaccine mRNA1273 is a COVID-19 vaccine candidate that encoded for the 'S' (spike) protein, was administered intramuscularly (IM) in two shots (Quintin *et al.*, 2012).

4.6. Immunity-trained Vaccines

Conventional vaccines provide pathogen-specific protection by eliciting the adaptive immune system. In similar lines, trained immunity-based vaccines (TibV) defend against unrelated infections by stimulating the innate immune system (O'Connor *et al.*, 2020; Angelidou *et al.*, 2020). Repurposing tuberculosis vaccine Bacille Calmette-Guerin (BCG) against COVID-19 for trained immunity needs further investigation, and was currently being clinically evaluated (Gao *et al.*, 2020). Even though BCG vaccine was successful in preventing COVID-19, the other issues to address are, i) having global standards for its manufacturing that vary between nations currently, and ii) the specific quality standards necessary to offer protection against COVID-19 is not apparent (Wang *et al.*, 2020).

4.7. Adjuvants in Inactivated and Vector-Based Vaccines for Enhanced Immunogenicity

To trigger an antigen-specific immune response, the antigen must be recognised by the innate immune system as a foreign object. Recombinant protein antigens and inactivated viruses often have low immunogenicity levels that need to be enhanced through adjuvant provision. Adjuvant is not a necessity for bacterial or viral vectors based vaccines. $Al(OH)_3$ was the adjuvant used in SinoVac's COVID-19 inactivated vaccine candidate (Kool *et al.*, 2008). Popularly known as 'alum', aluminium salts (like $Al(OH)_3$) were used as adjuvant in human vaccines that were sold even in the 1930s, and are still used in about 80% of the adjuvanted vaccines till date (Kool *et al.*, 2008).

The insoluble alum particles activate the inflammasome when NLRP3 is injected, that triggers the cascade 1 in turn. This leads to the downstream release of proinflammatory cytokines IL-1β, IL18 and IL-33 (Eisenbarth *et al.*, 2008; Mannhalter *et al.*, 1985; Ulanova *et al.*, 2001). The monocytes are drawn to the injection site by alum that migrate to become $CD11c^+$ MHC class II^+

peritoneal dendritic cells (DCs) in the draining lymph node. These monocytic DC precursor cells take charge to prepare naive $CD4^+$ T lymphocytes. Th_2 $CD4^+$ T cells differentiation facilitates B cells differentiation, brought about by the produced IL-1β that release IgG1 and IgE antibody isotopes.

The inefficacy of alum in eliciting cell-mediated immune responses (particularly cytotoxic T-cell response) could be explained by a Th2 response bias (Khurana *et al.*, 2018). A more promising adjuvant other than alum that was capable of generating stronger cellular immune response might help in designing an effective COVID-19 vaccine if particular antibodies alone are unable to do so. One such example of an adjuvant system is monophosphoryl lipid (MPL), which is a Toll-like receptor (TLR-4) agonist. TLR-4 activation enhances cellular immune response by promoting Th1-profile differentiation and IFN-γ production in CD4+ T cells (Didierlaurent *et al.*, 2009). CpG1808, AS-04 and AS-01B are few vaccine adjuvants used in human vaccines that could be further investigated and fine-tuned. The mRNA molecule itself in an mRNA vaccine is sometimes considered as 'self-adjuvant' as it possesses inherent immunogenicity similar to that of an RNA virus. Proinflammatory reactions to mRNA vaccinations could arise from both the mRNA molecules themselves and the carrier/delivery agents like the LNPs. The proinflammatory properties of the mRNA molecules and both the delivery system and the mRNA condensing lipids (that might inadvertently produce proinflammatory reactions) could be altered through chemical modifications (Scheel *et al.*, 2004).

4.8. Viral Vector Vaccines: Balancing the Scaled Up Costing and Quality

Viral vectors based vaccines do not replicate as these do not have the necessary elements for the virus to multiply in a healthy cell (Edwards *et al.*, 2017). During the manufacturing, the virus is cloned in a cell line that is complemented with the missing elements. The lacking components are complemented in the cell lines by dividing into three or four plasmids to ensure that the replication-competent viruses are not produced (Dudek *et al.*, 2006). Despite the fact that viral vectors are being produced commercially for decades for gene therapy, the complexity of viruses necessitates product optimisation to meet cost (commercial) efficiency and quality. The scaling-up of viral production capacity is an obstacle in manufacturing viral vectors (Dull *et al.*, 1998; Faust *et al.*, 2018). The production of good quality and cheaper virus vector-based vaccine requires striking the best balance between the economics, high recovery rate (yield) and purification which remains a seemingly difficulty proposition (Clément *et al.*, 2016).

Although adherent cell lines like HEK293T are transiently transfixed to conventionally produce viral vectors, the production capacity of this approach is limited (Vellinga *et al.*, 2014). Its scaling up could be accomplished by substituting adherent cells cultivated in cell stacks with a suspension expression system cultured in a bioreactor set-up (Moleirinho *et al.*, 2020). Virus particles are purified from the media in subsequent processing steps. However, further difficulties could be there in the suspension systems where the virus particles and cells mix in the liquid. Viral particles attach themselves on the cell detritus (cell 225). The selected filter membranes during clarification to clean the contaminants (like proteins and DNA) from the host cell may lead to the loss of the infection particle itself if the corresponding pore size is small or the process-related impurities to be insufficiently removed if the corresponding pore size is sufficiently large (Terova *et al.*, 2018).

Thus, downstream process optimisation is necessary to ensure efficient impurity removal and high recovery so that the dosage cost could be reduced. Downstream processing techniques typically include centrifugation, clarification, size-exclusion chromatography, ion-exchange chromatography, DNA digestion and tangential flow filtration (Hernandez *et al.*, 2019). Although the majority of the materials for these procedures are commercially available, the bioprocess is labour-intensive and time-intensive as the product needs optimisation that satisfies the set international quality standards. An associated difficulty in suspended viral generation process is the removal of leftover host cell proteins and DNA that might firmly cling to the viral particles and coelute during chromatography (Bandeira *et al.*, 2012). It is therefore important to account for the biophysical characteristics of each virus type as well as the interactions between process steps while designing and validating the manufacturing process. For instance, the LVV is susceptible to temperature, pressure and shear force. Due to the high force generated during the tangential flow filtering process, it could harm LVV cupids and create viral aggregation. It could lead to a low recovery yield as the filter membrane clogs due to the aggregated LVV during the ensuing filtration procedure.

4.9. Ensuring Global Distribution of Vaccines: Thermostability As A Massive Obstacle

A vaccine is ideally supplied in ready-to-use dosage form (in vials) and keeps well at room temperature for a designated extended time period (shelf-life). However, a few advanced vaccines such as the mRNA vaccines needed a dedicated cold supply chain (Fig. 6), that could have logistics and shelf-life compromises. As a timely equated delivery of the vaccines to the intended region/location is as important as the vaccine production itself, this aforementioned issue is critical which needs to be addressed.

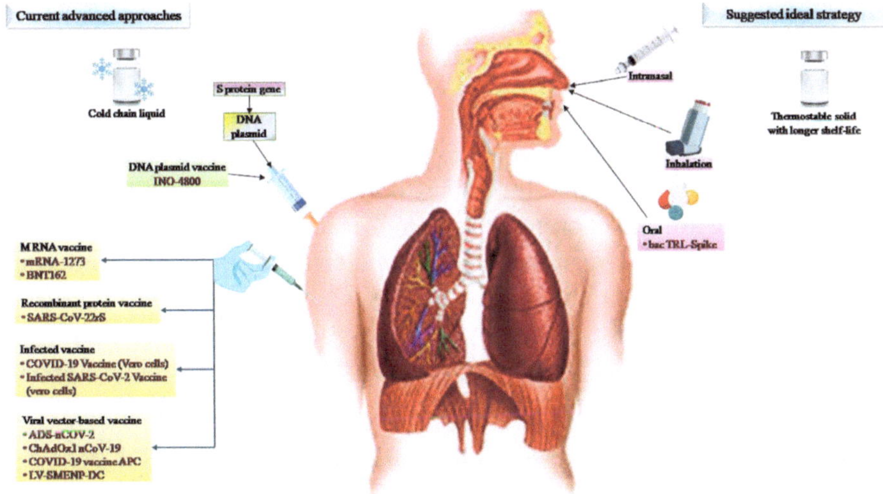

Fig. 6: Comparative best practices and ideal strategies in vaccinology during the COVID-19

As most of the regularly used vaccines these days need refrigeration storage between +2 and +8°C, the prevailing situation is far from optimal (Gramer *et al.*, 2014). However, certain biologics need even lower temperatures for stability and an extended shelf-life. For instance, ZOLGENSMA® is an AAV gene therapeutant that needs −60°C for storage. However, maintaining the vaccines in cold chain especially in low and middle-income countries is a difficult proposition (Murhekar *et al.*, 2013; Hanson *et al.*, 2017).

The cold supply chain alone is estimated to be up to 80% of the vaccination expenses, and sometimes the vaccines are frequently temperature abused at about below +2°C during the storage and transport due to the lack of proper information flow about the vaccines (Matthias *et al.*, 2007). As slow freezing greatly stresses the colloids, liquid-formulated vaccine should not be frozen. When the solutes or particles are forced into tiny spaces between icing crystals as water tends to nucleate during freezing, it produces irreversible aggregation (Niu *et al.*, 2017; Pastorino *et al.*, 2015). Although equipment issues and cold chain capabilities are outside the scope of the manufacturer, thermostability of vaccine could be improved by adopting a modified formulation process. The pH, ionic strength and redox potential of the solution in the liquid formulation influence the antigen's chemical stability and suspension's colloidal stability. To stabilise the product better, these parameters could be altered suitably by increasing the stabiliser content. To prevent aggregation in a protein formulation, argentine is a frequently used stabiliser. Sugar is used as a cryoprotectant in live-attenuated vaccines often to preserve the viability during lyophilisation of solid-formulated vaccine (Zhang *et al.*, 2005). The modified surface of LNP mutable delivery vehicle could stabilise a vaccine particle. PEG generates satiric repulsion and water dispensability in nanomedicine thereby preventing aggregation and improving penetration across biological barriers (Acar *et al.*, 2005). Thimerosal, phenol and 2-phenoxyethanol are some other preservatives used in vaccines (Offit *et al.*, 2003). It is important to bear in mind that the majority of these are still chosen with an empirical knowledge about them and without proper scientific justification, *e.g.*, the effect of the long-term usage of argentine as a product stabiliser is poorly known (Tischer *et al.*, 2010). Systematic techniques like Quality by Design (QbD) are frequently employed to determine the appropriateness of an excipient and the concentration (Baynes *et al.*, 2005).

5. Regulatory Approval and Usage Recommendation

Covaxin was the first indigenous Indian vaccine against coronavirus (SARS-CoV-2), created by BBIL in collaboration with NIV of the ICMR. The development team used the vero cell-line platform to create and manufacture the vaccine that would deliver the inactivated coronavirus strain isolated from an asymptomatic patient. Covaxin was approved 'for restricted use in clinical trial mode in emergency situations as a plentiful precaution in public interest' on 3 January 2021 (Mehrotra *et al.*, 2024), though numerous concerns were raised by the scientific community (Biswas *et al.*, 2021). Vaccine provision for the public at the earliest supported by extensive efficacy and safety data was urgent and a strong moral obligation then. As a result, the approval of the partially researched vaccine was expedited based on the results of the Phases I and II clinical trials (Ella *et al.*, 2021).

The lack of sufficient efficacy data for peer review raised more issues than it answered. Only until the safety and efficacy were confirmed in Phase III clinical trial, that is often planned and carried out in accordance with the specifications and guidelines of regulatory bodies and dedicated committees, an 'emergency use' authorisation was extended. While clinical trial continues, the approval may be extended in rare instances if there are substantial evidence supporting both the safety and efficacy. The term 'restricted use' mentioned in such cases referring to vaccines, that is usually referred to therapeutic pharmaceutical products, could be confusing. Similarly, the term 'clinical trial mode' creates even more uncertainty due to its imprecise connotation. Thus, the regulatory approval process, the terminologies and the recommended usage aspects need to be further streamlined ensuring that those are universal in deciphering, global in applicability and simple to follow-up.

Acknowledging the volunteers' consent and ensuring the necessary follow-up are necessary for an ongoing clinical study (under the Phase III clinical trial). Further, the volunteers participating in a clinical trial usually do not know if they received the vaccine or a placebo. The laid-down criteria to determine who gets vaccinated and who gets a placebo are also blurred. India could proudly view the country's innovative vaccine research and development as a huge accomplishment, although transparency to the concerns of the allies and winning over the public confidence are necessary. The information on the process and outcome may need to be exchanged especially in situations where the public faith in a domestic vaccine, the manufacturer, the regulators and the research partners are low. In case of Covaxin, the initial dented public trust due to media misinformation took a lot of time to regain. The public was worried about the lack of necessary thoroughness and conscientiousness for a confirmatory clinical investigation. Vaccine mistrust could increase anxiety and trigger domino effect of vaccine hesitancy, which might lead to the resurgence of virus and the pandemic becoming uncontrollable (Pallett *et al.*, 2020).

6. Monitoring the Safety after the Approval (pharmacovigilance)

As the majority of COVID-19 vaccines were certified on an urgency by concerned approval agencies for 'emergency use' only, these typically had temporary albeit moderate adverse effects, including injection site discomfort and swelling, fever, chills, exhaustion, joint pain, nausea, muscle soreness and headache. Further, many peculiar side-effects were seen during the clinical trials of exclusively particular vaccines, *e.g.*, neutropenia in case of CoviShield of AstraZeneca/Oxford (Bhopa *et al.*, 2021), heart palpitations in Sputnik V and vomiting in CanSino (Zhu *et al.*, 2020). Clinical trial data of many COVID-19 vaccines were favourable and exhibited good safety ratings. It triggered wider assessment of the COVID-19 vaccines in the ongoing Phase III trials with the majority regulatory bodies of various countries extending 'emergency use' approval (Voysey *et al.*, 2021; Logunov *et al.*, 2021). The side-effects of the licensed vaccines that were commonly encountered during clinical trials were compiled and documented. The vaccine safety must be closely monitored and documented to improve safety profiles and retain public trust.

The surveillance programmes for vaccine-associated adverse events and reactions in volunteers and the general public for vaccination are documented in 'spontaneous volunteer reporting system', combining with the Division of Immunisation (as in Canada). The crucial components included standardised causality assessment by the interdisciplinary experts' team and independent case reports (Collet *et al.*, 2000). The WHO's Programme for International Drug Monitoring compiled a safety surveillance handbook for COVID-19 vaccines. It stipulated a number of standards to fulfil to consider a vaccine as safe (Soldatos *et al.*, 2018). To ensure vaccination safety, pharmacovigilance of COVID-19 vaccines overseen by the designated national and regional centres was crucial (Paudyal *et al.*, 2020). Pharmacovigilance is a systematic identification, reporting, evaluation, comprehension and avoidance of adverse reactions to guarantee that a COVID-19 vaccine was safe (Shrestha *et al.*, 2020). Scientists worldwide collaborated to create safe and efficient vaccines.

Vaccine hesitancy was exacerbated by worries about the safety of COVID-19 vaccines due to the unexpectedly rapid growth in the sector. In a scoping analysis to determine the reasons behind the reluctance to get COVID-19 vaccinated even among the healthcare workers, worries over the efficacy, the safety and possible negative consequences were the primary reasons (Ullah *et al.*, 2021). Addressing such issues by offering evidence-based information from reputable regulatory and public health organisations is crucial. Using communication techniques effectively, framing the minor adverse consequences with a positive outlook and rectifying the information falsification regarding vaccine adverse effects are some of the steps to reduce worries about vaccine side-effects (Biswas *et al.*, 2021). Healthcare professionals could take initiative, paying attention to public concerns on vaccination programmes and responding appropriately. It was advisable to monitor vaccine safety away from the spotlight to prevent the dissemination of misinformation that would inflate vaccine hesitancy among the public (Rief *et al.*, 2021; Motta *et al.*, 2021).

7. Future Trends and Prospects

There are a lot of unsolved concerns regarding the SARS-CoV-2 including the protective immunity. Different vaccines may be required for different age-groups, like babies and young ones, expecting mothers and people with a compromised immunity. Also, the vaccination was seen to have critical side-effects and also breakthrough infections. All of these were because the bulk of the vaccines developed were intended for healthy population, mainly the adults in 18–55 age groups. A safe regulatory framework was needed to be established to vaccinate the immunocompromised, pregnant women and children. The recent outbreaks of measles and pertussis during the pandemic in countries where they were under control earlier meant that the scheduled vaccination programmes cannot be taken for granted and needed to be effectively continued without disruption. The long-term residual effect, altered disease epidemiology and decreased vaccination compliance could potentially derail the estimated initial impact of the vaccination programme. The post-commercialisation surveillance to document the adverse events should be religiously carried out. Pre-clinical testing must be conducted carefully considering all the critical parameters ensuring that the vaccine is efficient and safe with no serious side-effects. Global institutions and finding agencies like the Bill and Melinda Gates Foundation, WHO, CEPI and GAVI need to collaborate to guarantee sufficient funding for vaccine research and development. in an effort to contain the pandemic, COVID-19 vaccines were expected to be accessible globally by mid-2021. The efficacy of licensed vaccines even against the emerging mutant strains (variants) discovered in South Africa, the United Kingdom, India, the US and elsewhere is yet to be investigated. A possible reduced mortality strategy is to vaccinate the high-risk communities first with a nucleic acid-based priming vaccine followed by a booster dose of protein-based vaccine. Stronger and more reassuring second-generation vaccine could be created simultaneously (as next-generation vaccine) to counter the emerging and reemerging genetically-altered viral forms.

8. Recommendations and Conclusion

COVID-19 vaccine's research and development has yielded priceless insights into every step of the procedure including clinical testing, regulatory approval, pharmacovigilance and the emerging trends. One most important lesson learnt was the value of a simplified safety-first approach for regulatory approval. COVID-19 vaccines were authorised on fast-track bases, thanks to the Emergency Use Authorisation (EUA) procedures, demonstrating that vaccines may be created and licensed swiftly without compromising with the strict safety standards. Pharmacovigilance, the continued monitoring of vaccine safety following the approval, was essential to maintain public faith and addressing any inadvertent safety concerns that were encountered. Sturdy post-approval surveillance initiatives, like the Vaccine Adverse Event Reporting System (VAERS), provide real-time monitoring and prompt adverse event response. To ensure that the systems continued to function well, advanced data analytics could be added. To guarantee that a vaccine is safe and effective in different groups, clinical evaluation (testing of the vaccines on human subjects) must continue rigorously and inclusively involving wider range of demography. This step could lead to finding appropriate doses, efficacies and safety profiles. The proof-of-concept and the pre-clinical stages needed significant funding to promote innovation and to create new technologies. The efficacy of mRNA vaccines against COVID-19 highlights the possibility of the cutting-edge technology to contribute more to vaccine development. Future trends point to the necessity of developing adaptable vaccines to combat newly emerging infectious illnesses and their variants. Flexible processing platform that guarantees vaccination fairness and tackling vaccine hesitancy in line with the ongoing international cooperation and public outreach initiatives shall be essential. COVID-19 vaccine creation has shown the value of a meticulous and well-rounded regulatory approval strategy, strict pharmacovigilance, comprehensive clinical evaluation, and flexible proof-of-concept tactics. The vaccines to be developed in future could be more durable, effective and sensitive to the needs of global community health by combining these various components.

References

Acar HY, Garaas RS, Syud F, Bonitatebus P, and Kulkarni AM, 2005. Superparamagnetic nanoparticles stabilized by polymerized PEGylated coatings. J. Magn. Magn. Mater., 293(1): 1–7. doi: 10.1016/j.jmmm.2005.02.008.

Ahmed SF, Ahmed AQ, and Matthew RM, 2020.Preliminary identification of potential vaccine targets for the COVID-19 coronavirus (SARS-CoV-2) based on SARS-CoV immunological studies. Viruses, 12(3): 254. doi: 10.3390/v12030254.

Andersen KG, Andrew R, Ian WI,Edward CH, and Robert FG, 2020.The proximal origin of SARS-CoV-2. Nat. Med., 26(4): 450–452. doi: 10.1038/s41591-020-0820-9

André FE, 2001.The future of vaccines, immunisation concepts and practice. Vaccine, 19(17-19): 2206–2209.doi: 10.1016/s0264-410x(00)00546-6.

Angelidou A, Conti MG, Diray-Arce J, Benn CS, Shann F, Netea MG, Liu M, Potluri LP, Sanchez-Schmitz G, Husson R, and Ozonoff A, 2020. Licensed BacilleCalmette-Guérin (BCG) formulations differ markedly in bacterial viability, RNA content and innate immune activation. Vaccine, 38(9): 2229–2240. doi: 10.1016/j.vaccine.2019.11.060

Bandeira V, Peixoto C, Rodrigues AF, Cruz PE, Alves PM, Coroadinha AS, and Carrondo MJ, 2012. Downstream processing of lentiviral vectors: releasing bottlenecks. Hum. Gene Ther. Methods, 23(4): 255–263. doi: 10.1089/hum.2011.061.

Baynes BM, Wang DI, and Trout BL, 2005. Role of arginine in the stabilization of proteins against aggregation. Biochemistry, 44(12): 4919–4925. doi: 10.1021/bi047481p.

Begum J, Mir NA, Dev K, Buyamayum B, Wani MY, and Raza M, 2021. Challenges and prospects of COVID-19 vaccine development based on the progress made in SARS and MERS vaccine development. Transbound. Emerg. Dis., 68(3): 1111–1124. doi: 10.1111/tbed.13889.

Bhopal SS, Olabi B, and Bhopal R, 2021. Vaccines for COVID-19: learning from ten phase II trials to inform clinical and public health vaccination programmes. Public Health, 193: 57–60. doi: 10.1016/j.puhe.2021.01.018.

Biswas N, Mustapha T, Khubchandani J, and Price JH, 2021. The nature and extent of COVID-19 vaccination hesitancy in healthcare workers. J. Community Health, 46: 1244–1251. doi: 10.1007/s10900-021-00984-3.

Biswas S, 2021. Covaxin: What was the rush to approve India's homegrown vaccine. Available online at: https://www.bbc.com/news/world-asia-india-55534902, Accessed on 15th September 2024.

Bolles M, Deming D, Long K, Agnihothram S, Whitmore A, Ferris M, Funkhouser W, Gralinski L, Totura A, Heise M, and Baric RS, 2011. A double-inactivated severe acute respiratory syndrome coronavirus vaccine provides incomplete protection in mice and induces increased eosinophilic proinflammatory pulmonary response upon challenge. J. Virol., 85(23): 12201–12215. doi: 10.1128/JVI.06048-11.

Bompart F, 2019. Healthy volunteers for clinical trials in resource-poor settings: national registries can address ethical and safety concerns. Cambridge Q Healthc. Ethics, 28(1): 134–143. doi: 10.1017/S0963180118000425.

Bullen CK, Hogberg HT, Bahadirli-Talbott A, Bishai WR, Hartung T, Keuthan C, Looney MM, Pekosz A, Romero JC, Sillé FC, and Um P, 2020. Infectability of human BrainSphere neurons suggests neurotropism of SARS-CoV-2. ALTEX, 37(4): 665–671. doi: 10.14573/altex.2006111.

Busquet F, Hartung T, Pallocca G, Rovida C, and Leist M, 2020. Harnessing the power of novel animal-free test methods for the development of COVID-19 drugs and vaccines. Arch. Toxicol., 94(6): 2263–2272. doi: 10.1007/s00204-020-02732-0.

Calina D, Docea AO, Petrakis D, Egorov AM, Ishmukhametov AA, Gabibov AG, Shtilman MI, Kostoff R, Carvalho F, Vinceti M, and Spandidos DA, 2020. Towards effective COVID-19 vaccines: Updates, perspectives and challenges. Int. J. Mol. Med., 46(1): 3–16. doi: 10.3892/ijmm.2020.4596.

Casadevall A, and Pirofski LA, 2020. The convalescent sera option for containing COVID-19. J. Clin. Invest., 130(4): 1545–1548. doi: 10.1172/JCI138003.

Chalkias S, Schwartz H, Nestorova B, Feng J, Chang Y, Zhou H, Dutko FJ, Edwards DK, Montefiori D, Pajon R, and Leav B, 2022. Safety and immunogenicity of a 100 μg mRNA-1273 vaccine booster for severe acute respiratory syndrome coronavirus-2 (SARS-CoV-2). medRxiv. doi: 10.1101/2022.01.18.21268059.

Chen WH, Hotez PJ, and Bottazzi ME, 2020. Potential for developing a SARS-CoV receptor-binding domain (RBD) recombinant protein as a heterologous human vaccine against coronavirus infectious disease (COVID)-19. Hum. Vaccin. Immunother., 16(6): 1239–1242. doi: 10.1080/21645515.2020.1740564.

Chen WH, Wei J, Kundu RT, Adhikari R, Liu Z, Lee J, Versteeg L, Poveda C, Keegan B, Villar MJ, and de Araujo Leao AC, 2021. Genetic modification to design a stable yeast-expressed recombinant SARS-CoV-2 receptor binding domain as a COVID-19 vaccine candidate. Biochim. Biophys. Acta. Gen. Subj., 1865(6): 129893. doi: 10.1016/j.bbagen.2021.129893.

Clément N, and Grieger JC, 2016. Manufacturing of recombinant adeno-associated viral vectors for clinical trials. Mol. Ther. Methods Clin. Dev., 3: 16023. doi: 10.1038/mtm.2016.23.

Collet JP, MacDonald N, Cashman N, and Pless R, 2000. Monitoring signals for vaccine safety: the assessment of individual adverse event reports by an expert advisory committee. Bull. World Health Organ., 78: 178–185.

Corey L, Mascola JR, Fauci AS, and Collins FS, 2020. A strategic approach to COVID-19 vaccine R&D. Science, 368(6494): 948–950. doi: 10.1126/science.abc5312.

Craven J, 2021. COVID-19 vaccine tracker. Regul. Affairs Prot. Soc., 29.

Delany I, Rappuoli R, and De Gregorio E, 2014. Vaccines for the 21st century. EMBO Mol. Med., 6(6): 708–720. doi: 10.15252/emmm.201404866.

Detmer A, and Glenting J, 2006. Live bacterial vaccines–a review and identification of potential hazards. Microb. Cell Fact., 5: 1–12. doi: 10.1186/1475-2859-5-23.

Dhama K, Patel SK, Pathak M, Yatoo MI, Tiwari R, Malik YS, Singh R, Sah R, Rabaan AA, Bonilla-Aldana DK, and Rodriguez-Morales AJ, 2020. An update on SARS-CoV-2/COVID-19 with particular reference to its clinical pathology, pathogenesis, immunopathology and mitigation strategies. Travel. Med. Infect. Dis., 37: 101755. doi: 10.1016/j.tmaid.2020.101755.

Dhama K, Sharun K, Tiwari R, Dadar M, Malik YS, Singh KP, and Chaicumpa W, 2020. COVID-19, an emerging coronavirus infection: advances and prospects in designing and developing vaccines, immunotherapeutics, and therapeutics. Hum. Vaccin. Immunother., 16(6): 1232–1238. doi: 10.1080/21645515.2020.1734794.

Didierlaurent AM, Morel S, Lockman L, Giannini SL, Bisteau M, Carlsen H, Kielland A, Vosters O, Vanderheyde N, Schiavetti F, and Larocque D, 2009. AS04, an aluminum salt- and TLR4 agonist-based adjuvant system, induces a transient localized innate immune response leading to enhanced adaptive immunity. J. Immunol., 183(10): 6186–6197. doi: 10.4049/jimmunol.0900321.

Docea AO, Gofita E, Calina D, Ioan ZS, Valcea DI, and Mitrut P, 2016. Autoimmune disorders due to double antiviral therapy with peginterferon and ribavirin in patients with hepatitis C virus infection. Farmacia, 64(4).

Docea AO, Tsatsakis A, Albulescu D, Cristea O, Zlatian O, Vinceti M, Moschos SA, Tsoukalas D, Goumenou M, Drakoulis N, and Dumanov JM, 2020. A new threat from an old enemy: Re-emergence of coronavirus. Int. J. Mol. Med., 45(6): 1631–1643. doi: 10.3892/ijmm.2020.4505.

Dudek T, and Knipe DM, 2006. Replication-defective viruses as vaccines and vaccine vectors. Virology, 344(1): 230–239. doi: 10.1016/j.virol.2005.09.030.

Du L, Zhao G, He Y, Guo Y, Zheng BJ, Jiang S, and Zhou Y, 2007. Receptor-binding domain of SARS-CoV spike protein induces long-term protective immunity in an animal model. Vaccine, 25(15): 2832–2838. doi: 10.1016/j.vaccine.2006.11.034.

Du L, Zhao G, Lin Y, Sui H, Chan C, Ma S, He Y, Jiang S, Wu C, Yuen KY, and Jin DY, 2008. Intranasal vaccination of recombinant adeno-associated virus encoding receptor-binding domain of severe acute respiratory syndrome coronavirus (SARS-CoV) spike protein induces strong mucosal immune responses and provides long-term protection against SARS-CoV infection. J. Immunol., 180(2): 948–956. doi: 10.4049/jimmunol.180.2.948.

Dull T, Zufferey R, Kelly M, Mandel RJ, Nguyen M, Trono D, and Naldini L, 1998. A third-generation lentivirus vector with a conditional packaging system. J. Virol., 72(11): 8463–8471. doi: 10.1128/JVI.72.11.8463-8471.1998.

Edwards DK, Jasny E, Yoon H, Horscroft N, Schanen B, Geter T, Fotin-Mleczek M, Petsch B, and Wittman V, 2017. Adjuvant effects of a sequence-engineered mRNA vaccine: translational profiling demonstrates similar human and murine innate response. J. Transl. Med., 15: 1–18. doi: 10.1186/s12967-017-1373-2.

Eisenbarth SC, Colegio OR, O'Connor W, Sutterwala FS, and Flavell RA, 2008. Crucial role for the Nalp3 inflammasome in the immunostimulatory properties of aluminium adjuvants. Nature, 453(7198): 1122–1126. doi: 10.1038/nature06939.

Ella R, Vadrevu KM, Jogdand H, Prasad S, Reddy S, Sarangi V, Ganneru B, Sapkal G, Yadav P, Abraham P, and Panda S, 2021. Safety and immunogenicity of an inactivated SARS-CoV-2 vaccine, BBV152: a double-blind, randomised, phase 1 trial. Lancet Infect. Dis., 21(5): 637–646. doi: 10.1016/S1473-3099(21)00003-0.

Fang M, Cheng H, Dai Z, Bu Z, and Sigal LJ, 2006. Immunization with a single extracellular enveloped virus protein produced in bacteria provides partial protection from a lethal orthopoxvirus infection in a natural host. Virology, 345(1): 231–243. doi: 10.1016/j.virol.2005.09.027.

Funk CD, Laferrière C, and Ardakani A, 2020. A snapshot of the global race for vaccines targeting SARS-CoV-2 and the COVID-19 pandemic. Front. Pharmacol., 11: 937. doi: 10.3389/fphar.2020.00937.

Gao Q, Bao L, Mao H, Wang L, Xu K, Yang M, Li Y, Zhu L, Wang N, Lv Z, and Gao H, 2020. Development of an inactivated vaccine candidate for SARS-CoV-2. Science, 369(6499): 77–81. doi: 10.1126/science.abc1932.

Gorbalenya AE, Baker SC, Baric RS, de Groot RJ, Drosten C, Gulyaeva AA, Haagmans BL, Lauber C, Leontovich AM, Neuman BW, and Penzar D, 2020. The species severe acute respiratory syndrome-related coronavirus: classifying 2019-nCoV and naming it SARS-CoV-2. Nat. Microbiol., 5(4): 536–544. doi: 10.1038/s41564-020-0695-z.

Gramer MJ, 2014. Product quality considerations for mammalian cell culture process development and manufacturing. In: W Zhou, A Kantardjieff (eds) Mammalian Cell Cultures for Biologics Manufacturing, Springer, Berlin, Heidelberg: 139: 123–166. doi: 10.1007/10_2013_214

Gunneri SR, Yerroju V, Mogulla R, Turaga K, Kyasani M, Manoharan SK, Medigeshi G, Singh J, and Shaman H, 2022. Evaluation of safety and immunogenicity of receptor-binding domain-based COVID-19 vaccine (Corbevax) to select the optimum formulation in open-label, multicentre, and randomised phase-1/2 and phase-2 clinical trials. EBioMedicine, 83: 104217. doi: 10.1016/j.ebiom.2022.104217

Hanson CM, George AM, Sawadogo A, and Schreiber B, 2017. Is freezing in the vaccine cold chain an ongoing issue? A literature review. Vaccine, 35(17): 2127–2133. doi: 10.1016/j.vaccine.2016.09.070

Haynes BF, Corey L, Fernandes P, Gilbert PB, Hotez PJ, Rao S, Santos MR, Schuitemaker H, Watson M, and Arvin A, 2020. Prospects for a safe COVID-19 vaccine. Sci. Transl. Med., 12(568): eabe0948. doi: 10.1126/scitranslmed.abe0948.

Heaton PM, 2020. The Covid-19 vaccine-development multiverse. N. Engl. J. Med., 383(20): 1986–1988. doi: 10.1056/NEJMe2025111.

Henao-Restrepo AM, Camacho A, Longini IM, Watson CH, Edmunds WJ, Egger M, Carroll MW, Dean NE, Diatta I, Doumbia M, and Draguez B, 2017. Efficacy and effectiveness of an rVSV-vectored vaccine in preventing Ebola virus disease: final results from the Guinea ring vaccination, open-label, cluster-randomised trial (Ebola Ça Suffit!). Lancet, 389(10068): 505–518. doi: 10.1016/ S0140-6736(16)32621-6.

Hernandez Bort JA, 2019. Challenges in the downstream process of gene therapy products. Am. Pharm. Rev., 22(4): 25. Available online at: https://www.americanpharmaceuticalreview.com/Featured-Articles/362178-Challenges-in-the-Downstream-Process-of-Gene-Therapy-Products/, Accessed on 20th September 2024.

He Y, Zhou Y, Liu S, Kou Z, Li W, Farzan M, and Jiang S, 2004. Receptor-binding domain of SARS-CoV spike protein induces highly potent neutralizing antibodies: implication for developing subunit vaccine. Biochem. Biophys. Res. Commun., 324(2): 773–781. doi: 10.1016/j.bbrc.2004.09.106

Hotez PJ, Bottazzi ME, and Corry DB, 2020. The potential role of Th17 immune responses in coronavirus immunopathology and vaccine-induced immune enhancement. Microbes Infect., 22(4-5): 165–167. doi: 10.1016/j.micinf.2020.04.005.

Hotez PJ, Corry DB, and Bottazzi ME, 2020. COVID-19 vaccine design: the Janus face of immune enhancement. Nat. Rev. Immunol., 20(6): 347–348. doi: 10.1038/s41577-020-0323-4.

Hotez PJ, Corry DB, Strych U, and Bottazzi ME, 2020. COVID-19 vaccines: neutralizing antibodies and the alum advantage. Nat. Rev. Immunol., 20(7): 399–400. doi: 10.1038/s41577-020-0358-6.

Hotez PJ and Bottazzi ME, 2020. Developing a low-cost and accessible COVID-19 vaccine for global health. PLoS Negl. Trop. Dis., 14(7): e0008548. doi: 10.1371/journal.pntd.0008548.g001.

IqbalYatoo, M., Hamid, Z., Parray, O.R., Wani, A.H., UlHaq, A., Saxena, A., Patel, S.K., Pathak, M., Tiwari, R., Malik, Y.S. and Sah, R., 2020.COVID-19-Recent advancements in identifying novel vaccine candidates and current status of upcoming SARS-CoV-2 vaccines. Hum. Vaccines Immunother., 16(12): 2891–2904. doi: 10.1080/21645515.2020.1788310

Jahanafrooz Z, Baradaran B, Mosafer J, Hashemzaei M, Rezaei T, Mokhtarzadeh A, and Hamblin MR, 2020. Comparison of DNA and mRNA vaccines against cancer. Drug Discov. Today, 25(3): 552–560. doi: 10.1016/j.drudis.2019.12.003.

Jiang S, Zhang X, Yang Y, Hotez PJ, and Du L, 2020. Neutralizing antibodies for the treatment of COVID-19. Nat. Biomed. Eng., 4(12): 1134–1139.

Kaur SP, and Gupta V, 2020. COVID-19 Vaccine: A comprehensive status report. Virus Res., 288: 198114. doi: 10.1038/s41551-020-00660-2.

Khurana S, Coyle EM, Manischewitz J, King LR, Gao J, Germain RN, Schwartzberg PL, Tsang JS, and Golding H, 2018. AS03-adjuvanted H5N1 vaccine promotes antibody diversity and affinity maturation, NAI titers, cross-clade H5N1 neutralization, but not H1N1 cross-subtype neutralization. npj Vaccines, 3(1): 40. doi: 10.1038/s41541-018-0076-2.

Kool M, Pétrilli V, De Smedt T, Rolaz A, Hammad H, Van Nimwegen M, Bergen IM, Castillo R, Lambrecht BN, and Tschopp J, 2008. Cutting edge: alum adjuvant stimulates inflammatory dendritic cells through activation of the NALP3 inflammasome. J. Immunol., 181(6): 3755–3759. doi: 10.4049/jimmunol.181.6.3755.

Kool M, Soullié T, Van Nimwegen M, Willart MA, Muskens F, Jung S, Hoogsteden HC, Hammad H, and Lambrecht BN, 2008. Alum adjuvant boosts adaptive immunity by inducing uric acid and activating inflammatory dendritic cells. J. Exp. Med., 205(4): 869–882. doi: 10.1084/jem.20071087.

Kowalski PS, Rudra A, Miao L, and Anderson DG, 2019. Delivering the messenger: advances in technologies for therapeutic mRNA delivery. Molecular Therapy, 27(4): 710–728. doi: 10.1016/j.ymthe.2019.02.012.

Lakdawala SS, and Menachery VD, 2020. The search for a COVID-19 animal model. Science, 368(6494): 942–943. doi: 10.1126/science.abc6141.

Lee J, Liu Z, Chen WH, Wei J, Kundu R, Adhikari R, Rivera JA, Gillespie PM, Strych U, Zhan B, and Hotez PJ, 2021. Process development and scale-up optimization of the SARS-CoV-2 receptor-binding domain–based vaccine candidate, RBD219-N1C1. Appl. Microbiol. Biotechnol., 105: 4153–4165. doi: 10.1007/s00253-021-11281-3.

Le TT, Andreadakis Z, Kumar A, Román RG, Tollefsen S, Saville M, and Mayhew S, 2020. The COVID-19 vaccine development landscape. Nat. Rev. Drug Discov., 19(5): 305–306. doi: 10.1038/d41573-020-00073-5.

Logunov DY, Dolzhikova IV, Shcheblyakov DV, Tukhvatulin AI, Zubkova OV, Dzharullaeva AS, Kovyrshina AV, Lubenets NL, Grousova DM, Erokhova AS, and Botikov AG, 2021. Safety and efficacy of an rAd26 and rAd5 vector-based heterologous prime-boost COVID-19 vaccine: an interim analysis of a randomised controlled phase 3 trial in Russia. Lancet, 397(10275): 671–681. doi: 10.1016/ S0140-6736(21)00234-8.

Mannhalter JW, Neychev HO, Zlabinger GJ, Ahmad R, and Eibl MM, 1985. Modulation of the human immune response by the non-toxic and non-pyrogenic adjuvant aluminium hydroxide: effect on antigen uptake and antigen presentation. Clin Exp Immunol., 61(1): 143.

Matthias DM, Robertson J, Garrison MM, Newland S, and Nelson C, 2007. Freezing temperatures in the vaccine cold chain: a systematic literature review. Vaccine, 25(20): 3980–3986. doi: 10.1016/j.vaccine.2007.02.052.

Mehrotra N, and Manchikanti P, 2024. Emergency Approval Mechanisms for Human Vaccines in India. Pharma. Med., 38: 121–132. doi: 10.1007/s40290-023-00513-8.

Mohapatra RK, Azam M, Mohapatra PK, Sarangi AK, Abdalla M, Perekhoda L, Yadav O, Al-Resayes SI, Jong-Doo K, Dhama K, and Ansari A, 2022c. Computational studies on potential new anti-COVID-19 agents with a multi-target mode of action. J. King Saud Univ. Sci., 34(5): 102086. doi: 10.1016/j.jksus.2022.102086.

Mohapatra RK, Dhama K, El-Arabey AA, Sarangi AK, Tiwari R, Emran TB, Azam M, Al-Resayes SI, Raval MK, Seidel V, and Abdalla M, 2021a. Repurposing benzimidazole and benzothiazole derivatives as potential inhibitors of SARS-CoV-2: DFT, QSAR, molecular docking, molecular dynamics simulation, and in-silico pharmacokinetic and toxicity studies. J. King Saud Univ. Sci., 33(8): 101637. doi: 10.1016/j.jksus.2021.101637

Mohapatra RK, Kandi V, Tuli HS, Chakraborty C, and Dhama K, 2022b. The recombinant variants of SARS-CoV-2: concerns continue amid COVID-19 pandemic. J. Med. Virol., 94(8): 3506. doi:10.1002/jmv.27780

Mohapatra RK, Kuppili S, Kumar Suvvari T, Kandi V, Behera A, Verma S, Biswal SK, Al-Noor TH, El-Ajaily MM, Sarangi AK, and Dhama K, 2022a. SARS-CoV-2 and its variants of concern including Omicron: a never-ending pandemic. Chem. Biol. Drug Des., 99(5): 769–788. doi: 10.1111/cbdd.14035.

Mohapatra RK, Mishra S, Azam M, and Dhama K, 2021b. COVID-19, WHO guidelines, pedagogy, and respite. Open Med., 16(1): 491-493. doi:10.1515/med-2021-0266

Mohapatra RK, Mishra S, Kandi V, Branda F, Ansari A, Rabaan AA, and Kudrat-E-Zahan M, 2023a. Analyzing the emerging patterns of SARS-CoV-2 Omicron subvariants for the development of next-gen vaccine: An observational study. Health Sci. Rep., 6(10): e1596. doi:10.1002/hsr2.1596

Mohapatra RK, Pintilie L, Kandi V, Sarangi AK, Das D, Sahu R, and Perekhoda L, 2020. The recent challenges of highly contagious COVID-19, causing respiratory infections: Symptoms, diagnosis, transmission, possible vaccines, animal models, and immunotherapy. Chem. Biol. Drug Des., 96(5): 1187–1208. doi: 10.1111/cbdd.13761.

Mohapatra RK, Verma S, Kandi V, Sarangi AK, Seidel V, Das SN, Behera A, Tuli HS, Sharma AK, and Dhama K, 2023b. The SARS-CoV-2 Omicron variant and its multiple sub-lineages: transmissibility, vaccine development, antiviral drugs, monoclonal antibodies, and strategies for infection control–a review. ChemistrySelect, 8(9): e202201380. doi:10.1002/slct.202201380.

Moleirinho MG, Silva RJ, Alves PM, Carrondo MJ, and Peixoto C, 2020. Current challenges in biotherapeutic particles manufacturing. Expert Opin. Biol. Ther., 20(5): 451–465. doi: 10.1080/14712598.2020.1693541.

Montel Mendoza G, Pasteris SE, Otero MC, and Fatima Nader-Macías ME, 2014. Survival and beneficial properties of lactic acid bacteria from raniculture subjected to freeze-drying and storage. J. Appl. Microbiol., 116(1): 157–166. doi: 10.1111/jam.12359

Motta M, Sylvester S, Callaghan T, and Lunz-Trujillo K, 2021. Encouraging COVID-19 vaccine uptake through effective health communication. Front Polit Sci., 3: 630133.

Murhekar MV, Dutta S, Kapoor AN, Bitragunta S, Dodum R, Ghosh P, Swamy KK, Mukhopadhyay K, Ningombam S, Parmar K, and Ravishankar D, 2013. Frequent exposure to suboptimal temperatures in vaccine cold-chain system in India: results of temperature monitoring in 10 states. Bull. World Health Organ., 91: 906–913. doi: 10.2471/BLT.13.119974.

Nitulescu GM, Paunescu H, Moschos SA, Petrakis D, Nitulescu G, Ion GND, Spandidos DA, Nikolouzakis TK, Drakoulis N, and Tsatsakis A, 2020. Comprehensive analysis of drugs to treat SARS-CoV-2 infection: mechanistic insights into current COVID-19 therapies. Int. J. Mol. Med., 46(2): 467–488. doi: 10.3892/ijmm.2020.4608

Niu L, and Panyam J, 2017. Freeze concentration-induced PLGA and polystyrene nanoparticle aggregation: imaging and rational design of lyoprotection. J. Control Release, 248: 125–132. doi: 10.1016/j.jconrel.2017.01.019.

Offit PA, and Jew RK, 2003. Addressing parents' concerns: do vaccines contain harmful preservatives, adjuvants, additives, or residuals?. Pediatrics. 112(6): 1394–1397. doi: 10.1542/peds.112.6.1394.

Ou X, Liu Y, Lei X, Li P, Mi D, Ren L, Guo L, Guo R, Chen T, Hu J, and Xiang Z, 2020. Characterization of spike glycoprotein of SARS-CoV-2 on virus entry and its immune cross-reactivity with SARS-CoV. Nat Commun., 11(1): 1620. doi: 10.1038/s41467-020-15562-9.

O'Connor E, Teh J, Kamat AM, and Lawrentschuk N, 2020. Bacillus Calmette-Guérin (BCG) vaccination use in the fight against COVID-19–what's old is new again?. Future Oncol., 16(19): 1323–1325. doi: 10.2217/fon-2020-0381.

Pallett SJ, Rayment M, Patel A, Fitzgerald-Smith SA, Denny SJ, Charani E, Mai AL, Gilmour KC, Hatcher J, Scott C, and Randell P, 2020. Point-of-care serological assays for delayed SARS-CoV-2 case identification among health-care workers in the UK: a prospective multicentre cohort study. Lancet Respir. Med., 8(9): 885–894. doi: 10.1016/ S2213-2600(20)30315-5

Pang J, Wang MX, Ang IYH, Tan SHX, Lewis RF, Chen JIP, Gutierrez RA, Gwee SXW, Chua PEY, Yang Q, and Ng XY, 2020. Potential rapid diagnostics, vaccine and therapeutics for 2019 novel coronavirus (2019-nCoV): a systematic review. J. Clin. Med., 9(3): 623. doi: 10.3390/jcm9030623.

Pardi N, Hogan MJ, Porter FW, and Weissman D, 2018. mRNA vaccines—a new era in vaccinology. Nat. Rev. Drug Discov., 17(4): 261–279. doi: 10.1038/nrd.2017.243

Pastorino B, Baronti C, Gould EA, Charrel RN, and de Lamballerie X, 2015. Effect of chemical stabilizers on the thermostability and infectivity of a representative panel of freeze dried viruses. PLoS One., 10(4): e0118963. doi: 10.1371/journal.pone.0118963.

Patel SP, Patel GS, and Suthar JV, 2021. Inside the story about the research and development of COVID-19 vaccines. Clin. Exp. Vaccine Res., 10(2): 154. doi: 10.7774/cevr.2021.10.2.154.

Paudyal V, Al-Hamid A, Bowen M, Hadi MA, Hasan SS, Jalal Z, and Stewart D, 2020. Interventions to improve spontaneous adverse drug reaction reporting by healthcare professionals and patients: systematic review and meta-analysis. Expert Opin. Drug Saf., 19(9): 1173–1191. doi: 10.1080/14740338.2020.1807003.

Pino M, Abid T, Pereira Ribeiro S, Edara VV, Floyd K, Smith JC, Latif MB, Pacheco-Sanchez G, Dutta D, Wang S, and Gumber S, 2021. A yeast-expressed RBD-based SARS-CoV-2 vaccine formulated with 3M-052-alum adjuvant promotes protective efficacy in non-human primates. Science Immunol., 6(61): eabh3634. doi: 10.1126/sciimmunol.abh3634.

Plotkin SA, and Caplan A, 2020. Extraordinary diseases require extraordinary solutions. Vaccine, 38(24): 3987. doi: 10.1016/j.vaccine.2020.04.039

Pollet J, Chen WH, Versteeg L, Keegan B, Zhan B, Wei J, Liu Z, Lee J, Kundu R, Adhikari R, and Poveda C, 2021. SARS CoV-2 RBD219-N1C1: A yeast-expressed SARS-CoV-2 recombinant receptor-binding domain candidate vaccine stimulates virus neutralizing antibodies and T-cell immunity in mice. Hum. Vaccines Immunother., 17(8): 2356–2366. doi: 10.1080/21645515.2021.1901545.

Pollet J, Strych U, Chen WH, Versteeg L, Keegan B, Zhan B, Wei J, Liu Z, Lee J, Kundu R, and Adhikari R, 2022. Receptor-binding domain recombinant protein on alum-CpG induces broad protection against SARS-CoV-2 variants of concern. Vaccine, 40(26): 3655–3663. doi: 10.1016/j.vaccine.2022.05.007.

Pronker ES, Weenen TC, Commandeur H, Claassen EH and Osterhaus AD, 2013. Risk in vaccine research and development quantified. PloS One, 8(3): e57755. doi: 10.1371/journal.pone.0057755.

Quintin J, Saeed S, Martens JH, Giamarellos-Bourboulis EJ, Ifrim DC, Logie C, Jacobs L, Jansen T, Kullberg BJ, Wijmenga C, and Joosten LA, 2012. Candida albicans infection affords protection against reinfection via functional reprogramming of monocytes. Cell Host & Microbe, 12(2): 223–232. doi: 10.1016/j.chom.2012.06.006

Rammensee HG, and Pascolo S, 2004. Immunostimulating capacities of stabilized RNA molecules. Eur. J. Immunol., 34(2): 537–547. doi: 10.1002/eji.200324198.

Rego GN, Nucci MP, Alves AH, Oliveira FA, Marti LC, Nucci LP, Mamani JB, and Gamarra LF, 2020. Current clinical trials protocols and the global effort for immunization against SARS-CoV-2. Vaccines, 8(3): 474. doi: 10.3390/vaccines8030474.

Rief W, 2021. Fear of adverse effects and COVID-19 vaccine hesitancy: recommendations of the treatment expectation expert group. JAMA Health Forum, 2(4): e210804–e210804. doi:10.1001/jamahealthforum.2021.0804.

Rostami-Nejad M, Yazdi MH, Nikfar S, Rezaie A, and Abdollahi M, 2020. Potential vaccines for treating Crohn's disease. Iran. Biomed. J., 24(1): 1. doi: 10.29252/ibj.24.1.1.

Safety NIH, 2020. Immunogenicity study of 2019-nCoV vaccine (mRNA-1273) for prophylaxis of SARS-CoV-2 infection (COVID-19). N Engl J Med., 383: 2427–2438.

Saif LJ, 2020. Vaccines for COVID-19: perspectives, prospects, and challenges based on candidate SARS, MERS, and animal coronavirus vaccines. Euro. Med. J. doi: 10.33590/emj/200324

Sarangi AK, Salem MA, Younus MD, El-Haroun H, Mahal A, Tripathy L, Mishra R, Shabil M, Alhumaydhi FA, Khatib MN and Bushi G, 2024. Advanced biomaterials for regenerative medicine and their possible therapeutic significance in treating COVID-19: a critical overview. Int. J. Surg., 110(12):7508-27. doi: 10.1097/JS9.0000000000002110

Satapathy BS, Pattnaik G, Sahoo RN, Pattanaik S, Sarangi AK, Kandi V, Mishra S, Rabaan AA, Mohanty A, Sah R and Mohapatra RK, 2023. COVID□19 vaccines and their underbelly: Are we going the right way?. Health Sci. Rep., 6(9):e1540. doi: 10.1002/hsr2.1540

Shang, W, Yang, Y., Rao, Y. and Rao, X., 2020. The outbreak of SARS-CoV-2 pneumonia calls for viral vaccines. npj Vaccines, 5(1): 18. doi: 10.1038/s41541-020-0170-0.

Sharpe HR, Gilbride C, Allen E, Belij-Rammerstorfer S, Bissett C, Ewer K, and Lambe T, 2020. The early landscape of coronavirus disease 2019 vaccine development in the UK and rest of the world. Immunology, 160(3): 223–232. doi: 10.1111/imm.13222.

Shrestha S, Danekhu K, Kc B, Palaian S, and Ibrahim MIM, 2020. Bibliometric analysis of adverse drug reactions and pharmacovigilance research activities in Nepal. Ther. Adv. Drug Saf., 11: 2042098620922480. doi: 10.1177/2042098620922480.

Silva LPAD, and Rapini MS, 2023. Suitability of two WHO research and development initiatives for COVID-19 to promote equitable innovation: the Access to COVID-19 Tools Accelerator and COVID-19 Technology Access Pool. Revista Panamericana de Salud Pública, 46: e194. doi.org/10.26633/RPSP.2022.194

Soldatos TG, Taglang G, and Jackson DB, 2018. In silico profiling of clinical phenotypes for human targets using adverse event data. High-throughput, 7(4): 37. doi: 10.3390/ht7040037.

Stokes EK, 2020. Coronavirus disease 2019 case surveillance—United States, January 22–May 30, 2020. Morb. Mortal Wkly. Rep., 69(24): 759–765. doi: 10.15585/mmwr.mm6924e2.

Terova O, Soltys S, Hermans P, De Rooij J and Detmers F, 2018. Overcoming downstream purification challenges for viral vector manufacturing: enabling advancement of gene therapies in the clinic. Cell Gene Ther. Insights, 4(2): 101–111. doi: 10.18609/CGTI.2018.017

Thi EP, Mire CE, Lee AC, Geisbert JB, Zhou JZ, Agans KN, Snead NM, Deer DJ, Barnard TR, Fenton KA, and MacLachlan I, 2015. Lipid nanoparticle siRNA treatment of Ebola-virus-Makona-infected nonhuman primates. Nature, 521(7552): 362–365. doi: 10.1038/nature14442.

Tischer A, Lilie H, Rudolph R, and Lange C, 2010. L-Arginine hydrochloride increases the solubility of folded and unfolded recombinant plasminogen activator rPA. Protein Science, 19(9): 1783–1795. doi: 10.1002/pro.465.

Torequl Islam M, Nasiruddin M, Khan I.N, Mishra SK, Kudrat-E-Zahan M, Alam Riaz T, Ali ES, Rahman MS, Mubarak MS, Martorell M, and Cho WC, 2020. A perspective on emerging therapeutic interventions for COVID-19. Front. Public Health, 8: 281. doi: 10.3389/fpubh.2020.00281.

Tsatsakis A, Petrakis D, Nikolouzakis TK, Docea AO, Calina D, Vinceti M, Goumenou M, Kostoff RN, Mamoulakis C, Aschner M, and Hernández AF, 2020. COVID-19, an opportunity to reevaluate the correlation between long-term effects of anthropogenic pollutants on viral epidemic/pandemic events and prevalence. Food Chem. Toxicol., 141: 111418. doi: 10.1016/j.fct.2020.111418.

Ulanova M, Tarkowski A, Hahn-Zoric M, and Hanson LA, 2001. The common vaccine adjuvant aluminum hydroxide up-regulates accessory properties of human monocytes via an interleukin-4-dependent mechanism. Infect. Immun., 69(2): 1151–1159. doi: 10.1128/iai.69.2.1151-1159.2001.

Ullah I, Khan KS, Tahir MJ, Ahmed A, and Harapan H, 2021. Myths and conspiracy theories on vaccines and COVID-19: Potential effect on global vaccine refusals. Vacunas, 22(2): 93–97. doi: 10.1016/j.vacun.2021.01.001.

Ura T, Okuda K, and Shimada M, 2014. Developments in viral vector-based vaccines. Vaccines, 2(3): 624–641. doi: 10.3390/vaccines2030624.

van Doremalen N, Haddock E, Feldmann F, Meade-White K, Bushmaker T, Fischer RJ, Okumura A, Hanley PW, Saturday G, Edwards NJ, and Clark MH, 2020. A single dose of ChAdOx1 MERS provides protective immunity in rhesus macaques. Science Advances, 6(24): eaba8399. doi: 10.1126/sciadv.aba8399.

van Riel D, and de Wit E, 2020. Next-generation vaccine platforms for COVID-19. Nature Materials, 19(8): 810–812. doi: 10.1038/s41563-020-0746-0.

Vellinga J, Smith J.P, Lipiec A, Majhen D, Lemckert A, van Ooij M, Ives P, Yallop C, Custers J, and Havenga M, 2014. Challenges in manufacturing adenoviral vectors for global vaccine product deployment. Human Gene Therapy, 25(4): 318–327. doi: 10.1089/hum.2014.007.

Velásquez G, 2022. Vaccines, medicines and COVID-19: How can WHO be given a stronger voice? Nature. doi: 10.1007/978-3-030-89125-1.

Voysey M, Clemens SAC, Madhi SA, Weckx LY, Folegatti PM, Aley PK, Angus B, Baillie VL, Barnabas SL, Bhorat QE, and Bibi S, 2021. Safety and efficacy of the ChAdOx1 nCoV-19 vaccine (AZD1222) against SARS-CoV-2: an interim analysis of four randomised controlled trials in Brazil, South Africa, and the UK. The Lancet, 397(10269): 99–111. doi: 10.1016/ S0140-6736(20)32661-1

Wang J, Peng Y, Xu H, Cui Z, and Williams R.O, 2020. The COVID-19 vaccine race: challenges and opportunities in vaccine formulation. AAPS Pharm. Sci. Tech, 21(6): 225. doi: 10.1208/s12249-020-01744-7.

Wu F, Zhao S, Yu B, Chen YM, Wang W, Song ZG, Hu Y, Tao ZW, Tian JH, Pei YY, and Yuan ML, 2020. A new coronavirus associated with human respiratory disease in China. Nature, 579(7798): 265–269. doi: 10.1208/s12249-020-01744-7.

Yu J, Tostanoski LH, Peter L, Mercado NB, McMahan K, Mahrokhian SH, Nkolola JP, Liu J, Li Z, Chandrashekar A and Martinez D.R, 2020. DNA vaccine protection against SARS-CoV-2 in rhesus macaques. Science, 369(6505): 806–811. doi: 10.1126/science.abc6284.

Yung-Fang T, Chien C.S, Yarmishyn A.A, Yi-Ying L, Yung-Hung L, Yi-Tsung L, Wei-Yi L, De-Ming Y, Chou S.J, Yang Y.P and Wang M.L, 2020. A review of SARS-CoV-2 and the ongoing clinical trials. Int. J. Mol. Sci., 21(7): 2657. doi:10.3390/ijms21072657.

Zhang Y, and Zhang J, 2005. Surface modification of monodisperse magnetite nanoparticles for improved intracellular uptake to breast cancer cells. J. Colloid Interface Sci., 283(2): 352–357. doi: 10.1016/j.jcis.2004.09.042.

Zhang Y, Zeng G, Pan H, Li C, Hu Y, Chu K, Han W, Chen Z, Tang R, Yin W, and Chen X, 2021. Safety, tolerability, and immunogenicity of an inactivated SARS-CoV-2 vaccine in healthy adults aged 18–59 years: a randomised, double-blind, placebo-controlled, phase 1/2 clinical trial. Lancet Infect. Dis., 21(2): 181–192. doi: 10.1016/ S1473-3099(20)30843-4

Zhou P, Yang XL, Wang XG, Hu B, Zhang L, Zhang W, Si HR, Zhu Y, Li B, Huang CL, and Chen HD, 2020. A pneumonia outbreak associated with a new coronavirus of probable bat origin. Nature, 579(7798): 270–273. doi: 10.1038/s41586-020-2012-7

Zhou QA, Kato-Weinstein J, Li Y, Deng Y, Granet R, Garner L, Liu C, Polshakov D, Gessner C, and Watkins S, 2020. Potential therapeutic agents and associated bioassay data for COVID-19 and related human coronavirus infections. ACS Pharmacol. Transl. Sci., 3(5): 813–834. doi: 10.1021/acsptsci.0c00074?ref=pdf

Zhu FC, Guan XH, Li YH, Huang JY, Jiang T, Hou LH, Li JX, Yang BF, Wang L, Wang WJ, and Wu SP, 2020. Immunogenicity and safety of a recombinant adenovirus type-5-vectored COVID-19 vaccine in healthy adults aged 18 years or older: a randomised, double-blind, placebo-controlled, phase 2 trial. Lancet, 396(10249): 479–488. doi: 10.1016/ S0140-6736(20)31605-6

Zhu N, Zhang D, Wang W, Li X, Yang B, Song J, Zhao X, Huang B, Shi W, Lu R, and Niu P, 2020. A novel corona virus from patients with pneumonia in China, 2019. N. Engl J. Med., 382(8): 727–733. doi: 10.1056/NEJMoa2001017

3

mRNA Vaccines for Viral Diseases Challenges and Opportunities

Subrat Kumar[1*], Ritesh Pattnaik[1], Subhra Subhadra[2] Basavaraj Mathapati[3]

[1]School of Biotechnology, Campus-XI, KIIT Deemed University, Patia Bhubaneswar -751 024, Odisha, India
[2]Virology lab (VRDL), ICMR- Regional Medical Research Center Bhubaneswar – 751 023, Odisha, India
[3]ICMR- NIV Dibrugarh Unit, Dibrugarh – 786 001, Assam, India

Abstract

Messenger RNA (mRNA) vaccine was the first authorised vaccine developed using mRNA vaccine production technology, against SARS-CoV-2. Well accepted by the population, it proved to be a major life saving intervention during the COVID-19 pandemic. This article discusses the mRNA vaccine technology and its major advantages, and provides an update on the various ongoing and completed clinical trials on the leading mRNA vaccines against various viral diseases. It also delves into the prospects and the technical challenges associated with the manufacturing of mRNA vaccine and the issues with its deployment in the low- and middle-income countries around the world. Despite the already available classical vaccine candidates, the persistent interest and continuous research in mRNA vaccine technology and the related storage, immunogenicity and lipid nanoparticles delivery aspects have helped in expanding and upgrading the vaccinology arsenals to counter diseases. The technology holds promises in opening new vistas to protect against infectious diseases and the associated complications, where safe and effective immunisations are currently lacking. Furthermore, as mRNA vaccines evolve, they offer new hope against neglected and reemerging diseases like rabies, Zika, and Nipah viruses. The flexibility and rapid adaptability of this platform underscore its potential to address unmet medical needs, laying the groundwork for universal and multi-pathogen vaccines, vital in averting future pandemics. Enhanced by advancements in nanotechnology and innovative delivery systems, mRNA vaccines are poised to revolutionise infectious disease prevention, cancer treatment, and genetic disorders, marking a new era in vaccinology and offering hope for global health challenges through continued investment in research and infrastructure.

Keywords: virus, vaccine, vaccinology, public health, community health, immunisation, infectious disease

1. Introduction

Infectious diseases are the major cause of human morbidity and mortality (Mohapatra *et al.*, 2024). With COVID-19 pandemic by the viral pathogen SARS-CoV-2 that is seemingly ongoing, the emergence and reemergence of pathogens have always been a public health concern (Mohapatra et al., 2020; Mohapatra et al., 2021; Mohapatra *et al.*, 2023a; Mishra *et al.*, 2024; Sarangi *et al.*, 2024). Respiratory viral infections, arboviral infections and zoonotic viral infections continue to pose severe threat, and safe and effective methods to control them need to be developed and deployed (Rauch *et al.*, 2018; Mohapatra *et al.*, 2023b). Vaccines have proven their remarkable efficacy in preventing viral infections and have saved millions of lives over the years (Plotkin and Plotkin, 2011; Satapathy et al. 2023; Mohapatra *et al.*, 2023c). Meticulous and extensive implementation of vaccine campaigns over the last few decades have not only eliminated disease like smallpox (and polio is following the suit) but also brought down the incidence of viral diseases like polio, measles, etc. (Plotkin, 2009). Vaccination plays critical role in preventing more than two million deaths annually from bacterial (like pertussis and tetanus) and viral (like influenza and measles) infections each year, as per WHO reports (Chaudhary *et al.*, 2021).

Conventional vaccines have several disadvantages that restrict its usefulness in treating and preventing diseases. For instance, peptide vaccines show MHC restrictions and lead to selective T-cell activation, thus increasing the risk of the aetiological agent escaping the immunity. DNA vaccines pose the risk of genome alteration, long-term expression and auto-antibody generation (Kennedy *et al.*, 2020). The process of developing live or attenuated vaccines is intricate and complex, while the development of dendritic cell vaccines is labour intensive and time consuming. So, selecting a dependable vaccine format that has tremendous potential to treat and prevent infectious disease more effectively is of utmost importance. In light of these, mRNA vaccines seem to be advantageous.

Messenger RNA (mRNA) is a single nucleotide sequence that carries genetic information and guides the synthesis of protein. It plays a critical role in translating and expressing the genetic information of DNA into protein as may be needed to carry-out the numerous cellular activities. It is appropriate to state that mRNA molecule has multifunctional role in regulating the genetic and other cellular functions (Kloc *et al.*, 2011). The idea of using mRNA as therapeutic molecule was first conceptualised about three decades ago when naked mRNA encoding transgene demonstrated the subsequent expression of the functional proteins when injected into the skeletal muscle of mice (Wolff *et al.*, 1990). This groundbreaking finding was later confirmed when various studies demonstrated that the administered viral and cancer antigens encoded *in vitro* transcribed the mRNA and elicited antigen specific immune responses (Fig. 1; Conry *et al.*, 1995; Hoerr *et al.*, 2000). Despite offering promising results, mRNA vaccine platform was not pursued further for vaccine development particularly owing to the major shortcomings associated with mRNA synthesis and stability (Sahin *et al.*, 2014).

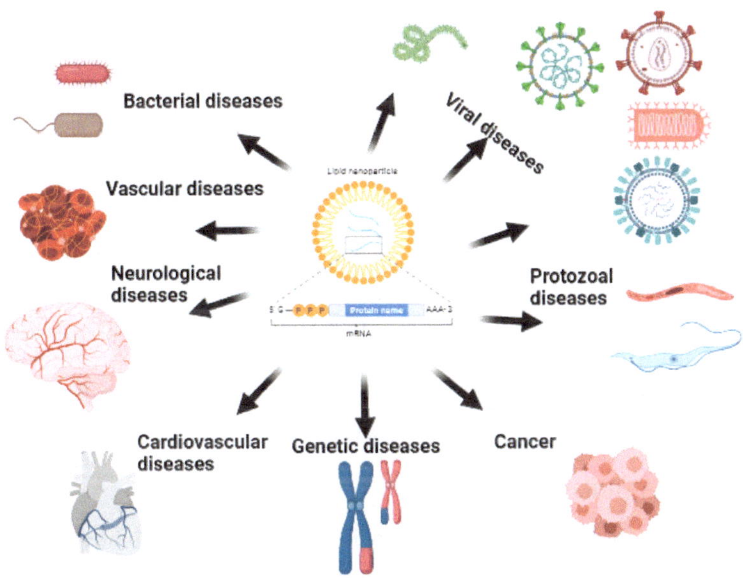

Fig. 1: Various potential applications of mRNA-based vaccines

An mRNA vaccine possesses many beneficial features over a conventional vaccine. While conventional vaccine is relatively time-consuming and expensive to manufacture, mRNA vaccine could be designed and synthesised faster, thereby offering an unprecedented response time to deal with emerging infectious diseases or evolving mutants (Maruggi *et al.*, 2019). Further, mRNA helps in mediating the expression of various transient therapeutic proteins with no risk of getting integrated to the genome. Also, mRNA therapeutics offers expanded successful treatment options for other diseases by altering the DNA template sequence (Beck *et al.*, 2021). All such advantages have propelled research on mRNA which has taken a new trajectory. The major challenges that hinder the success of mRNA vaccine are thermal instability, sensitivity to nuclease and poor *in vivo* expression (Sahin *et al.*, 2014). Although the *in vitro* transcription (IVT) process is relatively simple, producing high-quality therapeutic mRNA that does not induce inflammation remains a key challenge (Sahin *et al.*, 2014). Technological advancements have resolved majority of the issues over the last decade, like incorporating modified nucleosides, removing contaminants from IVT synthesised mRNA, optimising antigen coding and untranslated regions, optimising the length of poly (A) tail, improved capping analogues and developing safe and effective delivery mechanisms (Andries *et al.*, 2015; Karikó *et al.*, 2008, 2011; Asrani, 2018; Vaidyanathan *et al.*, 2018; Maruggi *et al.*, 2019).

Numerous vaccines were developed during the SARS-CoV-2 pandemic, and one among them was mRNA vaccine. COVID-19 mRNA vaccine attracted deeper research interests due to its disease prevention efficacy. Later, this vaccine became the first mRNA vaccine ever licensed for human use (Ye *et al.*, 2023). This successful development and deployment opened exciting new opportunities to develop similar strategies to combat healthcare challenges posed by the HIV-1, Nipah and Zika viruses. However, it is not quite clear as to whether mRNA vaccine could achieve similar results which time will unravel. As mRNA-based vaccine currently is evolving at a tremendous pace, understanding the various ongoing developments in mRNA engineering is important. Apart from discussing various types of mRNA-based vaccine for viral diseases, this article sheds light on the challenges and opportunities in mRNA as a safe and effective vaccine lying ahead.

2. mRNA Vaccines Against Viral Diseases

Vaccination has impacted tremendously the human and animal health and wellbeing. After the successful development and authorisation (for emergency use) of mRNA vaccine against SARS-CoV-2 virus, vaccine technology is revolutionised by this novel platform. This section is about the various mRNA vaccines either developed or are under investigation to treat the neglected and emerging viral diseases (Table 1).

2.1. mRNA Vaccines for Neglected Viral Diseases

Neglected tropical diseases (NTDs) are classified as those neglected diseases that are highly prevalent in various tropical and subtropical regions worldwide which affect over 1.6 billion people annually (WHO). The global report on neglected diseases released by the WHO in December 2023 lists a group of 21 bacterial, viral, parasitic and fungal diseases as NTDs. Amongst these 21 diseases, three (dengue, chikungunya and rabies) are viral. NTDs resulted in 26.06 million DALYs, *i.e.*, disability adjusted life years and contributed immensely to the social and economic burden, as per the study on global burden for diseases in 2010.

However, many of these NTDs are preventable. Improved sanitation, safe hygienic practices, vector control and access to safe and nutritionally-balanced food are some currently recommended non-medical interventions and strategies that could help reduce the disease burden through community participation alongside the local, regional and international healthcare agencies. Despite these efforts, limited access to healthcare services and lack of awareness in affected regions continue to hinder progress. Strengthening public health infrastructure and fostering collaborations among governments, NGOs, and the private sector are crucial for effective intervention. Additionally, the development of affordable vaccines and diagnostics tailored for low-resource settings can play a transformative role. Innovations in mRNA vaccine technology offer a promising avenue to target viral NTDs more efficiently. By integrating community-based programs with scientific advancements, a significant reduction in the prevalence and impact of NTDs can be achieved.

Both dengue and chikungunya are arboviral diseases spread by *Aedes* group of mosquitoes. Chikungunya infection is reported in over 40 countries, which is clinically presented with very high fever, intense joint pain (polyarthralgia) and rash. The infection is self-limiting and acute symptoms usually resolve in 1-2 weeks. However, joint pain recurs in 30-40% of the affected individuals and reportedly persists for years (Schwartz and Albert, 2010). Analgesics and corticosteroids are used as pain control to treat Chikungunya. Although attempts have been made to develop inactivated and attenuated chikungunya vaccine, these were low on immunogenicity and had adverse effects (Harrison *et al.*, 1971, White *et al.*, 1972). USFDA approved the first chikungunya vaccine called Ixchiq in November 2023 for adults (18 years or older) at high risk of virus exposure (Yin *et al.*, 2023).

Table 1: The ongoing and completed clinical trials of mRNA vaccine worldwide against the various viral diseases

Infection	Developer	Formulation	Clinical trial stage	Administration route	Type of UTP	Performance claimed	NCT no.
SARS-CoV2	BioNTech (BNT162b1)	LNP-mRNA	1/Completed	Intramuscular	Modified	Safe, no side-effects	04523571
	CureVac (CVnCoV)	LNP-mRNA	1/Completed	Intramuscular	Unmodified	Safe, immunogenic, induces neutralising antibodies	04449276
	ModernaTX (mRNA-1273)	LNP-mRNA	3/ Completed	Intramuscular	Modified	Safe, protects against asymptomatic infection	04470427
	BioNTech/Pfizer (BNT162b1, BNT162b2)	LNP-mRNA	2/3/ Completed	Intramuscular	Modified	Induces dose-dependent neutralising antibody	04368728
	CureVac (CVnCoV)	LNP-mRNA	2/Completed	Intramuscular	Unmodified	Induces high neutralising antibody levels	04515147
	ModernaTX (mRNA-1273)	LNP-mRNA	1/ Completed	Intramuscular	Modified	Induces humoral and cellular immune responses	04283461
	ModernaTX (mRNA-1273)	LNP-mRNA	2/Completed	Intramuscular	Modified	Safe, immunogenic, induces broad and neutralising antibodies by 28th day	04405076
	BioNTech SE (ARCT-021)	LNP-mRNA	1/2/ Completed	Intramuscular	Unmodified	Single-dose is immunogenic, low neutralising antibodies	04480957
	CureVac (CVnCoV)	LNP-mRNA	3/Terminated	Intramuscular	Unmodified	Low protection, shows side-effects	04860258
	Walvax Biotechnology Co. Ltd. (SARS-CoV-2)	LNP-mRNA	3/Ongoing	Intramuscular	Modified	Booster dose increases the neutralising antibodies, enhanced memory B-cells	04847102

Infection	Developer	Formulation	Clinical trial stage	Administration route	Type of UTP	Performance claimed	NCT no.
	AIM Vaccine Co. Ltd. (LVRNA009)	LNP-mRNA	1/Completed	Intramuscular	Modified	Safe, no side-effects, produces anti-S proteins and neutralising antibodies	05364047
Nipah virus	NIAID/Moderna TX (mRNA -1215)	LNP-mRNA	1/Ongoing	Intramuscular	Modified	Ongoing	05398796
HIV-1	National Institute of Allergy and Infectious Diseases, Massachusetts (PARC002)	Naked mRNA	1/2/ Completed	Intradermal	Modified	Induces CD4 proliferation, low IL-12p70 levels	00833781
	Fundacion Clinic per a la Recerca Biomédica (iHIVARNA-01)	Naked mRNA	1/Completed	Intranodal	Unmodified	Safe, tolerated well; moderate T-cell response	02413645
	Erasmus Medical Center (iHIVARNA-01)	Naked mRNA	2/Terminated	Intranodal	Unmodified	Insufficient immunity compared to placebo	02888756
	International AIDS Vaccine Initiative (mRNA-1644)	LNP-mRNA	1/Incomplete	Intraperitoneal	Unmodified	Safe and tolerated well	05414786
	McGill University Health Centre (AGS-004)	LNP-mRNA	1/2/ Completed	Intradermal	Modified	2-fold increase in T-cells, suboptimal HIV antigen presented *in vivo* by DCs	00381212
	Argos Therapeutics, National Institute of Allergy and Infectious Diseases (AGS-004)	Naked mRNA	1/Completed	Intradermal	Modified	Safe, immunogenic in participants with ART, low and inconsistent HIV-specific immune response	02042248

Infection	Developer	Formulation	Clinical trial stage	Administration route	Type of UTP	Performance claimed	NCT no.
Rabies	CureVac (CV7201)	Cationic protamine	1/Completed	Intradermal or intramuscular	Unmodified	Safe, tolerable; administered needle-free, generates protective antibodies	02241135
	GlaxoSmithKline (RG SAM (CNE) vaccine (GSK3903133A))	Self-amplified mRNA in cationic nano-emulsion	1/Completed	Intramuscularly	Unmodified	Safe, tolerated well; immunogenic	04062669
	Curevac (CV7202)	LNP-mRNA	1/Completed	Intramuscular	Unmodified	Safe, tolerated well; high innate immunity response	03713086
Zika	ModernaTX (mRNA-1325)	LNP-mRNA	1/Completed	Intramuscular	Modified	Safe, tolerated well; high innate immunity response	03014089
	ModernaTX (mRNA-1893)	LNP-mRNA	1/Completed	Intramuscular	Modified	Safe, tolerated well; high innate immunity response	04064905
	ModernaTX (mRNA-1893)	LNP-mRNA	2/Ongoing	Intramuscular	Modified	Ongoing	04917861
Influenza	ModernaTX (VAL-506440)	LNP-mRNA	1/Completed	Intramuscular or Intradermal	Modified	Safe, tolerated well; robust humoral response	03076385
	ModernaTX (VAL-339851)	LNP-mRNA	1/Completed	Intradermal	Modified	safe reactogenicity; elicits robust humoral immune response	03345043
	ModernaTX (mRNA-1010)	LNP-mRNA	1/2/ Completed	Intramuscular	Unmodified	Safe, no adversities; Single-dose elicits haemagglutination inhibition titer	04956575

Infection	Developer	Formulation	Clinical trial stage	Administration route	Type of UTP	Performance claimed	NCT no.
	ModernaTX (mRNA-1030 mRNA-1020 mRNA-1010)	LNP-mRNA	1/2/Complete	Intramuscular	Unmodified	Safe, dose-dependent reactogenicity boost; robust Anti-NA & Anti-HA titres	05333289
	ModernaTX (mRNA-1010)	LNP-mRNA	3/Complete	Intramuscular	Unmodified	Safe, well tolerated; superior seroconversion rates	05415462
Ebola	University of Oxford, Centre Hospitalier Universitaire le Dantec (CHUD), Dakar, Senegal (ChAd3-EBO Z)	Viral vector	1/Completed	Intramuscular	Unmodified	Safe, well tolerated; high cellular and humoral immune responses	02485912
hMPV/PIV3	Moderna (mRNA-1653)		1/Completed	Intramuscular	Modified	-	04144348 03392389
Chikungunya	ModernaTX (mRNA-1944)	LNP-mRNA	1/Completed	Intravenous	Modified	Well tolerated, favourable safety profile; induces neutralising antibodies	03829384
	ModernaTX (VAL-181388)	LNP-mRNA	1/Completed	Intramuscular	Modified	Safe, well tolerated across dose levels, immunogenic	03325075
RSV	ModernaTX (mRNA-1345)	LNP-mRNA	1/Ongoing	Intramuscular	Modified	Rise in neutralising abs after a month, min level is maintained till 6 months	04528719
	ModernaTX (mRNA-1273, mRNA-1010, mRNA-1345, mRNA-1647)	LNP-mRNA	1/Ongoing	Intramuscular	Modified	Ongoing	05397223

Infection	Developer	Formulation	Clinical trial stage	Administration route	Type of UTP	Performance claimed	NCT no.
	ModernaTX (mRNA-1010, mRNA-1345, mRNA-1273.214)	LNP-mRNA	1/Ongoing	Intramuscular	Modified	Ongoing	05585632
	ModernaTX (mRNA-1345)	LNP-mRNA	2/3/Ongoing	Intramuscular	Modified	94% reduction in severe RSV disease in the vaccinated, 83% overall efficacy	05127434
	ModernaTX (mRNA-1345)	LNP-mRNA	3/Ongoing	Intramuscular	Modified	Ongoing	06067230
	ModernaTX (mRNA-1345 and FluZone)	LNP-mRNA	3/Ongoing	Intramuscular	Modified	Ongoing	06060457
	Sanofi Pasteur (LNP CL-0059 or LNP CL-0137)	LNP-mRNA	1/2/Ongoing	Intramuscular	Modified	Ongoing	05639894
	ModernaTX (mRNA-1345 and mRNA-1273.214)	LNP-mRNA	3/Ongoing	Intramuscular	Modified	Ongoing	05330975
CMV	ModernaTX (mRNA-1647, mRNA-1443)	LNP-mRNA	1/Completed	Intramuscular	Modified	Enhances HCMV-specific IgG; robust neutralisation & high ADCC responses	03382405
	ModernaTX (mRNA-1647)	LNP-mRNA	2/Ongoing	Intramuscular	Modified	Ongoing	04232280
	ModernaTX (mRNA-1647)	LNP-mRNA	3/Ongoing	Intramuscular	Modified	Ongoing	05085366

Abbreviations used: The type of uridine-5′-triphosphate (UTP) used: modified means N1-methylpseudouridine-5′-triphosphate, and wild-type is non-modified uridine-5′-triphosphate found in native mRNA; CMV: human cytomegalovirus; HIV-1: human immunodeficiency virus-1; RSV: respiratory syncytial virus; hMPV: human metapneumovirus; PIV: parainfluenza virus; mRNA: messenger RNA; LNP: lipid nanoparticle; ADCC: antibody-dependent cellular cytotoxicity

Liu *et al.* (2023) constructed a chikungunya vaccine using mRNA platform that expressed the structural protein of the virus. They observed that the vaccine could induce higher titre of the neutralising antibodies but had low cellular response. Ge *et al.* (2022) evaluated a chikungunya E2-E1 antigen-expressing mRNA-lipid nanoparticle (LNP) vaccine, and found better neutralising antibody response magnitude and greater cellular (especially CD8+T-cell) immune response. August *et al.* (2021) evaluated the pharmacology and safety of a LNP encapsulated mRNA encoding the chikungunya specific (heavy and light chains) neutralising monoclonal antibody through randomised, placebo-controlled human trial. Mild to moderate side-effects were observed in few participants, which didn't worsen further after the second dose. This vaccine candidate is currently under further evaluation. Kose *et al.* (2019) evaluated another LNP encapsulated chikungunya antibody encoding mRNA and observed the virus-neutralising antibody protected both the immuno-compromised and the immuno-competent mice against the lethal challenge and joint pain. Such studies suggest that such mRNA vaccine immunisation is feasible and human clinical trials need be continued further.

It is estimated that 3.6 billion people are at risk of developing dengue infection in the tropics and the subtropics. As per WHO, about 500,000 clinically progressive severe dengue cases are confirmed each year, which record 2.5% deaths. As no effective treatment is currently available for the disease, it relies on supportive care of analgesics, increased fluid intake and rest. Managing dengue is critical as critical patients may need platelets or whole blood cells transfusion. Roth *et al.* (2019) engineered a modified LNP-encapsulated mRNA vaccine encoding for conserved and antigenic epitopes from the NS3, NS4B and NS5 regions of dengue virus serotype-1. They evaluated the vaccine in Human HLA Class 1 transgenic mice and observed a significant protection after two injections (Roth *et al.*, 2019). Zhang *et al*, (2020) designed and evaluated three nucleotide modified mRNA vaccine encoding for prME, E80 and NS1 proteins. mRNA with E80 alone or in combination with E80 and NS1 induced higher neutralising antibody levels and elucidated antigen specific T-cell response. Complete protection against dengue virus serotype-2 was also achieved in immune-competent mice (Zhang *et al.*, 2020). Wollner *et al.* (2021) evaluated another LNP encapsulated modified mRNA vaccine encoding for membrane proteins and envelope proteins of dengue virus serotype-1, and observed high levels of antiviral neutralising antibodies (CD4+ and CD8+T-cells) cells. The vaccine provided protection to the immuno-compromised mice against lethal dengue virus challenge. He *et al.* (2022) developed and evaluated novel mRNA-LNP dengue vaccine encoding viral E-DIII and NS1 proteins. This multi-target vaccine induced robust neutralising antibody titre and blocked the infections by all the four dengue virus types *in vitro*.

A fatal zoonotic disease reported from around the world, Rabies is caused by the Rabies virus (RABV). It is transmitted by bites of infected animal and kills about 55,000–70,000 annually, mainly in south Asia. Pre-exposure prophylaxis for high-risk individuals like animal handlers and veterinarians in endemic countries and lab technicians is recommended. WHO also recommends post-exposure prophylaxis like wound management and a course of anti-rabies vaccine, and immunoglobulins may be administered to high-risk cases. Although vaccine against rabies infection is commercially available, it is expensive and need multiple dosages. Studies to develop and evaluate mRNA vaccine candidates that express rabies virus surface glycoprotein (RABV-G) are being conducted as mRNA vaccine platform can overcome such challenges (Schnee *et al.*, 2016). Schnee *et al.* (2016) developed a lyophilised, thermostable mRNA vaccine CV7201 where the mRNA encoded the glycoprotein RABV-G. The vaccine induced humoral and cellular immunity in mice when administered intradermally in a dose-dependent manner. When tested on newborn pigs, the vaccine induced protective neutralising antibody (Schnee *et al.*, 2016). The candidate mRNA vaccine retained its immunogenicity and protective action after storing for prolonged period (up to several months) and even after being temperature-abused at as high as 70°C. The mice immunised with CV7201 vaccine remained protected with lethal rabies virus challenge in animal study (Stitz *et al.*, 2017). After such promising results, CureVac conducted human clinical trials of CV7201 and CV7202 (Alberer *et al.*, 2017; Aldrich *et al.*, 2021). While it was reasonably safe and well tolerated, the needle-free intradermal administration induced protective neutralising antibody levels. This candidate vaccine showed high reactogenicity as compared to rabipur, and double-dose shot was enough to elicit neutralising antibodies as compared to the usual three doses for other approved vaccines (Aldrich *et al.*, 2021). Hellergen *et al.* (2023) investigated the same mRNA vaccine in non-human primates and reported similar observations.

Li *et al.* (2022) assessed LVRNA001, a codon-optimised RABV-G-expressing mRNA vaccine construct. Tested for its immunogenicity and protective ability in animal subjects (mice and dogs), it was observed that the vaccine induced high neutralising antibody levels, and showed strong Th1 response in mice. It was also able to protect both mice and dogs when challenged with 50-fold lethal dose of rabies virus. Li *et al.* (2023) evaluated RV021, a non-replicating RABV-G-encoding mRNA vaccine, for immunogenicity and protective efficacy in mice. It induced long-lasting neutralising antibodies and effectively protected challenged animals even at lower dose. Long *et al.* (2023) developed LNP encapsulated RABV-G-encoding mRNA vaccine, and tested its efficacy on mice and dogs. Its double-dose was highly immunogenic and induced robust cellular immune response in mice thereby protecting it. A rapid and long-term protective antibody response in mice and dogs was induced even with a single dose as compared to the inactivated counterparts. Being a liquid formulation, the mRNA-B-LNP vaccine could be stored conveniently at 2–8°C for up to 2 months. Bai *et al.* (2023) developed a single-dose nucleoside-modified rabies mRNA-LNP vaccine in a dose-dependent manner that induced potent and persistent immune response. It protected the vaccinated mice against lethal doses of rabies virus. Differing from earlier approaches, Wan *et al.* (2023) developed RABV-G-expressing mRNA rabies vaccine with LPP (lipopolyplex) system. This LPP-encapsulated mRNA vaccine had a linear ssRNA having a 5' cap (untranslated region; UTR), the antigen-coding region and a 3' poly(A) tail. It showed favourable biodistribution pattern when administered intramuscularly with least accumulation in the liver or other major bodily organs. It indicates that LPP encapsulation facilitated better adsorption and had less toxicity compared to LNP encapsulation which may need validation.

2.2. mRNA vaccines Against Emerging and Remerging Viral Diseases

Emerging and reemerging viral diseases are also a cause of concern apart from NTDs. Majority of such pathogens are vector-borne zoonotic infections and could potentially lead to a deadly pandemic. Some such etiological agents are Ebola, Nipah, Influenza, Zika, MERS and SARS viruses.

Severe acute respiratory syndrome (SARS), novel coronavirusdisease (COVID-19) and middle east respiratory syndrome (MERS) belong to family *Coronaviridae* and have caused major pandemic in 2003, 2012 and 2019 (Zhou *et al.*, 2020). Alongside humans, coronavirus reportedly affects multiple animal species like bats, pigs, cows, camel, cats and dogs. Spillage of certain coronaviruses from their animal reservoirs to humans became a public health threat that needed rapid interventions to mitigate its further spread (Shi and Hu, 2008). Studies have revealed that the receptor binding domain (RBD) that is present in spike protein subunit-1 is immunogenic and can produce neutralising antibodies. Thus, it could be a potential vaccine development target (Greaney *et al.*, 2021). Due to this, researchers developed and evaluated LNP-formulated trimerized RBD-encoding mRNA vaccine (Sahin *et al.*, 2020; Mulligan *et al.*, 2020; Greaney *et al.*, 2021). Some of these are currently under Phase III clinical trials (Baden *et al.*, 2021; Kremsner *et al.*, 2022).

Another respiratory virus of concern is influenza virus which circulates in multiple animal species and causes the contagious respiratory disease. Apart from causing seasonal epidemic, influenza could potentially become pandemic. Due to viral re-assortment and varying antigens, vaccine composition is needed to be annually altered to achieve protection against the virus. Researchers use the mRNA vaccine platform to develop influenza vaccine as this vaccine platform has advantage to accommodate multiple antigens. In such a study, a multivalent mRNA vaccine that expressed conserved viral antigens HA, NA, M2 and NP provided broad-spectrum immune response and protection against all influenza virus strains (Freyn *et al.*, 2020). After the tremendous success of mRNA vaccine (mRNA-1273) during COVID-19, Moderna Biotech initiated a phasic clinical trial for mRNA-1010 vaccine, a quadrivalent mRNA vaccine against seasonal influenza. It showed similar or higher immune response as compared to the approved counterparts with no safety concerns (Lee *et al.*, 2023). The immunogenicity, reactogenicity and safety of vaccine are being evaluated in 18 years or older adults, now under the Phase III clinical trial (NCT05827978). Moderna Biotech has developed a combination mRNA vaccine (mRNA-1083) against influenza and COVID-19, which has entered the Phase III clinical trial (NCT06097273). Similarly, Pfizer developed an mRNA influenza vaccine which is undergoing the Phase III clinical trial (NCT05540522).

Belonging to the Flaviviridae family, Zika virus (ZIKV) spreads through arthropod vector. Majority of the mRNA vaccines for flaviviruses have encoded for proteins prM and ENV as major antigens. Due to this, same regions were also used to develop Zika virus mRNA vaccine. One such study evaluated LNP-encapsulated mRNA vaccine in mice. The ZIKV mRNA encoded for prM/ENV proteins with modified 1-methyl pseudo-uridine. It provided complete protection in immuno-competent as well as immuno-compromised mice (Richner *et al.*, 2017). Upon infection, no antibody-dependent enhancement (ADE) was observed in the immunised mice. Compared to inactivated ZIKV vaccine, the mRNA vaccine could produce higher levels of antigen-specific CD8+ and CD4+ T-cell responses, and thus could control ZIKV infection. Data from Phase I/II clinical trials showed that mRNA-1893 vaccine against ZIKV encoding the structural proteins prME induced over 90% of sero-conversion with prime-boost vaccination at 10 μg dose (Patnaik *et al.*, 2020). Meyer *et al.* (2018) developed two novel LNP-encapsulated mRNA vaccines encoding ebolavirus glycoprotein based on the technology used by Richner *et al.* (2017), They observed in animal testing that only two doses were effective, and successfully protected animals against lethal virus challenge.

3. Understanding mRNA Vaccines

3.1. What is an mRNA Vaccine?

Vaccines are prophylactics for infections by producing antibodies against them and preparing the body for the combat. Many vaccines work on the principle of introducing specific benign antigenic pieces of target etiological agents in to the host to trigger immune responses. Thus, it is immunogenic but avirulent in nature. However, mRNA vaccines gained extensive attention during the recent COVID-19 pandemic as a promising technology that can be explored for developing vaccines. mRNA vaccines have emerged as potential candidates making their way to Phase I clinical trials. The working principle of mRNA vaccines is to introduce a short mRNA piece that corresponds to the viral protein. The immune system, as a general phenomenon, recognises the introduced viral protein as a foreign entity and produces specialised proteins (antibodies) that aids in protecting the body against infection. The functioning of mRNA vaccines is attributed to administering a miniature mRNA encoding for a specific protein (often a fragment of viral outer membrane protein). When immune system of the host discovers the foreign protein (antigen), it responds and produces antibodies. In the event of reintroduction of the same antigen, there exists an interesting mechanism in the body that memorises the earlier antigenic encounter and help trigger rapid immune responses. Researchers have aided in increasing the feasibility of use of mRNA-based products while reducing the inflammatory reactions and have contributed towards the progress, development and stabilisation of mRNA vaccines (Rijkers *et al.*, 2021).

3.2. How does mRNA vaccine Work?

An mRNA vaccine works by introducing a mRNA fragment coding for a viral protein (Fig. 2). mRNA vaccine typically contains two vital components, mRNA and a complementing delivery system. Both the components are the primary requisites for the encoded antigens to express in the host body, and also to induce adaptive immune response. mRNA encoding the desired proteins initially helps in providing the molecular basis to induce pathogen-specific immunity. Studies reported that the mRNA encoding antigens are usually the surface proteins of the pathogens against which the vaccine works. For instance, the mRNA encodes for spike (S) protein present on the surface of SARS-CoV-2 in the mRNA-1273 vaccine candidate (NCT04283461). Thus, the induced antibodies help prevent infection by inhibiting the spike protein from binding to the host cell (ACE2) receptors, whereas other antibodies opsonise the virus to promote rapid removal from the host body. Contrastingly, the mRNA vaccine against cancer encodes for the antigens that are either overexpressed or encode for specific mutated protein or neo-epitope, generally presented by MHC (major histocompatibility complex) molecules. Based on technical information from numerous researches, mRNA vaccines are ideally manufactured through *in vitro* transcription using T7 RNA polymerase from a DNA template (Xu *et al.*, 2020). Usually, mRNA requires optimisation of 5' cap, 3' and 5' untranslated regions, various nucleotide modifications and poly(A) tail to efficiently translate. Purification is additionally performed using high-performance liquid chromatography (HPLC) to yield high-purity mRNA that could be used to produce vaccine.

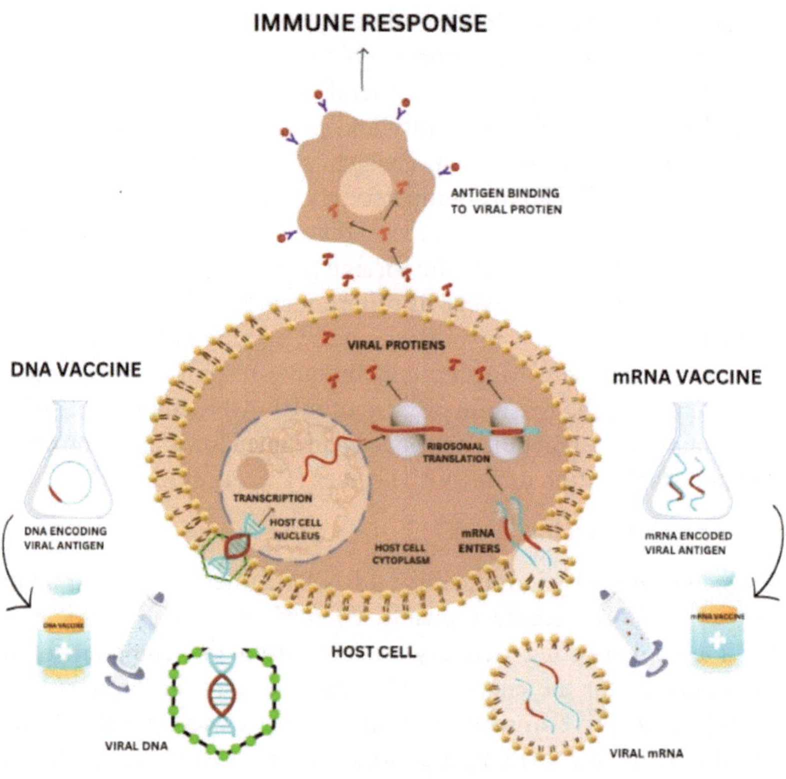

Fig. 2: Difference between conventional vaccine and mRNA vaccine

Likewise, a delivery system for the vaccine that plays a critical role in clinical applications of mRNA in human body is a key component (Aldosari *et al.*, 2021). It not only facilitates the entry of mRNA into the cytosol of the antigen-presenting cells (APCs) and encoded antigen expression, but also helps protect the mRNA from extracellular degradation. Importantly, efforts are made towards optimising mRNA in particular and its delivery systems in general.

Optimisation helps facilitate mRNA vaccine to adapt well to various clinical applications in future. The *in vivo* mRNA delivery is usually based on lipids, exosomes and polymers. Studies have reported lipid nanoparticles (LNPs) as the most advanced carriers for *in vivo* administration of mRNA vaccines. LNPs were applied successfully in SARS-CoV-2 mRNA vaccine. LNPs have four components, cholesterol, helper lipid, ionisable/cationic lipid and polyethylene glycol (PEG)-conjugated lipid. Ionisable/cationic lipid is the major component among the four that determines the delivery and efficient expression of mRNA vaccine. On the other hand, cholesterol and helper lipid contribute towards the stability and fusion of LNP membrane. With limited progress made in clinical application so far, efforts to apply PEG-modified lipid, polymers and exosomes as effective delivery systems for mRNA vaccines are constantly underway.

3.3. Advantage mRNA vaccines Over Conventional Vaccines

Considering the various aspects, mRNA vaccine technology offers various advantages as discussed earlier which highlight it as quite a promising alternative to traditional and DNA-based vaccines. Unlike inactivated or attenuated vaccines, mRNA is precise in expressing specific sequence to help elicit immune response. It promotes cellular and humoral-innate mediated immunity both (Maruggi *et al.*, 2019). As compared to the DNA-based, mRNA vaccines seem to be highly effective and safer as mRNA expression does not involve nuclear entry and any risk of integration of the random genome (Sullenger and Nair, 2016). Also, mRNA exhibits faster degradation by the host cellular processes usually within 3-5 days making the coded antigen expression transient in nature (Steinle *et al.*, 2017). The manufacturing process of mRNA vaccine is easier due to flexible feature of the platform particularly as the altered encoded antigens significantly alter and/or affect physicochemical traits of mRNA (Pardi *et al.*, 2018), and thus allow production standardisation. Further, because of the *in vitro* cell-free transcription-based process there are no safety concerns related to viral contaminants and cell-derived impurities during production.

4. Successes In Clinical Trials

4.1. Encouraging trial Stage Scenario

Before a vaccine is commercially released, it undergoes clinical evaluation across numerous clinical trial stages. Vaccine development may consume several years. However, the duration is often curtailed especially to address emergency health situations (with the benefit of doubt rested) as was witnessed during the COVID-19 pandemic. In the US, Moderna and Pfizer both received

Emergency Use Authorisation (EUA) in quite a short period (less than even a year). Similar was the case with Covaxin and Covishield in India too. Many mRNA vaccines are presently under investigation at various clinical trial stages that target infectious disease (like Zika, Nipah, SARS-CoV-2, Influenza A and B, RSV, etc.), genetic disorder and cancer. mRNA vaccine is especially promising as it elicits both the adaptive and the innate immune responses. Most vaccines that are currently under clinical trials use liposome (as carriers for targeting and efficacy enhancement) based technology. About 60-70% of the ongoing clinical trials focus on mRNA-based COVID-19 vaccines. Various mRNA-based vaccines that are either ongoing or have completed clinical trials are listed in Table 1. With only a handful into Phase III trials, most of these are in the early stages (Phase I or II trials) of development.

4.2. Successfully applied mRNA Vaccines

Based on manufacturing flexibility and versatility, mRNA is an excellent platform to develop both prophylactics and therapeutics against various infectious (such as viral and bacterial) and non-infectious (such as cancer) ailments. Moderna currently evaluates three single-dose mRNA vaccine for respiratory syncytial virus (RSV) infection. One of these is mRNA-1345 which encodes prefusion F viral glycoprotein to elicit neutralising antibodies. Clinical trials showed that it was well tolerated among children, adolescents and carrying women. Its II and III clinical trials for safety and efficacy evaluation are currently underway (NCT05127434) that are expected to be completed by November 2024. Moderna seeks to combine mRNA-1345 with the paediatric candidate mRNA-1653 targeting human metapneumovirus (hMPV) and human parainfluenza virus type 3 (hPIV3) to immunise children against three pathogenic ailments using single formula. mRNA-1647 against cytomegalovirus (CMV) human infection is another promising mRNA vaccine developed by Moderna. Specifically targeting women of child-bearing age group, it consists of five mRNAs coding for the membrane-bound pentamer complex and a sixth one coding for membrane-bound glycoprotein-B of CMV. With cheering Phase 1 and Phase 2 clinical trials results, this (mRNA-1647) vaccine currently undergoes Phase 3 clinical trials in healthy participants of 16–40 years. Initiated in October 2021 and registered as NCT05085366, the trial is expected to end by July 2025. mRNA-based vaccines are successfully tried for malaria (Scaria *et al.*, 2024), fungal (Bruch *et al.*, 2022), bacterial (Kon *et al.*, 2023), cancer (Heine *et al.*, 2021) and genetic ailments (Iyer *et al.*, 2024), apart from viral diseases.

5. Challenges to Address

After its success in combating the novel coronavirus during the COVID-19 pandemic, mRNA vaccinology has gained wider acceptance. However, this (mRNA-based vaccine) technology is mired with challenges like sequence optimisation, delivery of vector construct, and safety and efficacy of the vaccine as the major ones. These are discussed below.

5.1. Optimising the mRNA Sequence

mRNA vaccine has high programmability option thus making it a great tool compared to the traditional vaccines. It carries single-stranded nucleic acid sequence encoding for the desired target protein. Triggering strong innate response after entering host body, mRNA is prone to degradation by nucleases. Due to this, optimising mRNA bases during *in vitro* transcription (IVT) is essential to improve *in vivo* stability and reduces immunogenicity. Modification of 3' and 5' untranslated regions (UTRs) in the coding region is seen, which contributes to mRNA pharmacology immensely by providing stability and translation efficiency (Sahin *et al.*, 2014). The poly(A) tail and 5' cap provide protection to mRNA from premature degradation by nucleases. Studies have shown that deadenylation-dependant mRNA degradation can be controlled by increasing the length of poly(A) tail by adding about 120–150 nucleotides (Luo *et al.*, 2018). These apart, new strategies for co-transcriptional 5' capping to improve mRNA translation have evolved (Abbas *et al.*, 2017). Another strategy to bypass codon degeneracy is enriching the GC content, as this increases protein expression *in vivo* (Thess *et al.*, 2015). German company CureVac effectively set its entire mRNA vaccine platform on this concept. Higher antigen expression levels are achieved by adopting sequence optimisation strategy (Kudla *et al.*, 2009). Studies show that nucleoside-base mRNA modification can also reduce RNAse L activity, an enzyme responsible for mRNA cleavage and translation inhibition enzyme Protein kinase R (Nallagatia *et al.*, 2008; Anderson *et al.*, 2010). Due to this, majority of animal studies were conducted using modified mRNA as compared to unmodified mRNA.

5.2. mRNA Vaccine Delivery Challenges

A carrier material as vehicle to deliver the mRNA (bioactive) molecule is a critical step in vaccinology. Selecting suitable and effective vectors for successful delivery is needed. Due to its large size and possessing a net negative charge, it is difficult for a naked mRNA molecule to pass through host cell membrane. Additionally, naked mRNA molecule easily recognised by host immune system leading to interferon (IFN) secretion to degrade the foreign material (Linares *et al.*, 2020). A suitable mRNA delivery vehicle promotes cellular uptake of the exogenous mRNA and protects it from nuclease degradation to safely reach the cytoplasm to successfully translate to the desired proteins. Multiple approaches have been tried to deliver mRNA vaccines. A widely accepted strategy is employing self-assembled and biodegradable NPs involving amphiphilic molecules like lipid and polymers (Kowalski *et al.*, 2019).

Lipid-based delivery system (micelle, liposome and lipoplex) to deliver cargoes like mRNA in mice is in use since 1990s (Gonzalez *et al.*, 2007). However, these lipid nanostructures have reproducibility disadvantage that should be addressed to mass produce them (Ribeiro *et al.*, 2018). Also, these exhibit low encapsulation efficiency towards oligonucleotides and are less stable (Evers *et al.*, 2018). They have shown little success in various *in vivo* applications owing to these reasons. However, emerging technologies to formulate nanosized lipid NPs (LNPs) has made these the most common sought after vehicles for mRNA delivery (Wang *et al.*, 2023). Numerous formulation methods to efficiently assemble LNP-mRNA complexes have been developed (Aditya *et al.*, 2010; Otake *et al.*, 2006). Compared to the conventional methods of direct mixing and reverse phase evaporation, microfluidic hydrodynamic focusing seems quite promising (Huang *et al.*, 2017). In this, the lipid in solvent phase and mRNA in aqueous phase are allowed to swiftly diffuse in a continuous flow microfluidic device. This rapid mixing of the two phases forms micelles as the cationic lipid interacts with the anionic mRNA molecule. Although the performance of LNP-mRNA vaccines seems quite promising, further research into diverse delivery platform remains a priority.

5.3. Efficacy and Safety of mRNA Vaccine

The safety and efficacy are the two most critical factors for a vaccine that dictate its success. Studies revealed that the risk of developing venous thrombosis due to mRNA vaccine (by Pfizer, Jhonson and Jhonson, Moderna and AstraZeneca) during COVID-19 was high (Taquet *et al.*, 2021). The exposure of SARS-CoV-2 spike proteins to platelet factor 4 (PF4) produced anti-PF4 antibodies resulting in thrombocytopenia (Greinacher *et al.*, 2021). Apart from these safety concerns, mRNA vaccine must overcome certain other challenges, like requirement of low storage temperature, polyethylene glycol (PEG) allergy, anti-PEG antibody generation, intranasal administration, and the risk of myocarditis in the vaccinated (Uddin and Roni, 2021; Knop *et al.*, 2010; Hatziantoniou *et al.*, 2021; Ju *et al.*, 2022; Ramvikas *et al.*, 2017; Heymans and Cooper, 2021).

mRNA vaccines should produce proper and efficient immune responses to generate high neutralising antibodies titres against the infection. Numerous adjuvants modulate the mRNA vaccine induced immune response ensuring the therapeutic requirements of the latter. A clear characterisation of the adjuvants to be used in mRNA vaccination is lacking, and companies like CureVac focus on developing RNA-based (CV8102) and protamine-based adjuvants for stronger immune responses (Ziegler *et al.*, 2017). Safety of LNP-mRNA system improved with the development of novel biodegradable variants (Maier *et al.*, 2013). Developing thermostable vaccine, PEGylated compound alternative, carrier alternative and intranasal delivery of mRNA vaccine need further investigation for a safe and effective mRNA vaccine platform provision.

5.4. Bioprocessing and Scale-up Challenges

mRNA vaccine manufacturing is relatively simple that makes it advantageous over traditional vaccines. Manufacturing involves upstream and downstream processing. Enzymic synthesis of mRNA molecules is an upstream process and mRNA product purification is a downstream process. mRNA encoding the antigenic gene is produced using IVT enzymatic reaction, in a cell-free milieu. Multiple purifications steps are employed to achieve clinical standard mRNA that was generated enzymatically. Purification steps usually employed to purify mRNA includes (ion-exchange, size-exclusion, ion-pair reverse-phase, affinity base separation) chromatographies and tangential flow filtration (Akash and Rehman, 2020; Karikó *et al.*, 2011; Easton *et al.*, 2010). Each purification process has its own limitations and may need adaptation for large-scale mRNA purification while still being cost effective. Downstream processing involving purification is further complemented with LNP formulation, nuclease digestion and precipitation and the methodologies may vary depending on purpose (Kis *et al.*, 2021; Pardi *et al.*, 2018). The manufacturing cost and the dose cost depend on the exact set of process operations employed in vaccine production.

Existing IVT-based mRNA production methods need improvement for faster mRNA vaccine production complimenting with the high market demand (Kis *et al.*, 2021). The continuous processing may have process integration and facilitate automation to reduce the operation time and yield loss (Walther *et al.*, 2015; Kapoor *et al.*, 2021). It will ensure high productivity of high-quality product. *In situ* removal of product and substrate, and product recovery strategies to facilitate hassle-free process control, recirculation and material reuse need to be developed (Gruber *et al.*, 2017).

Ensuring an equitable access to mRNA vaccines that are manufactured by few companies only and sourcing it across international boundaries is another challenge to address. Limited supply to the low- and middle-income countries due to logistics issues is more complicated due to the low purchasing capacity which makes it challenging to make mRNA vaccines available there (Bajaj *et al.*, 2022). Even the humanitarian aid projects were unable to deliver the high demand of vaccine in various low- and middle-income countries during COVID-19 pandemic (Bajaj *et al.*, 2022). In this background, a robust and sustainable solution is to manufacture vaccine locally to cater to the local needs shall be an immense boost to these countries. The transfer of mRNA vaccine technology, capacity-building to manufacture the vaccine and a complementing supply chain management shall be useful in up-scaling the technical and manufacturing capacity over a period of time.

6. Future Prospects

6.1. mRNA Vaccine as a Strong 'New Generation' Vaccine Candidate

High potency, rapid production, low-cost process and relatively safe administration of mRNA vaccines make them promising alternatives against their traditional counterparts. The need of the moment during the COVID-19 pandemic was rapid development of vaccines and their widespread deployment. mRNA vaccines could make it possible. Infectious pathogens could potentially mutate and evade the existing immune system (Sah *et al.*, 2021; Mohapatra *et al.*, 2023d). Although conventional vaccines provide durable protection against pathogens, they lack the ability to rapidly produce and deploy, and also do not apply to non-infectious diseases like cancer.

Innovative technology and research in the last few decades have witnessed mRNA as a potent vaccine development tool. These vaccines are safe for usage as mRNA itself is non-infectious in nature. Also, the risk of insertional mutagenesis does not apply as mRNA provides a non-integrating platform. As normal cellular processes eventually degrade the mRNA, the *in vivo* half-life needs to be modulated which can done with ease (Thess *et al.*, 2015). Formulating the mRNA into carrier molecules renders the vaccine to be stable, swift in uptake and safely express in the host cell. mRNA vaccines need minimal or no genetic vector for delivery. Hence, the risk of anti-vector immunity in the host is greatly reduced.

Another advantage of mRNA vaccines is that these can be administered repeatedly with no seeming adversity. mRNA vaccine is enzymatically produced *in vitro* making the production relatively simple and fast compared to the traditional approach. Further, mRNA vaccines are bestowed with a rapid and relatively inexpensive easily-scalable manufacturing procedure. mRNA vaccine not only has the potential to address the challenges posed by infectious agents but could also address non-infectious ailments like cancer (Pardi *et al.*, 2018). Pre-clinical studies reported the prospects and multiple advantages of mRNA vaccines making them a strong candidate for the new-generation vaccines. Thus, mRNA vaccines offer a spectrum of biopharmaceutical solutions for the emerging and reemerging public health concerns.

6.2. mRNA nano-vaccine

The instability of the mRNA molecule and its susceptibility to degradation pose significant challenges in developing mRNA vaccines. In such state, nanotechnology is an innovative solution to amplifying the potential of mRNA vaccine development (Chen *et al.*, 2023). NPs not only stabilise a naked mRNA molecule, but also help in targeted delivery. The NPs encapsulate the mRNA thereby prevent their degradation and clearance by the host immune system. Nano-vaccines facilitate the mRNA infiltrate the targeted host site. Nano-vaccines reportedly improve mRNA capture by dendritic cells, amplify the effector T-cells activation and strengthen immune response. Various employed NPs are lipid-based nanostructure, inorganic NPs, polymer-based NPs, etc. LNPs to deliver mRNA in host cells are extensively being explored and used currently. LNPs are USFDA approved as carrier and are used to deliver the viral antigen encoding mRNA for proteins against viruses like rabies, HIV, CMV, Influenza, etc. mRNA-based nano-vaccines could focus on improved safety profile, improved stability even at high temperature and enhanced cellular penetration in future. Next-gen mRNA vaccine may use genetic engineering tools for personalised healthcare, allowing to explore their full potential.

6.3. Universal mRNA Vaccines

A single vaccine that provided protection against multiple pathogens or multiple strains of a particular pathogen sounds fantastic. Such a vaccine is called multi-epitope or universal vaccine. Viruses (like influenza and dengue) have multiple serotypes, so vaccine that targets a particular serotype may not extend cross-protection against other serotypes. Due to this, studies investigate developing a universal mRNA vaccine comprising of multiple conserved epitopes from all serotypes (Rcheulishvili *et al.*, 2023; Larkin, 2023; Uno and Ross, 2021). Single monovalent vaccine eliciting protective immunity against all the circulating serotypes seems an effective and economical strategy. Pathogens like SARS-CoV-2 and influenza undergo constant mutation and reassortment that lead to the rising number of mutants or new strains/variants that are resistant to available vaccines. An mRNA vaccine that contains multiple conserved epitopes could mitigate the associated problems with emerging strains. Another is single-vaccine approach protecting against two or more different or related pathogens. Vaccine manufacturing companies (like Pfizer and BioNTech) are investigating an mRNA-based vaccine designed to protect against both influenza and COVID-19. The vaccine is currently under Phase III clinical trial (Harris, 2023).

7. Conclusion

With tremendous success of mRNA vaccine against SARS-CoV-2 and its promising future, a renewed and sustained interest in mRNA-based vaccine platforms has been generated. The technology has the potential to overcome the constraints as encountered in conventional approaches that slowdown the desired fast-paced progress in vaccine development. Although it has its own inherent challenges, mRNA vaccine is poised as an effective tool and a significant player in preventive medicine to control various (especially the bacterial and viral) infectious diseases. The challenges include its stability, storage conditions, immunogenicity and vaccine side-effects (*e.g.*, certain LNPs components), that should be overcome through fine-tuned research and technologically advanced interventions. It is strongly believed that at least some of the mRNA vaccine candidates discussed herein should undergo clinical trials successfully and gain authorisation licenses. mRNA vaccine platforms shall shape the future of vaccinology, ultimately providing substantial and sustainable public health benefits, it is highly anticipated.

References

Abbasi J, 2021. Moderna's mRNA vaccine for seasonal flu enters clinical trials. JAMA, 326(14): 1365. doi: 10.1001/jama.2021.17499

Abbas YM, Laudenbach BT, Martínez-Montero S, Cencic R, Habjan M, Pichlmair A, Damha MJ, Pelletier J and Nagar B, 2017. Structure of human IFIT1 with capped RNA reveals adaptable mRNA binding and mechanisms for sensing N1 and N2 ribose 2'-O methylations. Proc. Natl. Acad. Sci., 114(11): E2106–E2115. doi: 10.1073/pnas.1612444114

Aditya NP, Patankar S, Madhusudhan B, Murthy RSR and Souto EB, 2010. Arthemeter-loaded lipid nanoparticles produced by modified thin-film hydration: Pharmacokinetics, toxicological and in vivo anti-malarial activity. Eur. J. Pharm. Sci., 40(5): 448–455. doi: 10.1016/j.ejps.2010.05.007

Akash MSH and Rehman K 2020. Column Chromatography. In: MSH A, Kanwal R (Eds). Essentials of Pharmaceutical Analysis, Singapore, Singapore: 167–174. doi: 10.1007/978-981-15-1547-7_13

Alberer M, Gnad-Vogt U, Hong HS, Mehr KT, Backert L, Finak G, Gottardo R, Bica MA, Garofano A, Koch SD and Fotin-Mleczek M, 2017. Safety and immunogenicity of a mRNA rabies vaccine in healthy adults: an open-label, non-randomised, prospective, first-in-human phase 1 clinical trial. Lancet, 390(10101): 1511–1520. doi: 10.1016/S0140-6736(17)31665-3

Aldosari BN, Alfagih IM and Almurshedi AS, 2021. Lipid nanoparticles as delivery systems for RNA-based vaccines. Pharmaceutics, 13(2): 206. doi: 10.3390/pharmaceutics13020206

Aldrich C, Leroux–Roels I, Huang KB, Bica MA, Loeliger E, Schoenborn-Kellenberger O, Walz L, Leroux-Roels G, von Sonnenburg F and Oostvogels L, 2021. Proof-of-concept of a low-dose unmodified mRNA-based rabies vaccine formulated with lipid nanoparticles in human volunteers: A phase 1 trial. Vaccine, 39(8): 1310–1318. doi: 10.1016/j.vaccine.2020.12.070

Anderson BR, Muramatsu H, Nallagatla SR, Bevilacqua PC, Sansing LH, Weissman D and Karikó K, 2010. Incorporation of pseudouridine into mRNA enhances translation by diminishing PKR activation. Nucleic Acids Res., 38(17): 5884–5892. doi: 10.1093/nar/gkq347.

Andries O, Mc Cafferty S, De Smedt SC, Weiss R, Sanders NN and Kitada T, 2015. N1-methylpseudouridine-incorporated mRNA outperforms pseudouridine-incorporated mRNA by providing enhanced protein expression and reduced immunogenicity in mammalian cell lines and mice. J. Controll. Release, 217: 337–344. doi: 10.1016/j.jconrel.2015.08.051

Asrani KH, Farelli JD, Stahley MR, Miller RL, Cheng CJ, Subramanian RR and Brown JM, 2018. Optimization of mRNA untranslated regions for improved expression of therapeutic mRNA. RNA Biol., 15(6): 756–762. doi: 10.1080/15476286.2018.1450054

August A, Attarwala HZ, Himansu S, Kalidindi S, Lu S, Pajon R, Han S, Lecerf JM, Tomassini JE, Hard M and Ptaszek LM, 2021. A phase 1 trial of lipid-encapsulated mRNA encoding a monoclonal antibody with neutralizing activity against Chikungunya virus. Nat. Med., 27(12): 2224–2233. doi: 10.1038/s41591-021-01573-6

Baden LR, El Sahly HM, Essink B, Follmann D, Neuzil KM, August A, Clouting H, Fortier G, Deng W, Han S and Zhao X, 2021. Phase 3 trial of mRNA-1273 during the Delta-variant surge. N. Engl. J. Med., 385(26): 2485–2487. doi: 10.1056/NEJMc2115597

Bai S, Yang T, Zhu C, Feng M, Zhang L, Zhang Z, Wang X, Yu R, Pan X, Zhao C and Xu J, 2023. A single vaccination of nucleoside-modified Rabies mRNA vaccine induces prolonged highly protective immune responses in mice. Front. Immunology, 13: 1099991. doi: 10.3389/fimmu.2022.1099991

Bajaj SS, Maki L and Stanford FC, 2022. Vaccine apartheid: global cooperation and equity. Lancet, 399(10334): 1452–1453. doi: 10.1016/S0140-6736(22)00328-2

Beck JD, Reidenbach D, Salomon N, Sahin U, Türeci Ö, Vormehr M and Kranz LM, 2021. mRNA therapeutics in cancer immunotherapy. Mol. Cancer, 20(1): 69. doi: 10.1186/s12943-021-01348-0

Bruch A, Kelani AA and Blango MG, 2022. RNA-based therapeutics to treat human fungal infections. Trends Microbiol., 30(5): 411–420. doi: 10.1016/j.tim.2021.09.007.

Chaudhary N, Weissman D and Whitehead KA, 2021. mRNA vaccines for infectious diseases: principles, delivery and clinical translation. Nat. Rev. Drug Discov., 20(11): 817–838. doi: 10.1038/s41573-021-00283-5

Chen S, Huang X, Xue Y, Álvarez-Benedicto E, Shi Y, Chen W, Koo S, Siegwart DJ, Dong Y and Tao W, 2023. Nanotechnology-based mRNA vaccines. Nat. Rev. Methods Primers, 3(1): 63. doi: 10.1038/s43586-023-00246-7

Conry RM, LoBuglio AF, Wright M, Sumerel L, Pike MJ, Johanning F, Benjamin R, Lu D and Curiel DT, 1995. Characterization of a messenger RNA polynucleotide vaccine vector. Cancer Res., 55(7): 1397–1400.

Easton LE, Shibata Y and Lukavsky PJ, 2010. Rapid, nondenaturing RNA purification using weak anion-exchange fast performance liquid chromatography. RNA, 16(3): 647–653. doi: 10.1261/rna.1862210

Evers MJ, Kulkarni JA, van der Meel R, Cullis PR, Vader P and Schiffelers RM, 2018. State□of□the□art design and rapid□mixing production techniques of lipid nanoparticles for nucleic acid delivery. Small methods, 2(9): 1700375. doi: 10.1002/smtd.201700375

Freyn AW, da Silva JR, Rosado VC, Bliss CM, Pine M, Mui BL, Tam YK, Madden TD, de Souza Ferreira LC, Weissman D and Krammer F, 2020. A multi-targeting, nucleoside-modified mRNA influenza virus vaccine provides broad protection in mice. Mol. Ther., 28(7): 1569–1584. doi: 10.1016/j.ymthe.2020.04.018

Gonzalez G, Pfannes L, Brazas R and Striker R, 2007. Selection of an optimal RNA transfection reagent and comparison to electroporation for the delivery of viral RNA. J. Virol. Methods, 145(1): 14–21. doi: 10.1016/j.jviromet.2007.04.013

Greaney AJ, Loes AN, Gentles LE, Crawford KH, Starr TN, Malone KD, Chu HY and Bloom JD, 2021. Antibodies Elicited by MRNA-1273 Vaccination Bind More Broadly to the Receptor Binding Domain than Do Those from SARS-CoV-2 Infection. Sci. Transl. Med., 13: eabi9915.

Greinacher A, Thiele T, Warkentin TE, Weisser K, Kyrle PA and Eichinger S, 2021. Thrombotic thrombocytopenia after ChAdOx1 nCov-19 vaccination. N. Engl. J. Med., 384(22): 2092–2101. doi: 10.1056/NEJMoa2104840

Gruber P, Marques MP, O'Sullivan B, Baganz F, Wohlgemuth R and Szita N, 2017. Conscious coupling: The challenges and opportunities of cascading enzymatic microreactors. Biotechnol. J., 12(7): 1700030. doi: 10.1002/biot.201700030

Harris E, 2023. Combined COVID-19, flu vaccine candidate headed to phase 3 trials. JAMA. 330(21): 2044. doi:10.1001/jama.2023.22353

Harrison VR, Eckels KH, Bartelloni PJ and Hampton C, 1971. Production and evaluation of a formalin-killed Chikungunya vaccine. J Immunol.,107(3): 643–647. doi: 10.4049/jimmunol.107.3.643

Hatziantoniou S, Maltezou HC, Tsakris A, Poland GA and Anastassopoulou C, 2021. Anaphylactic reactions to mRNA COVID-19 vaccines: a call for further study. Vaccine. 39(19): 2605–2607. doi: 10.1016/j.vaccine.2021.03.073

Heine A, Juranek S and Brossart P, 2021. Clinical and immunological effects of mRNA vaccines in malignant diseases. Mol. Cancer. 20: 52. doi: 10.1186/s12943-021-01339-1

Hellgren F, Cagigi A, Arcoverde Cerveira R, Ols S, Kern T, Lin A, Eriksson B, Dodds MG, Jasny E, Schwendt K and Freuling C, 2023. Unmodified rabies mRNA vaccine elicits high cross-neutralizing antibody titers and diverse B cell memory responses. Nat. Commun., 14(1): 3713. doi: 10.1038/s41467-023-39421-5

Heymans S and Cooper LT, 2022. Myocarditis after COVID-19 mRNA vaccination: clinical observations and potential mechanisms. Nat. Rev. Cardiol., 19(2): 75–77. doi: 10.1038/s41569-021-00662-w

Hoerr I, Obst R, Rammensee HG and Jung G, 2000. In vivo application of RNA leads to induction of specific cytotoxic T lymphocytes and antibodies. Eur. J. Immunol., 30(1): 1–7. doi: 10.1002/1521-4141(200001)30:1<1::AID-IMMU1>3.0.CO;2-%23

Huang X, Lee RJ, Qi Y, Li Y, Lu J, Meng Q, Teng L and Xie J, 2017. Microfluidic hydrodynamic focusing synthesis of polymer-lipid nanoparticles for siRNA delivery. Oncotarget, 8(57): 96826. doi: 10.18632/oncotarget.18281

Iyer VR, Praveen P, Kaduskar BD, Moharir SC and Mishra RK, 2024. mRNA biotherapeutics landscape for rare genetic disorders. J. Biosci., 49(1): 33. doi: 10.1007/s12038-023-00415-6

Ju Y, Lee WS, Pilkington EH, Kelly HG, Li S, Selva KJ, Wragg KM, Subbarao K, Nguyen TH, Rowntree LC and Allen LF, 2022. Anti-PEG antibodies boosted in humans by SARS-

CoV-2 lipid nanoparticle mRNA vaccine. Acs Nano, 16(8): 11769–11780. doi: 10.1021/acsnano.2c04543

Kapoor Y, Meyer RF, Meyer BK, DiNunzio JC, Bhambhani A, Stanbro J, Ploeger KJ, Guidry EN, Troup GM, Procopio AT and Templeton AC, 2021. Flexible manufacturing: the future state of drug product development and commercialization in the pharmaceutical industry. J. Pharm. Innov., 16: 2–10. doi: 10.1007/s12247-019-09426-z

Karikó K, Muramatsu H, Ludwig J and Weissman D, 2011. Generating the optimal mRNA for therapy: HPLC purification eliminates immune activation and improves translation of nucleoside-modified, protein-encoding mRNA. Nucleic Acids Res., 39(21): e142-e142. doi: 10.1093/nar/gkr695

Karikó K, Muramatsu H, Welsh FA, Ludwig J, Kato H, Akira S and Weissman D, 2008. Incorporation of pseudouridine into mRNA yields superior nonimmunogenic vector with increased translational capacity and biological stability. Mol. Ther., 16(11): 1833–1840. doi: 10.1038/mt.2008.200

Kennedy RB, Ovsyannikova IG, Palese P and Poland GA, 2020. Current challenges in vaccinology. Front. Immunol., 11: 1181. doi: 10.3389/fimmu.2020.01181

Kis Z, Kontoravdi C, Shattock R and Shah N, 2020. Resources, production scales and time required for producing RNA vaccines for the global pandemic demand. Vaccines, 9(1): 3. doi: 10.3390/vaccines9010003

Kloc M, Foreman V and Reddy SA, 2011. Binary function of mRNA. Biochimie, 93(11): 1955–1961. doi: 10.1016/j.biochi.2011.07.008

Knop K, Hoogenboom R, Fischer D and Schubert US, 2010. Poly (ethylene glycol) in drug delivery: pros and cons as well as potential alternatives. Angew. Chem., Int. Ed. Engl., 49(36): 6288–6308. doi: 10.1002/anie.200902672

Kon E, Levy Y, Elia U, Cohen H, Hazan-Halevy I, Aftalion M, Ezra A, Bar-Haim E, Naidu GS, Diesendruck Y and Rotem S, 2023. A single-dose F1-based mRNA-LNP vaccine provides protection against the lethal plague bacterium. Sci. Adv., 9(10): eadg1036. doi: 10.1126/sciadv.adg1036

Kose N, Fox JM, Sapparapu G, Bombardi R, Tennekoon RN, De Silva AD, Elbashir SM, Theisen MA, Humphris-Narayanan E, Ciaramella G and Himansu S, 2019. A lipid-encapsulated mRNA encoding a potently neutralizing human monoclonal antibody protects against chikungunya infection. Sci. Immunol., 4(35): eaaw6647. doi: 10.1126/sciimmunol.aaw6647

Kowalski, P.S., Rudra, A., Miao, L. and Anderson, D.G., 2019. Delivering the messenger: advances in technologies for therapeutic mRNA delivery. Mol. Ther., 27(4): 710–728. doi: 10.1016/j.ymthe.2019.02.012

Kremsner PG, Guerrero RAA, Arana-Arri E, Martinez GJA, Bonten M, Chandler R, Corral G, De Block EJL, Ecker L, Gabor JJ and Lopez CAG, 2022. Efficacy and safety of the CVnCoV SARS-CoV-2 mRNA vaccine candidate in ten countries in Europe and Latin America (HERALD): a randomised, observer-blinded, placebo controlled, phase 2b/3 trial. Lancet Infect. Dis., 22(3): 329–340. doi: 10.1016/S1473-3099(21)00677-0

Kudla G, Murray AW, Tollervey D and Plotkin JB, 2009. Coding-sequence determinants of gene expression in Escherichia coli. Sci., 324(5924): 255–258. doi: 10.1126/science.1170160

Larkin H, 2023. Twenty-strain "universal" mRNA flu vaccine effective in animal studies. JAMA, 329(2): 114–114. doi: 10.1001/jama.2022.23512

Lee IT, Nachbagauer R, Ensz D, Schwartz H, Carmona L, Schaefers K, Avanesov A, Stadlbauer D, Henry C, Chen R and Huang W, 2023. Safety and immunogenicity of a phase 1/2 randomized clinical trial of a quadrivalent, mRNA-based seasonal influenza vaccine (mRNA-1010) in healthy adults: interim analysis. Nat. Commun., 14(1): 3631. doi: 10.1038/s41467-023-39376-7

Li J, Liu Q, Liu J, Wu X, Lei Y, Li S, Zhao D, Li Z, Luo L, Peng S and Ou Y, 2022. An mRNA-based rabies vaccine induces strong protective immune responses in mice and dogs. Virol. J., 19(1): 184. doi: 10.1186/s12985-022-01919-7

Li M, Fang E, Wang Y, Shi L, Li J, Peng Q, Li X, Zhao D, Liu X, Liu X and Liu J, 2023. An mRNA vaccine against rabies provides strong and durable protection in mice. Front. Immunol., 14: 1288879. doi: 10.3389/fimmu.2023.1288879

Linares-Fernández S, Lacroix C, Exposito JY and Verrier B, 2020. Tailoring mRNA vaccine to balance innate/adaptive immune response. Trends Mol. Med., 26(3): 311–323. doi: 10.1016/j.molmed.2019.10.002

Liu J, Lu X, Li X, Huang W, Fang E, Li W, Liu X, Liu M, Li J, Li M and Zhang Z, 2023. Construction and immunogenicity of an mRNA vaccine against chikungunya virus. Front. Immunol., 14: 1129118. doi: 10.3389/fimmu.2023.1129118

Long J, Yu C, Cao Y, Miao Y, Sun H, Zhang Z, Mai J, Wang X, Mao Y, Li H and Yang J, 2023. A rabies mRNA vaccine provides a rapid and long-term immune response in mice. Nano Today, 53: 102038. doi: 10.1016/j.nantod.2023.102038

Luo Y, Na Z and Slavoff SA, 2018. P-Bodies: Composition, Properties, and Functions. Biochemistry, 57(17): 2424–2431. doi: 10.1021/acs.biochem.7b01162

Maier MA, Jayaraman M, Matsuda S, Liu J, Barros S, Querbes W, Tam YK, Ansell SM, Kumar V, Qin J and Zhang X, 2013. Biodegradable lipids enabling rapidly eliminated lipid nanoparticles for systemic delivery of RNAi therapeutics. Mol. Ther., 21(8): 1570–1578. doi: 10.1038/mt.2013.124

Maruggi G, Zhang C, Li J, Ulmer JB and Yu D, 2019. mRNA as a transformative technology for vaccine development to control infectious diseases. Mol. Ther., 27(4): 757–772. doi: 10.1016/j.ymthe.2019.01.020

Meyer M, Huang E, Yuzhakov O, Ramanathan P, Ciaramella G and Bukreyev A, 2018. Modified mRNA-Based Vaccines Elicit Robust Immune Responses and Protect Guinea Pigs from Ebola Virus Disease. J. Infect. Dis., 217(3): 451–455. doi: 10.1093/infdis/jix592

Mishra S, Mohapatra RK, Dash G, Mohanty A and Sah R, 2024. Countering the threatening surge in SARS-CoV-2 variants in China and its possible global implications: stocktaking in the ongoing FISU and the Asian Games vigilance. Ann. Med. Surg., 86(5):2373-5. doi: 10.1097/MS9.0000000000001811

Mohapatra RK, Das PK and Kandi V, 2020. Challenges in controlling COVID-19 in migrants in Odisha, India. Diabetes Metab Syndr., 14(6):1593-9. doi: 10.1016/j.dsx.2020.08.024

Mohapatra RK, Kandi V, Gaidhane AM, Zahiruddin QS, Rustagi S, Satapathy P, Mishra S and Tuglo LS, 2024. Global domination of the recently VoI-classified'JN. 1′ outcompeting other variants–Comparing the vaccines' efficacy. Clinical Infection in Practice, 22:100358. https://doi.org/10.1016/j.clinpr.2024.100358

Mohapatra RK, Mahal A, Mishra S, Dash G, Tuglo LS and Kandi V, 2023a. Current surge of severe acute respiratory syndrome coronavirus-2 (SARS-CoV-2) variants in China could be threatening as the Asian Games 2023 flags off in September: foolproof cautionary measures are suggested. Cureus. 15(9):e45591. doi: 10.7759/cureus.45591

Mohapatra RK, Mahal A, Mishra S, Kandi V and Obaidullah WJ, 2023c. SARS-CoV-2 variants BA. 2.86 and EG. 5.1 alongside scrub typhus and nipah in India during the ongoing cricket world cup 2023: threat perceptions and countermeasures. Cureus, 15(11):e48895. doi: 10.7759/cureus.48895

Mohapatra RK, Mishra S, Azam M and Dhama K, 2021. COVID-19, WHO guidelines, pedagogy, and respite. Open Med., 16(1):491-3. doi: 10.1515/med-2021-0266

Mohapatra RK, Mishra S, Kandi V, Branda F, Ansari A, Rabaan AA and Kudrat-E-Zahan M, 2023b. Analyzing the emerging patterns of SARS-CoV-2 Omicron subvariants for the development of next-gen vaccine: An observational study. Health Sci. Rep., 6(10):e1596. doi: 10.1002/hsr2.1596

Mohapatra RK, Verma S, Kandi V, Sarangi AK, Seidel V, Das SN, Behera A, Tuli HS, Sharma AK and Dhama K, 2023d. The SARS-CoV-2 Omicron variant and its multiple sub-lineages: transmissibility, vaccine development, antiviral drugs, monoclonal antibodies, and strategies for infection control–a review. ChemistrySelect., 8(9):e202201380. https://doi.org/10.1002/slct.202201380

Mulligan MJ, Lyke KE, Kitchin N, Absalon J, Gurtman A, Lockhart S, Neuzil K, Raabe V, Bailey R, Swanson KA and Li P, 2020. Phase I/II study of COVID-19 RNA vaccine BNT162b1 in adults. Nature, 586(7830): 589–593. doi: 10.1038/s41586-020-2639-4

Nallagatla SR and Bevilacqua PC, 2008. Nucleoside modifications modulate activation of the protein kinase PKR in an RNA structure-specific manner. RNA, 14(6): 1201–1213. doi: 10.1261/rna.1007408

Ningning Ge, Jin Sun, Zhihua Liu, Jiayi Shu, Huimin Yan, Zhihua Kou, Yu Wei and Xia Jin, 2022. An mRNA vaccine encoding Chikungunya virus E2-E1 protein elicits robust neutralizing antibody responses and CTL immune responses. Virol. Sin., 37(2): 266–276. doi: 10.1016/j.virs.2022.01.032

Otake K, Shimomura T, Goto T, Imura T, Furuya T, Yoda S, Takebayashi Y, Sakai H and Abe M, 2006. Preparation of liposomes using an improved supercritical reverse phase evaporation method. Langmuir, 22(6): 2543–2550. doi: 10.1021/la051654u

Pardi N, Hogan MJ, Porter FW and Weissman D, 2018. mRNA vaccines—a new era in vaccinology. Nat. Rev. Drug Discov.,17(4): 261–279. doi: doi:10.1038/nrd.2017.243

Pattnaik A, Sahoo BR and Pattnaik AK, 2020. Current Status of Zika Virus Vaccines: Successes and Challenges. Vaccines, 8: 266. doi: 10.3390/vaccines8020266

Plotkin SA, 2009 Vaccines: The Fourth Century. Clin. Vaccine Immunol., 16: 1709–1719. doi: 10.1128/CVI.00290-09

Plotkin SA and Plotkin SL, 2011. The development of vaccines: how the past led to the future. Nat. Rev. Microbiol., 9: 889–893. doi: 10.1038/nrmicro2668

Ramvikas M, Arumugam M, Chakrabarti SR, Jaganathan KS 2017. Nasal vaccine delivery. In: Mariusz S and Istvan T (Eds) Micro and Nanotechnology in Vaccine Development, Elsevier: 279–301.

Rauch S, Jasny E, Schmidt KE and Petsch B, 2018. New vaccine technologies to combat outbreak situations. Front Immunol., 9: 1963. doi: 10.3389/fimmu.2018.01963

Rcheulishvili N, Mao J, Papukashvili D, Liu C, Wang Z, Zhao J, Xie F, Pan X, Ji Y, He Y and Wang PG, 2023. Designing multi-epitope mRNA construct as a universal influenza vaccine candidate for future epidemic/pandemic preparedness. Int. J. Biol. Macromol., 226: 885–899. doi: 10.1016/j.ijbiomac.2022.12.066

Ribeiro LNM, Couto VM, Fraceto LF and de Paula E, 2018 Use of nanoparticle concentration as a tool to understand the structural properties of colloids. Sci. Rep., 8(1): 982. doi: 10.1038/s41598-017-18573-7

Richner JM, Jagger BW, Shan C, Fontes CR, Dowd KA, Cao B, Himansu S, Caine EA, Nunes BT, Medeiros DB and Muruato AE, 2017. Vaccine mediated protection against Zika virus-induced congenital disease. Cell, 170(2): 273–283. doi: 10.1016/j.cell.2017.06.040

Rijkers GT, Weterings N, Obregon-Henao A, Lepolder M, Dutt TS, van Overveld FJ and Henao-Tamayo M, 2021. Antigen presentation of mRNA-based and virus-vectored SARS-CoV-2 vaccines. Vaccines, 9(8): 848. doi: 10.3390/vaccines9080848

Roth C, Cantaert T, Colas C, Prot M, Casadémont I, Levillayer L, Thalmensi J, Langlade-Demoyen P, Gerke C, Bahl K and Ciaramella G, 2019. A modified mRNA vaccine targeting immunodominant NS epitopes protects against dengue virus infection in HLA class I transgenic mice. Front. Immunol., 10: 1424. doi: 10.3389/fimmu.2019.01424

Sahin U, Karikó K and Türeci Ö, 2014. mRNA-based therapeutics—developing a new class of drugs. Nat. Rev. Drug Discov., 13(10): 759–780. doi:10.1038/nrd4278

Sahin U, Muik A, Derhovanessian E, Vogler I, Kranz LM, Vormehr M, Baum A, Pascal K, Quandt J, Maurus D and Brachtendorf S, 2020. COVID-19 vaccine BNT162b1 elicits human antibody and TH1 T cell responses. Nature, 586(7830): 594–599. doi: 10.1038/s41586-020-2814-7

Sah R, Khatiwada AP, Shrestha S, Bhuvan KC, Tiwari R, Mohapatra RK, Dhama K and Rodriguez-Morales AJ, 2021. COVID-19 vaccination campaign in Nepal, emerging UK variant and futuristic vaccination strategies to combat the ongoing pandemic. Travel Med. Infect. Dis., 41:102037. doi: 10.1016/j.tmaid.2021.102037

Sarangi AK, Salem MA, Younus MD, El-Haroun H, Mahal A, Tripathy L, Mishra R, Shabil M, Alhumaydhi FA, Khatib MN and Bushi G, 2024. Advanced biomaterials for regenerative medicine and their possible therapeutic significance in treating COVID-19: a critical overview. Int. J. Surg., 110(12):7508-27. doi: 10.1097/JS9.0000000000002110

Satapathy BS, Pattnaik G, Sahoo RN, Pattanaik S, Sarangi AK, Kandi V, Mishra S, Rabaan AA, Mohanty A, Sah R and Mohapatra RK, 2023. COVID-19 vaccines and their underbelly: Are we going the right way?. Health Sci. Rep., 6(9):e1540. doi: 10.1002/hsr2.1540

Scaria PV, Roth N, Schwendt K, Muratova OV, Alani N, Lambert LE, Barnafo EK, Rowe CG, Zaidi IU, Rausch KM and Narum DL, 2024. mRNA vaccines expressing malaria transmission-blocking antigens Pfs25 and Pfs230D1 induce a functional immune response. npj Vaccines 9: 9. doi: 10.1038/s41541-023-00783-y

Schnee M, Vogel AB, Voss D, Petsch B, Baumhof P, Kramps T and Stitz L, 2016. An mRNA Vaccine Encoding Rabies Virus Glycoprotein Induces Protection against Lethal Infection in Mice and Correlates of Protection in Adult and Newborn Pigs. PLoS Negl. Trop. Dis., 10(6): e0004746. doi: 10.1371/journal.pntd.0004746

Schwartz O and Albert M, 2010. Biology and pathogenesis of chikungunya virus. Nat. Rev. Microbiol., 8: 491–500. doi: 10.1038/nrmicro2368

Shi Z and Hu ZA, 2008 Review of Studies on Animal Reservoirs of the SARS Coronavirus. Virus Res., 133: 74–87. doi: 10.1016/j.virusres.2007.03.012

Steinle H, Behring A, Schlensak C, Wendel HP and Avci-Adali M, 2017. Concise review: application of in vitro transcribed messenger RNA for cellular engineering and reprogramming: progress and challenges. Stem Cells, 35(1): 68–79. doi: 10.1002/stem.2402

Stitz L, Vogel A, Schnee M, Voss D, Rauch S, Mutzke T, Ketterer T, Kramps T and Petsch B, 2017. A thermostable messenger RNA based vaccine against rabies. PLoS Negl. Trop. Dis., 11(12): e0006108. doi: 10.1371/journal.pntd.0006108

Sullenger BA and Nair S, 2016. From the RNA world to the clinic. Sci., 352(6292): 1417–1420. doi: 10.1126/science.aad8709

Taquet M, Husain M, Geddes JR, Luciano S and Harrison PJ, 2021. Cerebral venous thrombosis and portal vein thrombosis: a retrospective cohort study of 537,913 COVID-19 cases. EClinicalMedicine, 39. doi: 10.1016/j.eclinm.2021.101061

Thess A, Grund S, Mui BL, Hope MJ, Baumhof P, Fotin-Mleczek M and Schlake T, 2015. Sequence-engineered mRNA without chemical nucleoside modifications enables an effective protein therapy in large animals. Mol. Ther., 23(9): 1456–1464. doi: 10.1038/mt.2015.103

Uddin MN and Roni MA, 2021. Challenges of storage and stability of mRNA-based COVID-19 vaccines. Vaccines. 9(9): 1033. doi: 10.3390/vaccines9091033

Uno N and Ross TM, 2021. Universal dengue vaccine elicits neutralizing antibodies against strains from all four dengue virus serotypes. J. Virol., 95(4). doi: 10.1128/jvi.00658-20

Vaidyanathan S, Azizian KT, Haque AA, Henderson JM, Hendel A, Shore S, Antony JS, Hogrefe RI, Kormann MS, Porteus MH and McCaffrey AP, 2018. Uridine depletion and chemical modification increase Cas9 mRNA activity and reduce immunogenicity without HPLC purification. Mol. Ther. Nucleic Acids, 12: 530–542. doi: 10.1016/j.omtn.2018.06.010

Walther J, Godawat R, Hwang C, Abe Y, Sinclair A and Konstantinov K, 2015. The business impact of an integrated continuous biomanufacturing platform for recombinant protein production. J. Biotechnol., 213: 3–12. doi: 10.1016/j.jbiotec.2015.05.010

Wang MM, Wappelhorst CN, Jensen EL, Chi YCT, Rouse JC and Zou Q, 2023 Elucidation of lipid nanoparticle surface structure in mRNA vaccines. Sci. Rep., 13(1): 16744. doi: 10.1038/s41598-023-43898-x

Wan J, Yang J, Wang Z, Shen R, Zhang C, Wu Y, Zhou M, Chen H, Fu ZF, Sun H and Yi Y, 2023. A single immunization with core–shell structured lipopolyplex mRNA vaccine against rabies induces potent humoral immunity in mice and dogs. Emerg. Microbes Infect., 12(2): 2270081. doi: 10.1080/22221751.2023.2270081

White A, Berman S and Lowenthal JP, 1972. Comparative immunogenicities of chikungunya vaccines propagated in monkey kidney monolayers and chick embryo suspension cultures. Appl. Microbiol., 23(5): 951–952. doi: 10.1128/am.23.5.951-952.1972

Wolff JA, Malone RW, Williams P, Chong W, Acsadi G, Jani A and Felgner PL, 1990. Direct gene transfer into mouse muscle in vivo. Sci., 247(4949): 1465–1468. doi: 10.1126/science.1690918

Wollner CJ, Richner M, Hassert MA, Pinto AK, Brien JD and Richner, J.M., 2021. A dengue virus serotype 1 mRNA-LNP vaccine elicits protective immune responses. J. Virol., 95(12). doi: 10.1128/jvi.02482-20

Xu S, Yang K, Li R and Zhang L, 2020. mRNA vaccine era—mechanisms, drug platform and clinical prospection. Int. J. Mol. Sci., 21(18): 6582. doi: 10.3390/ijms21186582

Ye Z, Harmon J, Ni W, Li Y, Wich D and Xu Q, 2023. The mRNA vaccine revolution: COVID-19 has launched the future of vaccinology. ACS nano, 17(16): 15231–15253. doi: 10.1021/acsnano.2c12584

Yin P, Davenport BJ, Wan JJ, Kim AS, Diamond MS, Ware BC, Tong K, Couderc T, Lecuit M, Lai JR and Morrison TE, 2023. Chikungunya virus cell-to-cell transmission is mediated by intercellular extensions in vitro and in vivo. Nat. Microbiol., 8(9): 1653–1667. doi: 10.1038/s41564-023-01449-0

Zhang M, Sun J, Li M and Jin X, 2020. Modified mRNA-LNP vaccines confer protection against experimental DENV-2 infection in mice. Mol. Ther., Methods Clin. Dev., 18: 702–712. doi: 10.1016/j.omtm.2020.07.013

Zhou P, Yang XL, Wang XG, Hu B, Zhang L, Zhang W, Si HR, Zhu Y, Li B, Huang CL and Chen HD, 2020. A pneumonia outbreak associated with a new coronavirus of probable bat origin. Nature, 579(7798): 270–273. doi: 10.1038/s41586-020-2012-7

Ziegler A, Soldner C, Lienenklaus S, Spanier J, Trittel S, Riese P, Kramps T, Weiss S, Heidenreich R, Jasny E and Guzmán CA, 2017. A new RNA-based adjuvant enhances virus-specific vaccine responses by locally triggering TLR-and RLH-dependent effects. J. Immunol., 198(4): 1595–1605. doi: 10.4049/jimmunol.1601129

4

A 360° Understanding of Vaccine Design and Production Prospects and Challenges

Arindam Jana[1,2], Shreyashree Pal[1], Snehasish Mishra[1] and Rahul Modak[1,*]

[1]School of Biotechnology, Campus 11, KIIT Deemed University, Patia Bhubaneswar – 751 024, Odisha, India
[2]Bioprocess facility, KIIT - Technology Business Incubator (KIIT-TBI) KIIT Deemed University, Patia, Bhubaneswar – 751 024, Odisha, India

Abstract

Constantly emerging and reemerging vaccine-preventable infectious diseases recently around the globe challenged the health infrastructure and has been a critical concern for the medical fraternity. There are 21 other neglected tropical diseases, as classified and recently updated by the World Health Organisation, many of which are seemingly vaccine-preventable. The unprecedented scenario that the world encountered during the recent COVID-19 pandemic was also a 'silver lining in the dark cloud' for primarily the vaccinologists. The scientific world witnessed stupendous developments in vaccine development. One such instance was the cutting-edge mRNA vaccine development platform. Once a vaccine is successfully designed, the next step is scaling it up in a milieu that is conducive for its mass production. There are numerous ways to achieve it, from biological system (animal models like the chick embryo, mouse cell-lines, suspension-cultured tobacco cells) to the non-biological (bioreactor) settings. This chapter provides a comprehensive overview of the intricacies in vaccine development, from designing to large-scale manufacturing (mass production). It delves into key scientific guiding principles behind developing and formulating vaccines, adopting both the traditional and emerging bioprocessing and bioseparation engineering and technology. It also explores the technical and management challenges faced before and during scaling up, including maintaining product efficacy, ensuring high quality for human administration, and navigating regulatory landscapes, among others. The chapter offers a holistic understanding of bioprocessing continuum, to educate and inform the research (academia) and development (bioindustry) community for more promising and effective strategies in the future to optimise vaccine production, thus contributing to the global public healthcare initiatives.

***Keywords*:** vaccine, upstreaming, downstreaming, process design, scale-up, bioseparation

1. Introduction

The development and production scale-up of vaccines represent one of the most critical and complex aspects of modern medical biotechnology (Panda *et al.*, 2022). The new-age or modern vaccine development and manufacturing operates on a multifaceted landscape by integrating cutting-edge biotechnological advancements and scalable production strategies (Satapathy *et al.*, 2023; Mohapatra *et al.*, 2023; Dash et al., 2024). This chapter explores the critical stages of vaccine bioprocessing in line with the advent of novel vaccine development platforms like mRNA, viral vectors and recombinant protein technologies, from antigen design and optimisation to large-scale production and quality assurance. It highlights the necessity of robust and efficient bioprocesses to meet the global demand, particularly in the context of emerging infectious diseases and pandemics that needed immediate and expeditious healthcare attention. The discussion delves through the utilisation of advanced cell culture systems, bioreactor technologies and purification strategies, alongside the challenges of ensuring consistency, safety and the national and international regulatory compliances. The chapter also addresses the role of Quality by Design (QbD), continuous process approach, process analytical technologies (PAT) and challenges to address in enhancing process control and product yield (Gerzon *et al.*, 2022). By providing a comprehensive overview of the current state and future directions of vaccine bioprocessing, this chapter serves as an essential resource equally for the researchers, bioprocess engineers and policymakers dedicated to advancing global healthcare through innovative vaccine production solutions. Once a vaccine candidate is technically approved for public administration, it is imperative to establish a foolproof and standardised process for its development, verification and validation from time to time (Salalli *et al.*, 2023). It ensures that a consistently safe vaccine is produced at a scale that is seemingly sufficient to meet the global demand.

1.1. The Need for Process Standardisation

Standardisation of a scientific process and its validation is always essential for numerous reasons. Firstly, it ensures the reproducibility and repeatability of a process that is crucial to maintain a consistency on the efficacy and safety of the product for the end-user. The process followed from the development to mass production needs meticulous designing that should also include stringent quality control measures to detect a deviation or anomaly even as the process continues (rather than only the final product), and mitigate it. The critical steps in this context are verification and validation of the end-to-end foolproof process. Verification involves confirming that the process is capable of consistently producing the desired outcome, while validation ensures that the process does what it is intended to do, with respect to the designated parameters (U.S. FDA, 2011).

1.2. Verification and Validation

Verification and validation are neither one-time events nor continuous. These are continually evolving ongoing processes that span the entire lifecycle of the production of a vaccine. The verification and validation activities include rigorous analyses and testing at various stages of production, from raw material sourcing to final product packaging. The guidelines that are followed are in line with the Hazard Analysis Critical Control Point (HACCP). The analytical methods to test the stability and simulation studies of the process play pivotal roles in this. Regulatory agencies such as the FDA of the US and the EMA of the European Union provide guidelines and frameworks for these processes, underscoring their importance in the production pipeline (EMA, 2016; U.S. FDA, 2011). It is however necessary to note that, these guidelines mention what to do and not how to do (which need to be confirmed in-house).

1.3. Bioprocess Techniques for Production Scale-up

Bioprocess techniques for vaccine production scale-up are essential to translate laboratory research into commercial manufacturing. It involves optimising living systems like microbial, insect or mammalian cells, to enhance antigen production while preserving the integrity and potency of the product. Bioreactor systems are the conventional approaches to scale-up and mass-produce an economically significant material of biological origin. Advanced strategies like fed-batch, perfusion and continuous mode of bioprocessing are employed to maximise output and minimise the resource input requirements. Downstream processing, including sophisticated filtration, ultracentrifugation and chromatography techniques, is crucial in purifying the immunogen and removing impurities to meet the stringent regulatory standards for medical products meant for human use. However, bioreactor scale-up has its inherent unique challenges like shear stress management, maintaining cell viability, ensuring product homogeneity across batches and mitigating contamination risks. Beyond traditional bioreactor systems, several other bioprocess techniques are employed for increased production of biomaterials like vaccines (Fig. 1). The techniques that are usually employed in mass production of vaccines are as follows.

1.3.1. Animal Model

Pre-clinical evaluation is an essential phase prior to initiating a human clinical trial, using animal models. This step is critical as it is useful in elucidating the safety profile of the vaccine candidate, its immunogenic potential and its overall efficacy. Animal models like mice, rat, woodchuck, guinea pig, rabbit, ferret, pig, etc. are employed to qualify and quantify immune responses, vaccine formulation, optimising the vaccine delivery routes, determining the level of protection against the target infection and mitigating transmission, and assessing the potential toxicity and overall safety of the vaccine candidate (Kiros *et al.*, 2012; Mohapatra *et al.*, 2020).

1.3.2. Cell Culture System

Various cell culture systems, including mammalian cell-lines, insects and yeast cells are used especially for the production of recombinant vaccines. Each of these systems has its advantages and challenges based on the specific vaccine type, thus influencing the choice of the bioprocess scale-up system (Soler and Houdebine, 2007).

1.3.3. Microbial Fermentation

Microbial fermentation is a foundational process in vaccine manufacturing, particularly for vaccines in recombinant bacterial or yeast systems to produce antigens or recombinant proteins. In this method, microbes like *Escherichia coli* or *Saccharomyces cerevisiae* are genetically engineered to express target antigens, which are then mass-cultured, harvested and purified for vaccine formulation. The mass-culturing is typically undertaken in bioreactor, where growth conditions like temperature, pH, oxygen levels, and nutrient supply are precisely and optimally controlled to control microbial metabolism and protein expression. Microbial fermentation offers several advantages, including rapid growth rates, scalability, and cost-effectiveness, but it also presents challenges like managing endotoxin contamination and ensuring protein folding accuracy. These factors must be carefully managed to produce safe and effective vaccines. To mass-produce certain vaccines, microbial fermentation using bacteria or yeasts could be employed as an effective strategy. This method is often used to produce subunit vaccines and recombinant proteins (Cid and Bolívar, 2021).

1.3.4. Single-use Technologies

The adoption of single-use systems in bioprocessing has gained popularity owing to their flexibility, no need of sterilisation between batches (thus reducing the duration of a process cycle), reduced risk of cross-contamination, and lower initial capital investments such as the direct and indirect fixed capitals (Pollard and Pralong, 2018). Further, single-use system reduces the setting up duration, enhances production efficiency and supports faster scale-up, thereby making them highly attractive especially for bioindustries dealing with rapid vaccine manufacturing and deployment. Owing to their innumerable process advantages, adopting single-use (use-n-throw type) technological approaches in bioprocessing has significantly increased in recent years, particularly in vaccine production. These systems utilise disposable components like the bioreactor (in form of, say, bags), filters, tubing, and connectors which are used for a single batch and then discarded. Innovative approaches are being tried to recycle as many of the non-contact materials as possible for environmental reasons though. Such systems have reduced upfront capital need as compared to the conventional systems as they reduce the need for costly infrastructure associated with cleaning (CIP), (*in situ*) sterilisation, and process validation and verification. A reduced direct and indirect fixed capital cost requirements makes them particularly suitable for small- and medium-scale production set-up. These technologies are therefore especially advantageous for production at the small- and medium-scales.

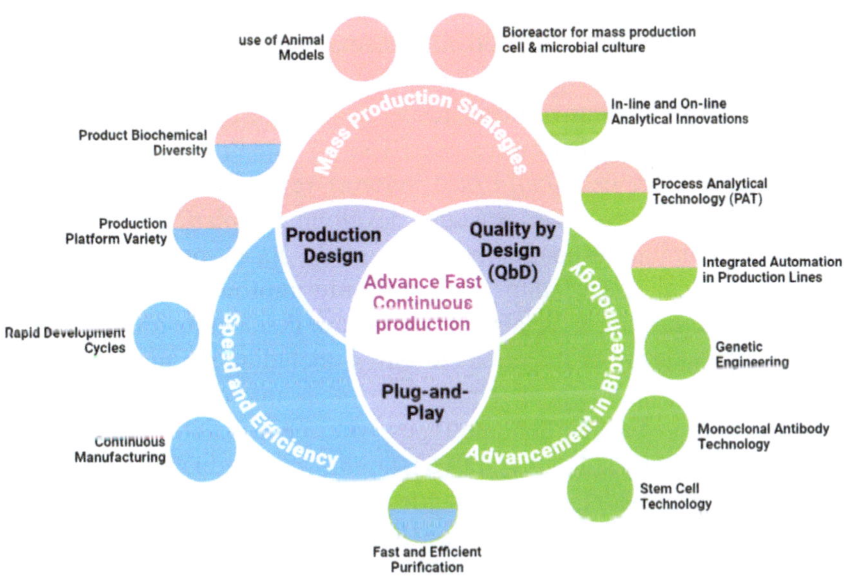

Fig. 1: The prospects of advanced process-optimised vaccine manufacturing strategies

1.3.5. Downstream Processing

Also termed as bioseparation engineering, this post-harvest step involves techniques like chromatography, ultrafiltration and centrifugation that are employed to purify and concentrate the desired vaccine product and purify it before the final formulation preparation. Meticulous planning of these series of steps are crucial to reduce the yield loss and streamlining the skill-set requirements while ensuring the purity and potency of the final product (Wolf and Reichl, 2011).

Although there are numerous challenges in the journey from designing of the vaccine to its large-scale production, a standardised and validated bioprocess strategy could mitigate many of these risks. By leveraging a combination of advanced bioprocess techniques, including animal models and various cell culture systems, the biopharmaceutical industries could enhance their capacity to mass produce vaccines more efficiently and safely (Buckland *et al.*, 2024). Continuous innovation and adherence to stringent regulatory standards are paramount for the successful development and scale-up of vaccines, ultimately ensuring global health and safety.

2. Biotechnology Advancements and Vaccinology

The field of biotechnology has witnessed transformative advancements over the past few decades, which has also significantly impacted vaccine development strategies. Cutting-edge research advances in genetic engineering, monoclonal antibody technology and applications of stem cells lead the vaccinology revolution from the front. These advancements have not only enhanced the effectiveness and specificity of vaccines but also have opened new vistas for therapeutic and preventive measures against numerous deadly infectious and contagious diseases that were otherwise threatening the human race. Also, integrated stem cell (cell-based system) research has expanded the possibilities to innovate novel vaccine development platforms that could mimic human immune responses more accurately during preclinical testing. These technological interventions have not only improved the efficacy and precision of vaccines but have also expanded the therapeutic and preventive options against an array of infectious diseases, including the many that were hitherto considered untreatable. Unlike the other microbial pathogens, all the viral forms are of seven genome-types. These are double-stranded DNA (dsDNA), single-stranded DNA (ssDNA), double-stranded DNA with reverse transcriptase (dsDNA-RT), single-stranded RNA with reverse transcriptase (ssRNA-RT), double-stranded RNA (dsRNA), positive sense single-stranded RNA, and negative sense single-stranded RNA. Table 1 outlines the key vaccines developed successfully during the past century, with a variety of host organisms and production strategies, from the traditional viral cultivation in cell-lines to the advanced recombinant DNA and mRNA technologies.

Table 1. A list of some path-breaking advancement in vaccine technology in a century

Vaccine	**Host**	**Production strategy**	**Source**
Smallpox	Cow	Virus grown in vero cells	Smith, 2011
Polio	Monkey kidney cell	Mass-scale growth in vero cells	Salk and Health, 1956
Influenza	Chicken egg	Vaccine developed by inoculating the virus in fertilised chicken egg	Kilbourne, 1973
Measles	chicken embryo	Both forms of Measles virus, formalin-inactivated and attenuated (live virus grown in embryonated chicken egg and fibroblasts until attaining acceptable level of attenuation)	Hedley-Whyte and Milamed, 2021
Hepatitis B	Yeast (*P. pastoris, S. cerevisiae*)	rDNA technology; Hepatitis B surface antigen (HBsAg) encoding gene inserted into yeast	Hilleman, 1987
HPV	Insect cell system (for Baculovirus)	Baculovirus-infected insect cells expressing L1 (HPV capsid) protein	McLemore, 2006
Rotavirus	Vero cells	Virus grown in vero cells in bioreactors	Ruiz-Palacios *et al.*, 2006
Zika	Vero cells	Cloning the pathogen antigen using DNA plasmid to generate DNA vaccines	Poland *et al.*, 2018
COVID-19 mRNA vaccine	Cell-free	mRNA synthesised via *in vitro* transcription (IVT); lipid nanoparticle formulated	Salian *et al.*, 2021
Dengue	Vero cells	Multivalent (four) chimeric vaccine from CYD-1, -2, -3 and -4 viruses, using vero cells	Thomas *et al.*, 2019
COVID-19 (viral vector)	Human cell-line (HEK293)	Adenovirus grown on HEK293 cells; gene encoding SARS-CoV-2 spike protein inserted	Cross *et al.*, 2021
Malaria (RTS,S)	Circumsporozoite protein (CSP) antigen	Recombinant protein (fused circumsporozoite and hepatitis B surface antigen proteins); produced in yeast	Nadeem *et al.*, 2022

Through the state-of-art innovative techniques like mRNA technology, viral vector platforms and nanoparticles-based delivery systems, molecular biotechnology and associated advancements have paved the way for the development of next-generation vaccines that were capable to combat multiple viral strains, including the rapidly mutating pathogens. Such advancements have also laid the platform for the new-generation vaccines that could effectively counter not only the target pathogen and its strains but also its numerous emerging and reemerging deadly variant lineages (as the virus mutates and evolves with time).

2.1. Genetic Engineering and Vaccine Development

Genetic engineering has significantly transformed vaccine development, particularly through the application of recombinant DNA technology (RDTech). A major advancement in recent years is the emergence of mRNA platforms to design and develop vaccines, such as the ones developed by Pfizer-BioNTech (BNT162b2) and Moderna (mRNA-1273) (Al Fayez *et al.*, 2023). These vaccines worked by delivering the messenger RNA (mRNA) that had the code for the viral antigen into the host cells, where it instructed the cellular machinery to produce the specified viral antigen protein that elicited the desired immune response. These vaccines were developed against the viral pathogen SARS-CoV-2 that was responsible for the infamous COVID-19 pandemic (Wang *et al.*, 2020).

mRNA vaccines have several advantages over traditional vaccine approaches. Some of the most encouraging factors are, these could be developed more quickly (a very critical benefit especially during a pandemic) and do not require the use of live or attenuated pathogens, thereby enhancing the safety feature of the vaccine.. Additionally, mRNA vaccines are highly adaptable, allowing for rapid updates to combat new viral variants, making them a versatile and potent tool in managing infectious diseases (Sahin *et al.*, 2014).

2.2. Monoclonal Antibody Technology

Monoclonal antibody (mAb) technology has emerged as a powerful tool in both therapeutic and prophylactic applications, transforming the landscape of vaccine development and infectious disease management. First developed in 1975 by Köhler and Milstein, monoclonal antibodies are highly specific proteins engineered to recognise and bind to a single antigenic epitope. This precise targeting makes them invaluable for pathogen neutralisation, enhancing immune responses, and offering passive immunity in cases where traditional vaccines are ineffective or slow to act. mAbs production begins with the fusion of antibody-producing B-cells with immortal myeloma cells to form hybridomas, which can be cultured indefinitely to produce a continuous supply of uniform antibodies. Recent advancements in recombinant DNA technology have enabled the development of fully human or humanised mAbs, reducing the risk of immunogenicity and adverse reactions in the subjects. Monoclonal antibodies (mAbs) are synthetic molecules engineered to replicate the immune system's natural ability to combat harmful pathogens. This technology facilitates the creation of highly specific and potent agents for vaccination (prophylactics) and medicines (therapeutics). Monoclonal antibodies (mAbs) could be tailored to bind selectively to specific antigens on a pathogen, offering a targeted and and effective defense system in the body. They have proven to be successful interventions in treating various infectious diseases, and are increasingly being investigated as an integral approach in vaccine development strategies. For instance, monoclonal antibodies (mAbs) have been employed in passive immunisation to provide expeditious protection against dreaded infectious diseases like Ebola and COVID-19 (Pavia and Wormser, 2021).

2.3. Reliance on the Live-Attenuated, Weakened and Toxoid Vaccines

Historically, live-attenuated, weakened and toxoid forms of vaccines were fundamental in combating infectious diseases. Live-attenuated vaccines contain weakened form of pathogen, designed to closely mimic natural infections, thereby eliciting robust and long-lasting immune responses. Notable examples include the measles, mumps and rubella (MMR) vaccine and the oral polio vaccine (OPV), both of which have played critical roles in the near-eradication of the corresponding diseases. Weakened pathogen forms are altered so they cannot manifest the disease in a healthy individual, but could still effectively stimulate the immune system. On the other hand, toxoid vaccines are based on inactivated toxins produced by certain bacteria, like *Corynebacterium diphtheriae* (causing diphtheria) and *Clostridium tetani* (causing tetanus), which are chemically altered to render them harmless while maintaining their ability to induce immunity. However, these conventional methods are often time-consuming, expensive, low in the quality assurance and need to be administered a number of times to generate the adequate level of sustained immunity in the body. Such conventional approaches to develop live-attenuated, weakened and toxoid vaccines have been successful against the frequently-occurring diseases that are considered 'simple' (with the minimal antigen variability to combat against) not meant to act against a substantially diverse antigens that might evade or misdirect the host immune response.

Live attenuated vaccines are developed by reducing the pathogenicity of a target pathogen, without compromising its viability. While they are less virulent than the normal and natural live counterpart, these are capable of generating an immune response upon being administered to a recipient. The immune response kind of mimics the protective immunity in the people who had survived an infection or have never been infected. These vaccines are highly effective and elicit a strong cellular and humoral response (Yadav *et al.*, 2020).

Inactivated or weakened vaccines consist of bacterins of one or several bacterial (microbial) species or killed viral strains. They are usually stable and are inexpensive at the production level. The killed versions of a target pathogen are obtained through numerous physical and/or chemical treatments that could damage the protein or the DNA. The inactivated antigen may be mixed with an adjuvant to increase its efficacy (Kallerup and Foged, 2014).

Toxoid is one of the best traditional vaccination strategies at the moment classified among the numerous conventional strategies. Such vaccines contain the inactivated native toxins (toxoids) along with adjuvants that prove to be efficient as compared to many other vaccine forms. However, there are certain limitations on the basis of their biosafety that could be overcome through recombinant toxoid vaccines, wherein they are produced in large quantities with low reactogenicity and toxicity (Kallerup and Foged, 2014).

2.4. Stem Cells as a Potential Therapeutics and Preventives Option

Using stem cells in biotechnology represents significant potential for advancing both therapeutics and preventive formulation strategies against numerous existing and emerging infectious diseases (Sarangi *et al.*, 2024). Stem cells possess the remarkable ability to differentiate into a wide range of cell types, making them a valuable resource in regenerative medicine. Emerging research indicates that stem cells may also contribute to the development of novel vaccines and treatments (personalised medicine).

Stem cells can be genetically modified to enhance the generation of immune cells or molecules that bolster body's capacity to combat an infection. Additionally, these could be utilised to create *in vitro* models of human tissues, enabling more precise testing of vaccines and therapeutic agents. Moreover, stem cell therapy offers the potential to repair and regenerate tissues that are damaged due to severe infections, providing a comprehensive approach to address both preventive and therapeutic interventions (Marcuzzi and Maximova, 2023).

3. Mass Production Strategies

Efficient and scalable production strategies are essential to meet the growing global demand for vaccines, both in quantity and range. Advances in cell culture technologies, bioreactor systems, and the strategic use of animal models have significantly transformed the vaccine manufacturing approaches, enhancing both consistency and quality. The latest strategies employed in large-scale vaccine production, Highlighting recent research and technological innovations are detailed below.

3.1. Cell Culture System

Cell culture system is fundamental to contemporary vaccine production. Mammalian, insect, and yeast cells are utilised in large-scale vaccine manufacturing processes that also ensure consistency, scalability, and stringent quality assurance (Soler and Houdebine, 2007). Mammalian cell lines of Chinese Hamster Ovary (CHO) are extensively used due to their abilities to produce complex proteins with accurate post-translational modifications, which are essential for the efficacy of numerous vaccines (Tihanyi and Nyitray, 2020). Insect cell lines like those derived from *Spodoptera frugiperda* (Sf9) are also useful especially to produce recombinant proteins and virus-like particles (VLPs) (Liu *et al.*, 2013). Yeast cells like *Saccharomyces cerevisiae* provide another reliable platform for vaccine production (Kumar and Kumar, 2019). The advantages of such platform are the rapid biomass growth of *S. cerevisiae*, and their easy genetic modification.

Recent technological advancements have further opened up windows to optimise these cell culture systems. Innovations like CRISPR/Cas9-mediated genome editing have improved cell line engineering, resulting in higher yields and enhanced product quality (Tavakoli *et al.*, 2021). Additionally, the integration of single-use bioreactors and perfusion systems into the cell culture processes have enabled continuous and scalable production while minimising the cross-contamination risk (Takao *et al.*, 2023; Pollard and Pralong, 2018).

3.2. Bioreactors

Bioreactors are crucial for scaling-up vaccine production from laboratory settings to the industrial-scale manufacturing. Modern bioreactors provide controlled environments with optimised cell culture growth and productivity parameters. These systems extend the facility to meticulously regulate some key parameters like temperature, pH, dissolved oxygen and the nutrient supply, which are essentially to ensure consistency and high-quality vaccine as the output.

Recent advances have led to the development of sophisticated bioreactor designs, like the single-use bioreactors (SUBs) and microcarrier-based systems (Szczypka *et al.*, 2014). SUBs have transformed vaccine bioprocessing by offering greater flexibility, cost-efficiency and ease of operation as compared to the conventional stainless-steel reusable bioreactors. Constructed from biocompatible plastics, pre-sterilised SUBs reduce the contamination risks and eliminate the need to clean and sterilize after every batch, thereby significantly reducing the operational costs and the downtime. From small laboratory units to large-scale production systems, the scalability of SUBs ensures seamless transitions from research to commercial manufacturing. Although concerns about plastic waste exist, majority of them as attachments could be recycled especially the ones that were not in direct contact with the production process. With advancements in recycling technologies helping to mitigate these concerns, SUBs may have environmental benefits through reduced wastage of water, used chemicals, and reagents.

Ongoing research in bioprocess operations has focused on improving sensor integration for real-time monitoring of critical parameters, enhancing mixing and oxygen transfer rates, and ensuring material compatibility through studies on leachables and extractables. Automated and integrated systems have further streamlined the bioprocess workflow, enhancing the scope of reproducibility and scalability (Busse *et al.*, 2017). However, challenges such as the lack of standardisation, capacity limitations, waste management and regulatory compliance remain. Efforts are being made to address these issues through industry-wide standardisation, advancements in biodegradable materials, and continuous collaborations between industry stakeholders and regulatory bodies. With continued innovation and collaboration, single-use bioreactors are expected to play a pivotal role in meeting the global vaccine demand in a shorter span.

Additionally, microcarrier-based systems have improved the cell growth and productivity by offering an expanded surface area for cell attachment and proliferation within a bioreactor system (Lembong *et al.*, 2020). The integration of process analytical technology (PAT) and real-time monitoring tools has further enabled the control and optimisation of the bioreactor conditions precisely (Gerzon *et al.*, 2022). These technologies facilitate the early detection of deviations and allow for immediate corrective actions, ensuring the consistency in product quality and reducing the likelihood of batch failures.

3.3. Novel Approaches in Bioseparation Engineering

Advancements in downstream processing of chimeric vaccines have been driven by the integration of innovative technologies aimed at improved product recovery and cost rationalisation. Traditional chromatographic methods like affinity chromatography, ion-exchange chromatography, gel permeation chromatography, size-exclusion chromatography, etc. continue to be the fundamentals in the downstream purification strategies. Affinity chromatography utilises the characteristic property of interaction specificity of the vaccine with ligands to achieve high selectivity and yield. Ion-exchange chromatography separates proteins based on their charge properties, while gel permeation chromatography and size-exclusion chromatography separate molecules by size, contributing as essential tools to refine the high-purity of the vaccine.

Emerging technologies are reshaping the downstream processing (bioseparation engineering) strategies. Aqueous two-phase extraction has shown potential due to its simplicity, scalability, and the ability to maintain protein integrity, making it a promising alternative during the initial vaccine recovery stages (Iqbal *et al.*, 2016). Additionally, design of experiments (DoE) methodologies enhance the optimization of the purification protocols by systematically analysing multiple factors and their dependency and interdependency, leading to more robust and reproducible results. Integrated downstream processing is another innovative approach that integrates the production process with the purification steps into a unified workflow, thus reducing the production cost, increasing the throughput, and improving the process efficiency (Mandenius and Brundin, 2008).

Recent research underscores the effectiveness of these advanced technologies in purifying chimeric vaccines, demonstrating their capacity to revolutionise vaccine bioprocessing. The strategic application of these techniques is crucial in achieving a scalable and cost-effective production process of high-purity chimeric vaccines, ultimately enhancing the community health outcomes.

3.4. Animal Models

Animal models, particularly laboratory animals, are essential in the vaccine development and production pipeline, as also the clinical trials. They are extensively utilised in preclinical testing to assess the safety, efficacy and immunogenicity of the vaccine candidates preceding the human clinical trials. The laboratory animals that are usually employed include the mice, rats, rabbits and non-human primates, each offering distinct advantages for the development of different vaccine types (Kiros *et al.*, 2012).

Due to their well-characterised immune systems and the availability of various genetically modified strains, mice are the most frequently employed animal models. Non-human primates are selected for their close immunological and physiological similarities with humans, making them crucial in evaluating the efficacy of vaccines that are especially intended for human administration.

Additionally, animal models are integral to pilot production runs, enabling the optimisation of the production processes and identification of potential issues to address before large-scale manufacturing (Mukherjee *et al.*, 2022).

Thus, evolution of mass production strategies for vaccines has been marked by the adoption of advanced cell culture systems, modern bioreactors and an extensive use of animal models. These innovations ensure high-quality, consistent and easily scalable production systems that meet the increasing global demand for vaccines in a time-bound (for emergency situations) and decentralised manner (for equitable distribution and timely availability). As research and technology progress further, the biopharmaceutical industries shall be better equipped to address even the emerging infectious diseases through robust and scalable vaccine production strategies.

4. Production Design

An effective designing of the production process is fundamental to successful vaccine manufacturing. Ideally, it considers the kind of the production platform employed and the biochemical diversity of the final vaccine product. Modern advancements in science and technology have facilitated the introduction of innovative approaches in vaccinology, like genetic engineering, bioreactor design and cell-free systems. These all have enhanced the efficiency, scalability and versatility of large-scale vaccine manufacturing (Garenne *et al.*, 2021; Sharma *et al.*, 2022). These advancements not only ensure the consistent production of high-quality vaccines but also enable expeditious response against the emerging infectious diseases. The sub-sections below discuss the biochemical diversity of vaccine products and the variety of production platforms, focusing objectively on the novel techniques, recent developments and emerging strategies in the sector.

4.1. Biochemical Diversity of Vaccines

Characterising the biochemical diversity of the final product (vaccines) is essential to ensure their broad immunogenicity and address the various target pathogenic forms (Zhang *et al.*, 2015). Biochemical diversity of vaccines is reflected by an array of biological components and molecular mechanisms employed to stimulate protective immune responses. Traditionally, vaccines were based on whole pathogens, either inactivated or attenuated, to mimic natural infections. However, advancements in immunology and biotechnology have led to the development of more refined vaccine types, including subunit, conjugate, DNA, mRNA, and viral vector vaccines. Each of these platforms represents a distinct biochemical approach. Subunit vaccines, for instance, use specific proteins or polysaccharides from a pathogen to provoke an immune response without introducing the whole organism. Conjugate vaccines, on the other hand, chemically link polysaccharides to proteins to enhance immunogenicity, particularly in cases where the antigen alone is weakly immunogenic, as seen in *Haemophilus influenzae* type B (Hib) vaccines. DNA and mRNA vaccines, recent innovations, employ nucleic acids to direct host cells to produce the target antigen, triggering both humoral and cellular immune responses. Viral vector vaccines utilise engineered viruses to deliver the genetic material of the antigen, offering a platform that combines strong immunogenicity with flexibility in design. This biochemical diversity allows for tailoring vaccines to specific pathogens and clinical needs, enhancing efficacy and safety. The diverse vaccine composition contributes to varied storage, handling and production requirements, influencing how these vaccines are implemented globally. Understanding this biochemical complexity is the key to advancing vaccine design, addressing challenges such as antigenic variability, and combating emerging infectious diseases. The vaccine types range from the traditional inactivated and live-attenuated vaccines to the more advanced recombinant protein subunit, conjugate, viral vector and nucleic acid (mRNA and DNA) vaccines. Each of these vaccine types has distinct biochemical properties and thus the production requirements.

4.1.1. Recombinant Protein Subunit Vaccine

Recombinant protein subunit vaccines represent a sophisticated immunisation approach using only specific proteins or antigens from a pathogen rather than the whole organism. These vaccines are produced using recombinant DNA technology, where the gene encoding a pathogen's antigen (like the viral surface protein) is inserted into a host cell (often yeast, bacteria or mammalian cells) to produce large quantities of the target protein. Once harvested and purified, these proteins are formulated into vaccines. Such vaccines utilise a target pathogenic antigen, like a protein, to elicit the desired immune response in the body of the recipient. Advancements in genetic engineering have enabled the production of highly purified and effective recombinant proteins. Techniques like codon optimisation and glycoengineering have facilitated the enhancement of protein expression and functionality, ensuring higher immunogenicity and stability in vaccine performance (Cid and Bolívar, 2021).

Unlike live-attenuated or inactivated vaccines, recombinant subunit vaccines are non-replicating and do not pose a risk of causing the disease, making them safer for especially the immunocompromised individuals. Examples include the hepatitis B vaccine and the more recent recombinant protein based COVID-19 vaccines. One of the key advantages of this approach is the ability to focus the immune response on specific antigens known to induce protective immunity, thereby minimising potential side-effects and increasing the safety. However, because recombinant protein subunit vaccines typically do not provoke a strong immune response on their own, they often require the use of adjuvants to boost immunogenicity. While the vaccines are highly effective, production of these could be complex requiring rigorous purification steps to ensure purity and consistency. Their development represents a critical advancement in vaccine technology, particularly for pathogens with complex structures or high mutation rates.

4.1.2. Conjugate Vaccine

Conjugate vaccines are a specialised subunit vaccines designed to enhance immune response towards the antigens. These are weakly immunogenic on their own, particularly the polysaccharides on the bacterial surface. In these vaccines, polysaccharides from the bacterial capsule are chemically linked or conjugated to a carrier protein, which is typically a strong immunogen (like the tetanus or diphtheria toxoids). These vaccines represent polysaccharide antigens linked to the carrier proteins, thereby improving their immunogenicity (Pichichero, 2013). Modern conjugation techniques like site-specific conjugation and click chemistry offer precise control over the conjugation process, resulting in more consistent and effective vaccine products.

4.1.3. Viral Vector Vaccine

Viral vector vaccines represent a novel and highly effective approach to immunisation by harnessing modified viruses to deliver genetic material that encodes antigens from a target pathogen. In this technology, a benign or attenuated virus is genetically engineered to carry and express a gene encoding a specific antigen from the target pathogen (such as a protein from a virus or bacterium). Once administered, the viral vector infects the host cell, which then produces the target antigen and triggers an immune response. This approach mimics a natural infection and stimulates both humoral and cellular immune responses. The viral vectors, like adenoviruses and lentiviruses are used to deliver the genetic material that encodes the antigen. Innovations in vector design including the use of non-replicating and tissue-specific vectors enhance the safety and efficacy of the vaccines. The use of viral vectors has been pivotal in the rapid evolution in vaccine development techniques, such as the COVID-19 vaccines of AstraZeneca and Johnson & Johnson (Deng *et al.*, 2022). The use of viral vectors allows to induce a strong and comprehensive immune response with a single dose that could be adopted for a wide range of pathogens.

4.1.4. Nucleic Acid Vaccine (mRNA and DNA)

Such types of vaccines utilise genetic materials to instruct the host cell to produce the antigen *in vivo*. Recent advancements in delivery systems like the lipid nanoparticles (LNPs) and designed plasmid have significantly improved the delivery efficiency of mRNA and DNA vaccines and their stability (Hajiaghapour Asr *et al.*, 2023). The success of mRNA vaccines like those of Pfizer-BioNTech and Moderna highlights the potential of this platform for rapid and scalable vaccine development.

4.2. The Range of Production Platforms

An array of vaccine development platforms is crucial to accommodate the varying biochemical characteristics of vaccines and forge an optimised production process. Modern techniques and platforms have enhanced the scalability, flexibility and the efficiency of production of an array of vaccines.

4.2.1. Microbial Production System

Bacteria and yeasts are commonly employed for the production of recombinant proteins and subunit vaccines. Bioprocess operations like the fed-batch and continuous culture improve the yield and consistency in production. For instance, the use of *Pichia pastoris* (a methylotrophic yeast) has been optimised for high-level protein expression, making it a popular choice (Karbalaei *et al.*, 2020).

4.2.2. Mammalian Cell Culture System

Mammalian cells, like CHO and HEK293 cells, are used for the production of complex proteins and viral vector vaccines (Tan *et al.*, 2021[a]). Advances in perfusion and single-use bioreactors technologies have streamlined the scaling up processes of these systems, reduced the contamination risks and the production costs, thereby rationalising the economics.

4.2.3. Insect Cell Culture Systems

Insect cells like Sf9 and Sf21 are used in the baculovirus expression vector system (BEVS) to produce recombinant proteins and VLPs. The baculovirus expression vector (BEV) platform offers rapid and high-yield protein production, which is particularly useful in case of vaccines that require complex post-translational modifications (Liu *et al.*, 2013).

4.2.4. Plant-based Production System

Plants can be genetically engineered to produce vaccine antigens. This platform offers several advantages, including low production costs and scalability. Techniques like transient expression and stable transformation have been optimised to enhance the protein yield and quality in plant systems (Lee and Ko, 2017).

4.2.5. Cell-free Expression System

These systems use cell extracts to produce proteins without living cells, offering rapid and scalable production (Garenne *et al.*, 2021). Recent advancements in cell-free systems include the use of modular and customisable reaction conditions, which allow for the efficient production of an array of proteins, including the vaccine antigens.

5. Quality by Design (QbD) Approach for Continuous Bioprocessing

The quality by design (QbD) approach has been the cornerstone in modern biopharmaceutical manufacturing, including vaccine production (Pramod *et al.*, 2016). In the context of continuous bioprocessing, QbD involves a systematic framework for identifying and controlling the critical quality attributes (CQAs) of a biopharmaceutical product, as well as the critical process parameters (CPPs) that influence these attributes. This approach relies on a thorough understanding of the process, including its variability and interactions, to ensure that the final product consistently meets predefined quality standards. QbD emphasises on understanding the processes and devising workable control mechanisms to ensure consistency in the product quality. By implementing QbD principles, manufacturers can enhance process robustness, reduce variability and improve the overall product quality. In continuous bioprocessing, QbD is complemented with the process analytical technology (PAT) and Advanced Analytical Innovations (Fig. 2). These facilitate real-time monitoring and control that would ensure enhanced consistency, efficiency and quality of the produced vaccine.

5.1. Process Analytical Technology (PAT)

Process Analytical Technology (PAT) is a framework developed by the USFDA to design (FDA, 2004), analyse and control pharmaceutical manufacturing processes through the real-time monitoring. PAT tools enable the continuous assessment of Critical Quality Attributes (CQAs) and Critical Process Parameters (CPPs) to ensure that the final product meets the predefined quality standards (Bondi Jr and Drennen III 2011).

5.1.1. Real-time Monitoring and Control

Real-time monitoring and control of the bioprocessing operation involves continuous data collection and analysis. Sensors and analytical instruments are integrated into the production line to measure the critical parameters like pH, temperature, dissolved oxygen, and the concentrations of critical metabolites. This real-time data acquisition allows for immediate adjustments in line with in-process quality assurance, ensuring that optimal operational conditions are maintained throughout the production process.

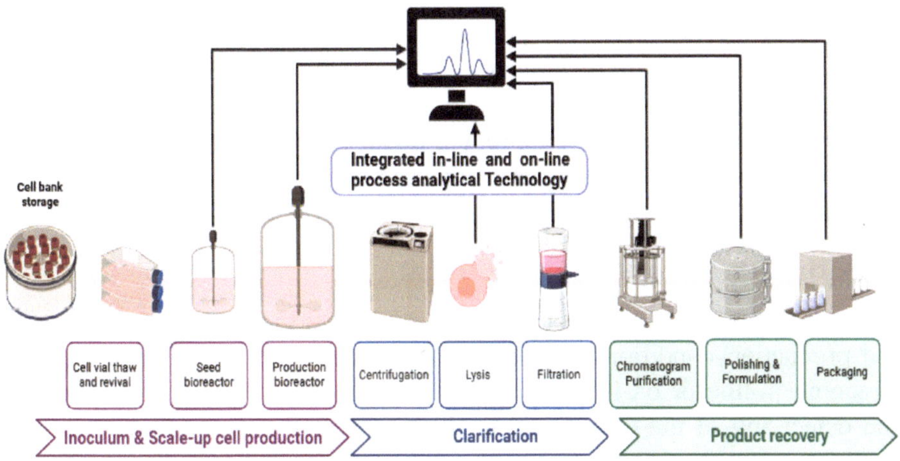

Fig. 2: The quality by design (QbD) approach in vaccine bioprocessing

5.1.2. Improving Consistency and Quality

By continuously monitoring the critical parameters, PAT reduces variability and enhances the consistency of vaccine production. For instance, near-infrared (NIR) spectroscopy and Raman spectroscopy are used to monitor the cell culture conditions and the product quality (Zhang *et al.*, 2015). These techniques provide real-time insights into the bioprocess operation, enabling proactive adjustments by monitoring and controlling the undesirable deviations and prevent any form of quality-compromise, thereby ensuring consistent product quality.

5.2. In-line and on-line Analytical Innovations

In-line and on-line integrated analytical techniques are integral components of the QbD approach, particularly in continuous bioprocessing (Gerzon *et al.*, 2022). Such techniques involve the direct integration of analytical instruments into the production process that facilitate real-time data acquisition and data analysis without interrupting the workflow.

5.2.1. Mass Spectrometry (MS)

Mass spectrometry is used for a detailed characterisation of vaccine components, including protein identification and quantification. In a continuous bioprocess operation, MS can be employed in-line to monitor the quality and purity of the intermediate and final products. This reduces the need for any sort of offline sample analysis and thereby accelerates the production process (Liu and Schulz, 2021).

5.2.2. Capillary Electrophoresis (CE)

Capillary electrophoresis is a powerful technique for the analysis of the purity and heterogeneity of biopharmaceuticals (van der Burg *et al.*, 2023). Integrating capillary electrophoresis on-line in the production process allows for real-time monitoring of the product quality, ensuring that impurities are detected in time and the issues are addressed immediately. This enhances the efficiency and reliability of vaccine production.

5.2.3. High-throughput Screening (HTS)

High-throughput screening methods are used for rapid screening of cell cultures and production conditions (Ayon, 2023). By incorporating high-throughput screening in-line or on-line, the manufacturers could expeditiously identify and detect any of the operational deviations from the desired process. This accelerates process development and ensures consistent production quality.

5.3. Integrated Automation in Production Lines

The integration of automation in production lines significantly reduces human error and increases efficiency. Automated systems control various aspects of a production process, from raw material handling to final product packaging, ensuring precision and consistency.

5.3.1. Reduced Human Errors

Automation minimises manual interventions, which are often sources of variability and error. Automated sampling, data acquisition and process adjustments enhance the reliability and reproducibility of vaccine production. For instance, automated bioreactors with integrated PAT tools could adjust culture conditions based on real-time data, ensuring optimal growth and productivity (Gerzon *et al.*, 2022).

5.3.2. Increasing Efficiency and Quality

Automation streamlines the production process, reduces the downtime and increases the throughput. Integrated systems can perform complex analyses and adjustments rapidly, maintaining continuous production without compromising the quality. This is particularly important in vaccine manufacturing, where demand can fluctuate significantly, and rapid scaling may often be required.

Supported by PAT and in-line/on-line analytical innovations, QbD approach has transformed continuous bioprocessing in vaccine production (Gerzon *et al.*, 2022). These technologies enable real-time monitoring and control, reducing variability, and enhancing product consistency and quality. By integrating automation, the production process could become more efficient and less prone to errors owing to human interventions, thus ensuring the supply of high-quality reliable vaccines.

6. Speed and Efficiency

The urgency of vaccine development and production, especially in response to global health emergencies, necessitates innovative approaches to enhance speed and efficiency. Advances in synthetic biology, computational modeling, continuous manufacturing and plug-and-play platforms have significantly accelerated vaccine development cycles, increased production yields, and rationalised the production costs. This segment of the chapter explores these advancements and their impact on vaccine production speed and efficacy.

6.1. Rapid Development Cycles

The swift development of vaccines within a short duration especially during human health emergency situations in response to the numerous emerging and reemerging infectious diseases is crucial. Synthetic biology and computational modeling have emerged as the two quite powerful tools in accelerating designing and testing phases during the development of vaccines.

6.1.1. Synthetic Biology

Synthetic biology enables the precise engineering of biological systems to create novel vaccines. Some of the cutting-edge techniques like gene synthesis, DNA assembly, and CRISPR/Cas9 genome editing allow for the rapid construction of vaccine candidates and optimisation of the process. By designing and synthesising genetic sequences *de novo*, researchers could expeditiously generate antigens and other vaccine components, significantly reducing the required time for the development in the initial phases (Kitney *et al.*, 2021).

6.1.2. Computational Modeling

Computational modeling techniques like *in silico* simulations and bioinformatics facilitate the process to rapidly identify a potential vaccine candidate and optimise and standardise the operation. These models could predict the structure and function of antigens, simulate immune responses and optimise the formulation of vaccines. Computational tools like multi-graft and multivalent scaffolding, codon optimisation and antibodyomics could be employed to identify and design the vaccine candidate *in silico*. It also enables to virtually screen large libraries of vaccine candidates and identify the most promising ones that could be further tested for confirmation (Sunita *et al.*, 2020). This approach accelerates the preclinical phase, thereby allowing for quicker transition to clinical trials.

6.2. Continuous Manufacturing

The transition from traditional batch processes to the continuous manufacturing operations has revolutionised the mass production of vaccines, ensuring higher yields and reducing the production time and costs significantly.

6.2.1. Higher Yield and Efficiency

A batch process operation typically requires a downtime between cycles for cleaning and setup (collectively termed as upstream activities). On the contrary, a continuous manufacturing process operates uninterrupted thus doing away with the time-lag between the production batches. Due to this, a continuous mode of operation maximises the temporal production capacity, ultimately leading to higher yields within a specified time period. Moreover, a continuous process could be more easily scaled up or scaled down to meet the fluctuating demand, thus enhancing the flexibility of vaccine production and responsiveness to the demand (Rathore *et al.*, 2015).

6.2.2. Reduced Production Time and Costs

Continuous manufacturing streamlines production the workflow, reducing the required duration to complete each batch of vaccine production. This could also efficiently translate into cost savings as fewer resources are needed for the maintenance and process validation. Further, a continuous process enables real-time process monitoring and control, which ensures the desired consistency in product quality and the reduced risk of 'batch' failures. The reduced need for the intermediate storage and handling of the final vaccine product also cuts down the overall production and logistics costs.

6.3. Plug-and-Play Platform

Establishing a plug-and-play platform for vaccine production by providing a standardised approach for purification and other critical processes could further enhance the speed and efficiency.

6.3.1. Fast and Efficient Purification

Plug-and-play platforms involve the use of the pre-validated modular components that could be easily integrated into the production process. These platforms standardise the purification steps including filtration and chromatography, ensuring consistent and efficient removal of the undesired artefact (impurities). The pre-validated modules reduce the need for an extensive process development and validation, thus curtailing the timeline and accelerating the production.

6.3.2. Scalability and Flexibility

Plug-and-play platforms are designed especially for scalability and flexibility which allows the manufacturers to adapt to different vaccine types and the production scales quickly. This approach is particularly beneficial in responding to sudden outbreaks as in case of the COVID-19 scenario, as it enables rapid switching between the different vaccine production processes with a bare minimum revalidation. The modular nature of plug-and-play systems also facilitates easy upgrading and integration of the novel technologies that emerge from time to time (Hong *et al.*, 2018).

Thus, the speed and efficiency of vaccine development and production could significantly be enhanced through the integration of synthetic biology, computational modeling, continuous manufacturing and plug-and-play platforms. Such integration of the advanced techniques and technologies would be able to reduce the development cycles, increase the yield and reduce the production costs, thereby ensuring a more rapid and effective response against the emerging and reemerging infectious diseases in due course. As these technologies continue to evolve, they hold the potential to further streamline vaccine manufacturing protocols, and ultimately help improve the global healthcare outcomes.

7. Personalised Vaccines

The emergence of mRNA and DNA vaccine technologies has transformed personalised medicine (both therapeutics and preventives), enabling the creation of vaccines customised to the genetic make-up of an individual. This innovation holds significant promise in the realm of cancer immunotherapy especially where vaccines can be tailored to target specific tumour antigens that are unique to each patient. This section of the chapter delves into the development and use of personalised vaccines adopting the molecular (mRNA and DNA) techniques, with a focus on their application particularly in treating cancers (Wang *et al.*, 2023; Leitner *et al.*, 1999).

7.1. mRNA and DNA Vaccines

mRNA and DNA vaccines represent a novel class of vaccines that utilise the genetic information of both the pathogen and the host to instruct the host cells to produce the desired immunogenic antigens. These antigens trigger an immune response, enabling the host body to recognise the pathogen as it enters and fight it off. These also target and eliminate the tumour cells in case of cancers. The rapid and adaptable nature of these technological platforms makes them particularly well-suited for the development of personalised vaccines.

7.1.1. Rapid Development

A major advantage of mRNA and DNA vaccines is their flexibility in approach and the ability to design and develop a specified vaccine rapidly. Traditional vaccine development often requires the cultivation of pathogens or the expression of proteins in a cell culture system, wherein both the processes are both complex and time-consuming. In contrast, mRNA and DNA vaccines are synthesised directly from the genetic sequences, thus dramatically reducing the development timeline.

7.1.2. mRNA Vaccine

These vaccines carry the genetic instructions in the mRNA for the production of the specific desired antigen, delivered into the body through the lipid nanoparticles (LNPs). The mRNA translates into the antigen once inside the cells, utilising the central dogma of the host cell and then prompt an immune response. The flexibility of mRNA technology allows to swiftly creating the desired vaccine candidate by simply modifying the genetic sequence encoded in the mRNA. This feature is especially beneficial in crafting personalised vaccines that are tailor-made to the unique form of mutations in the tumour of individual patients (Chehelgerdi and Chehelgerdi, 2023).

7.1.3. DNA Vaccine

DNA vaccines operate by delivering the plasmid DNA that encodes the antigen into the host cell, where it transcribes and translates into the desired antigen. Like the mRNA vaccines, DNA vaccines could be rapidly designed and produced based on the genetic profile of the tumour of individual patients

(Leitner *et al.*, 1999). Also, as compared to the mRNA vaccines, DNA vaccines also offer advantages in terms of stability as they are easier to store and transport.

7.2. Personalised Cancer Immunotherapy

Cancer immunotherapy approach seeks to engage the immune system of the body in the battle against cancer wherein personalised vaccines play a pivotal role by targeting the tumour-specific antigens, termed as neoantigens (Xie *et al.*, 2023). Neoantigens result from the unique mutations in each patient suffering from cancer.

7.2.1. Identifying the Neo-antigen

The first step in personalised cancer vaccine development involves the exact identification of the neoantigens. Advances in genome sequencing and bioinformatics tools have enabled rapid detection of these mutations in DNA within the tumour of a cancer patient. The neoantigen that is most likely to be recognised better by the patient's immune system is then predicted by employing computational tools (Xie *et al.*, 2023).

7.2.2. Designing the Vaccine and Its Production

After identifying the neoantigens, the mRNA or DNA sequences that encode these antigens are synthesised. These sequences are then incorporated into the vaccines that are administered to the patient (as personalised vaccines), training the immune system to recognise and attack the target cancer cells that express these neoantigens. This approach extends the scope for highly targeted therapies.

7.2.3. Clinical Applications and Efficacy

Personalised mRNA and DNA vaccines have demonstrated high promises across various cancer types, during the clinical trials. For instance, recent studies have shown that personalised mRNA vaccines could trigger strong immune responses and deliver the medical benefits to patients with melanoma and other such similar solid tumours (Li *et al.*, 2023). The ability to tailor-make vaccines with enhanced efficacy in individual patients while minimising the risk of the adverse side-effects seems to be the major advantages of these vaccines.

The advent of personalised mRNA and DNA vaccines represent a major advancement in cancer immunotherapy. These techniques that utilise genetic information to create customised vaccines offer a rapid and adaptable approach to target specific tumor antigens (neoantigens). As research and clinical trials advance further, personalised vaccines would have the potential to revolutionise cancer therapeutics and preventives, providing the human subject with highly specific and effective options.

8. Challenges

Despite the significant advancements in vaccine development and production, numerous challenges still remain (Salalli *et al.*, 2023). A major hurdle among the many is the availability of diverse technology platforms in manufacturing vaccines. Each of these platforms (whether mRNAs, viral vectors, protein subunits, etc.) has unique requirements, complexities and performance matrix. Standardising the underlying processes and validating the products across platforms is challenging but essential, as it necessitates harmonising the scaled-up process to ensure consistent quality and efficacy. This challenging situation is further compounded by the process scale-up difficulties, the laboratory-scale procedures to be translated into large-scale manufacturing, without compromising the product integrity. Ensuring the robustness of these processes through rigorous verification and validation is crucial in ensuring vaccine safety and efficacy.

Obtaining regulatory approval is another significant challenge as the vaccines must meet the stringent safety, efficacy and quality criteria before they can be approved for human (or even animal) use. Regulatory bodies like the FDA (of the US) and the EMA (of the European Union) have rigorous guidelines that require to carry out the numerous clinical trials followed with extensive documentation and data acquisition (U.S. FDA, 2011; EMA, 2016). Ethical concerns, particularly in the context of expedited vaccine development especially during a sudden pandemic outbreak (as during the COVID-19) play a critical role. This situation is primarily where a balance between a thorough testing and the rapid availability with equitable distribution are the matters of contention.

Equitable distribution that ensures equitable global access and mass administration of vaccines (through vaccination campaigns) pose additional challenges. Cold chain logistics that is essential to maintain the potency of vaccine during transport require substantial funds and resources, particularly in the low- and middle-income countries (LMICs), to develop the required infrastructure (Olawade *et al.*, 2024). Moreover, vaccine hesitancy that is fueled by the misinformation being floated through media that leads to the lack of trust further complicates the distribution efforts. Addressing these multifaceted challenges (Fig. 3) to ensure that the vaccines could be developed, produced and delivered efficiently and ethically calls for coordinated efforts across the scientific communities, regulatory bodies, the public in general and the healthcare personnel (Sinuraya *et al.*, 2024).

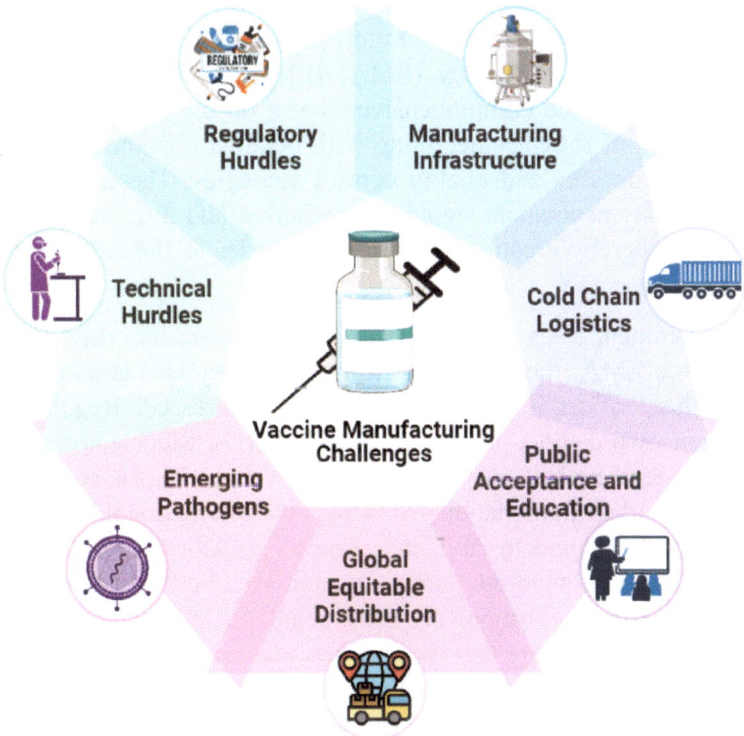

Fig. 3: Various challenges or hurdles in development and efficient distribution of vaccines that need to be addressed

8.1. Regulatory Hurdles

Developing a novel vaccine and its distribution is often significantly impeded by the global regulatory challenges. Approval processes for vaccines are a deliberate, detailed, and rigorous exercise, designed to guarantee that the vaccine in question meets the highest standards of safety and efficacy. While this thorough approach is vital to safeguard community health, it could potentially be a roadblock in expeditious introduction of novel vaccines in the market, especially during a global health emergency when rapid deployment becomes essential. The two major bodies that have a profound presence as global regulatory players in the approval processes are the USFDA and EMA that work in coordination with the World Health Organisation (WHO) of the

United Nations (UN).

The approval process (that is especially stringent for the food and pharma sectors) involves several stages that include the pre-clinical testings, multiple phases of clinical trials, and an in-depth review by the regulatory agencies such as the US Food and Drug Administration (USFDA) (U.S. FDA, 2011) and the European Medicines Agency (EMA) (EMA, 2016). Each of the stage demands a detailed and comprehensive dataset on the safety, immune response and efficacy of the vaccine, along with detailed documentation of the manufacturing processes and quality control strategies. These stringent requirements obviously necessitate significant resources and time that would delays the process, thereby creating a substantial barrier to the expeditious availability of novel vaccines.

In spite of the prominent roles played by the global players like the WHO, the USFDA and the EMA, the lack of uniform regulatory standards across countries is another critical issue that needs to be addressed. Regulatory agencies have their own distinct guidelines and criteria for vaccine approval, leading to inconsistent evaluation process (Salalli *et al.*, 2023), and non-compliance of the product trans-nationally (across the international borders). As the manufacturers struggle to navigate various regulatory landscapes to secure approval in different markets, such disparities could complicate global vaccine distribution efforts. Harmonising these standards and bringing them under a single umbrella to ensure that the vaccines can be distributed quickly and widely, particularly during a pandemic situation, is crucial. However, achieving a well-aligned global regulatory guideline is a complex and constant challenge that requires the sustained cooperation among the regulatory bodies, industry stakeholders and community healthcare organisations. In light of this, recent global initiatives like the International Council for Harmonisation (ICH; of Technical Requirements for Pharmaceuticals for Human Use) aim to streamline these processes and create common guidelines to evaluate the vaccines (Brennan *et al.*, 2004). International organisations like the WHO could play a crucial role in facilitating the promotion of converged regulatory standards.

8.2. Technical Hurdles

Technical hurdles such as stability issues and scale-up challenges pose significant obstacles in the development and production of vaccines, especially using novel vaccine development platforms such as the mRNA (Rosa *et al.*, 2021). Addressing these challenges calls for innovative approaches in formulating, manufacturing and regulatory compliance to ensure that the vaccines are both effective and globally accessible.

8.2.1. Stability Issues

One of the foremost technical challenges in vaccine development, as in the case of mRNA vaccines (Rosa *et al.*, 2021), is ensuring the stability with an extended shelf-life. mRNA vaccines, such as the ones developed during COVID-19, are inherently unstable which require stringent storage conditions to maintain the efficacy (Uddin and Roni, 2021). Unlike the conventional vaccines, which may remain stable at refrigerated temperatures, mRNA vaccines often need ultra-low storage temperature, typically around -70°C. Such a requirement poses significant logistics challenge, particularly in regions with limited access to cold chain infrastructure (as in case of the low- and medium-income countries). Ensuring the stability of mRNA vaccines throughout their shelf-life therefore could involve an optimised formulation, and an efficient delivery system (such as lipid nanoparticles) which could protect the mRNA from rapid degradation even before it reaches the target location or recipient. Advances in excipients as stabilizers and lyophilisation techniques are being explored to enhance the thermal stability of these vaccines and thus reduce their dependency on the cold-chain logistics.

8.2.2. Scale-up Challenges

Yet another major technical hurdle is transitioning from the laboratory-scale process standardisation and optimisation stage to the large-scale industrial manufacturing stage. The scale-up process involves replicating the self-contained controlled conditions in the laboratory to a larger industrial setting without compromising the quality and compliance levels. This transition is particularly challenging for biopharmaceutical products, where even a minor deviation in the production process could have a profound effect on the safety and efficacy of the final product. Scaled-up vaccine production must address several critical factors including the cell culture system optimisation, the 'bioreactor' efficiency, and a well-optimised purification process that is consistent in its performance to attain the bioindustrial manufacturing readiness level (BioMRL) (Smanski *et al.*, 2022).

8.2.2.1. Cell Culture Systems: For large-scale production and yield maximisation, it is essential to optimise the cell culture conditions while maintaining the product quality and consistency. The decision-making in this includes the selection of an appropriate cell line (*e.g.*, mammalian, insect or yeast cells), optimisation of the culture media, and the scope of scalability of the adopted cell culture technique.

8.2.2.2. Bioreactors: Modern bioreactors provide a due diligent controlled environment that is crucial for scaling up the vaccine production. However, transitioning from a small-scale operation to large-scale bioprocessing requires meticulous calibration and validation that would ensure that the cells produce the vaccine antigen at the desired levels of quality and quantity. It includes maintaining the optimal physicochemical conditions that are essential for a biological process throughout the production cycle, such as pH, temperature, and dissolved gas levels.

8.2.2.3. Purification Processes: Scaling up also necessitates efficient and scalable purification (downstream or bioseparation) techniques to ensure the removal of undesirable impurities and contaminants that might interfere in the performance of the vaccine. As for instance, filtration and chromatography systems must be capable of handling larger volumes without compromising the vaccine purity and potency.

Regulatory compliance and quality assurance become increasingly more complex at the industrial-scale operations. Therefore, each of the scaled-up process steps must be validated to meet the regulatory standards. This may require extensive testing and documentation. Implementing Process Analytical Technology (PAT) and Quality by Design (QbD) principles could help in monitoring and controlling the production process with quality consistency being ensured (Gerzon *et al.*, 2022; Pramod *et al.*, 2016).

8.3. Manufacturing Infrastructure

The establishment and maintenance of advanced manufacturing infrastructure for vaccine production involve significant financial investment and operational complexity. The high costs that are associated with developing a cutting-edge facility and the intricate management of the supply chains (for both raw materials and the finished product) present substantial challenges. Addressing these issues effectively is essential to ensure a constant availability and an equitable distribution of vaccines addressing the global healthcare needs.

8.3.1. High Costs

Setting up and maintaining a state-of-art vaccine production or manufacturing facility is capital-intensive. Any advanced biopharmaceutical manufacturing facility needs a very sophisticated infrastructure, including high-tech bioreactors, bioseparation set-up, analytical laboratories and quality assurance setting. The initial capital investments, such as the direct fixed capital (DFC) and the indirect fixed capital (IFC) for settingup these facilities, equipping them with the cutting-edge technology and implementing a rigorous validation framework could be substantial. Additionally, the maintenance of these facilities (including personnel training, equipment maintenance and compliance with the stringent regulatory standards) and calibrating the biotechnical instruments involves high level of recurring (operational) expenses. The financial bearings are particularly pronounced for the innovative novel vaccine development technologies (such as the mRNA and viral vector vaccines development platforms) which necessitate the need for specialised equipments and high level of expertise or skill-sets (Plotkin *et al.*, 2017). These high costs often could limit the ability of smaller companies, organisations and the economically-backward countries to enter the vaccine market, which could potentially affect innovation, healthy competition and decentralised operations.

8.3.2. Supply Chain Management

The complex vaccine manufacturing process involves multiple interdependent stages, each being dependent on a reliable supply of raw materials, intermediary process components, and warehousing of the final product (Gomez *et al.*, 2013). Thus, an effectively managed supply chain (logistics) ensures a robust vaccines production and distribution system in place. Managing this supply chain presents several challenges:

8.3.2.1. Raw Material: Vaccine production requires the supply of a diverse range of raw materials, including biological reagents, cell culture media and the downstream (purification) materials. Ensuring a consistent and high-quality supply of these materials is essential to maintain the integrity of the production process and ensuring a high-purity product with consistency in quality. Fluctuations in the availability or quality of raw materials could impact the product quality and production timelines.

8.3.2.2. Process Components: Vaccine manufacturing facilities must also manage the supply and timely delivery of process components such as the filters, chromatography columns and other consumables and replaceable components. Any delays or a shortage of supply in these components could disrupt the production schedules and affect the overall process efficiency (Ulmer *et al.*, 2006).

8.3.2.3. Equitable Distribution of Vaccines: Once manufactured, the vaccines must be distributed quickly, efficiently and equitably to ensure vaccine performance and a broader global access. This involves not only addressing the logistics challenges related to the transport and storage but also addressing the disparities in trans-national availability of vaccines across regions. An effective vaccine distribution requires robust logistics infrastructure, including cold chain systems (particularly for temperature-sensitive vaccines) and close coordination with the global and local healthcare agencies.

Integrating the advanced supply chain management practices such as real-time tracking, inventory optimisation and risk management strategies, would be critical in addressing these challenges. Ensuring a reliable supply chain needs collaboration and proactive involvement of the manufacturers, suppliers and the distributors, as well as sustained high investments in infrastructure to support the efficient management of logistics and the inventory.

8.4. Cold Chain Logistics

Addressing the challenges associated with the cold chain logistics involves improving the infrastructure, investing in advanced temperature-monitoring technologies and developing innovative solutions such as the formulation of thermostable vaccines that do not require ultra-cold storage conditions. Enhancing the collaboration and support at the global scale for cold chain logistics could also help mitigate these issues and ensure that the vaccines are distributed equitably and effectively (Pambudi *et al.*, 2022).

8.4.1. Storage and Transport

Cold chain logistics are essential for the effective storage and transportation of particularly the vaccines that need a stringent temperature regime (such as the mRNA vaccines). To ensure vaccine stability and efficacy, the cold chain involves maintaining end-to-end controlled temperature conditions from the point of manufacturing through to the point of vaccine administration (the recipient). Maintaining an ultra-cold condition (typically –70°C) for the highly sensitive mRNA vaccines, which could not tolerate high temperature fluctuations, is critical. Such preconditions present a significant logistics challenge, particularly in regions with skeletal (limited) infrastructure as is frequently encountered in the low- and medium-income countries. Inadequate cold chain infrastructure could lead to temperature abuse that might compromise the vaccine potency and safety, potentially rendering them ineffective or unsafe for use (Uddin and Roni, 2021).

Ensuring the integrity of the cold supply chain involves a combination of specialised equipments, including ultra-low temperature freezers, refrigerated transport vehicles and temperature-monitoring devices across the supply chain. Establishing and maintaining this infrastructure requires substantial investment and coordination among the various stakeholders, especially in the resource-limited settings (James, 2021). The logistics challenges of distributing vaccines to remote or underserved areas would further exacerbate the issue, as transportation networks may be insufficient to support the complex requirements of cold chain logistics.

8.4.2. Addressing Temperature Sensitivity

Temperature sensitive mRNA vaccines pose a significant barrier to their equitable distribution and preferential use. Unlike many traditional vaccines, which can be stored at standard refrigeration temperatures (2–8°C), mRNA vaccines require an ultra-cold storage for the sake of stability (Uddin and Roni, 2021). This requirement creates a bottleneck in regions where such storage and transport capabilities are not readily available.

8.4.2.1. Limited Infrastructure: The need for ultra-cold storage systems imposes additional logistics and financial burden, making it difficult to seamlessly engage in widespread equitable distribution, especially among the low- and middle-income countries. The cost of ultra-cold freezers and the need for specialised transport and handling protocols further complicate the efforts to ensure equitable distribution.

8.4.2.2. Impact on Distribution: The challenge of maintaining the necessary cold temperatures throughout the supply chain could lead to supply delays and management inefficiencies. For instance, power outages or equipment failures could result in temperature fluctuations, potentially impacting the vaccine quality and shelf-life. Effective cold chain management requires robust systems for monitoring and maintaining temperatures, which may not be feasible across regions worldwide (Pambudi *et al.*, 2022).

8.5. Education and Awareness to reduce hesitancy

The education and awareness, and acceptance of vaccination by the general public these days are challenging (especially during the large-scale 'emergency' vaccination during the COVID-19 pandemic), and these seem crucial for a successful vaccination drive. Overcoming vaccine hesitancy (Galagali *et al.*, 2022) and imparting accurate and optimal knowledge about the vaccines through targeted education and awareness initiatives are essential steps in achieving high vaccination coverage to protect public health. The awareness about direct protection (vaccinating the eligible individuals) and indirect protection (herd immunity for the individuals that are ineligible for direct vaccine administration) due to the vaccines is also critical and useful to reduce vaccine hesitancy.

8.5.1. Vaccine Hesitancy

Vaccine hesitancy that hinders the process of achieving high vaccination coverage to ensure community wellbeing remains a significant challenge. The hesitancy is often fueled by the misinformation that insanely float around, a lack of trust in the vaccines or the entities that promote them. Misinformation can spread rapidly through social media and other digital platforms, leading to widespread misconceptions about vaccine safety, efficacy and the necessity. For example, false claims about vaccines causing severe side-effects or containing harmful ingredients can deter an individual from getting vaccinated, even when the evidence overwhelmingly supports the safety and efficacy of the vaccine in question (Galagali *et al.*, 2022). Overcoming vaccine hesitancy requires addressing these misconceptions and fostering public trust through transparent communication and community engagement.

Building trust involves providing clear, accurate and evidence-based information about the vaccines. Health authorities, healthcare providers, non-government organisations and public healthcare organisations must actively engage with the communities to address concerns, clear their doubts, and counter misinformation. Efforts should include organising outreach programmes, public service announcements, and collaborations with trustworthy community leaders and influencers to effectively convey the benefits of vaccination and the risks associated with vaccine-preventable diseases.

8.5.2. Education and Awareness

Education and awareness are critical components in promoting acceptance of the vaccines and ensuring successful vaccination campaigns. Educating the general public about the safety and benefits of vaccines helps combat misinformation and build an environment of informed decision-making (Lip *et al.*, 2023). Comprehensive education programmes should address common questions and concerns, emphasising the rigorous testing and regulatory oversight that vaccines undergo before approval. Providing information on how a vaccine works, its benefits in preventing the target disease, and the potential negative consequences of the vaccine-preventable illnesses can help demystify the vaccination process and encourage participation.

Effective educational strategies include incorporating vaccines into routine health education curricula, leveraging various media platforms to disseminate accurate Information, and training the healthcare professionals to communicate effectively with the patients and their attendants about the vaccines. Ensuring that educational materials are accessible, culturally sensitive, and tailored to diverse audiences can enhance the overall impact. Additionally, engaging in community-based interventions and support programmes could help address specific concerns and barriers faced by the various population groups across age and ethnicity.

8.6. Global Equitable Distribution

The challenges of global equitable distribution of vaccines involve tackling issues related to affordability, access, and intellectual property. Ensuring that vaccines are accessible to all (like COVAX which was aimed at assuring equitable access to the COVID-19 vaccines around the globe) especially in low-income and middle-income countries (LMICs) required coordinated efforts from international organisations, local and national governments, and the private sector to overcome the economic and logistics barriers with regard to the public healthcare needs while delicately balancing the intellectual property rights (Yarlagadda *et al.*, 2022).

8.6.1. Access for the Developing Countries

Ensuring that the vaccines are affordable and accessible in low- and middle-income countries (LMICs) remains a global healthcare challenge significantly. The disparities between the high-income and LMICs with regard to the access to vaccines could be attributed to several factors including financial constraints, inadequate healthcare infrastructure, and logistics barriers. Vaccines, especially the novel and innovative ones, could be prohibitively expensive for many LMICs due to their limited purchasing power owing to the high production costs (Farlow *et al.*, 2023). This economic barrier prevents these countries from securing sufficient quantities of the vaccines, leading to inequitable access and exacerbated global healthcare disparities.

Efforts to improve the access to vaccines in the LMICs include initiatives like GAVI, the Vaccine Alliance, which works to provide vaccines at reduced prices through partnerships with manufacturers and governments (Kumraj *et al.*, 2022). Additionally, the introduction of tiered pricing models, where vaccines are sold at different prices based on the purchasing capacities of the various countries, aims to make vaccines more affordable even for the low-income nations. However, these approaches require sustained international support and coordination to ensure that they effectively address the needs of the most vulnerable populations and endemic regions.

8.6.2. Intellectual Property Issues

Balancing the intellectual property (IP) rights with the need for wider access to vaccines presents a complex challenge. IP protection like patents provides incentives for innovation by granting exclusive rights to vaccine developers. However, these protections can also lead to high pricing of the vaccine, thereby limiting the access in LMICs. The debate over IP rights often centers on finding a balance between rewarding innovation and ensuring that the vaccines are available to all who need them, regardless of their economic status.

The Agreement by the World Trade Organisation (WTO) on the Trade-Related Aspects of Intellectual Property Rights (TRIPS) allows for certain flexibilities, such as compulsory licensing, which enables governments to bypass patents under specific conditions to ensure access to essential medicines (Urias and Ramani, 2020). During the COVID-19 pandemic, there were calls for a temporary waiver of TRIPS provisions for COVID-19 vaccines to facilitate broader production and distribution. The TRIPS waiver proposal was an enabler of mass manufacturing and wider distribution by allowing countries to produce vaccines without facing IP constraints. While discussions on this waiver continue, it highlights the ongoing tension between IP protection and global health needs.

In addition to policy adjustments, collaborations between pharmaceutical companies, governments, and non-governmental organisations (NGOs) are crucial to address IP issues and promote equitable access to vaccines (Sung *et al.*, 2021). Public-private partnerships, such as those facilitated by organisations like GAVI and the Coalition for Epidemic Preparedness Innovations (CEPI), will play a key role in bridging the gap between vaccine innovation and distribution to LMICs.

8.7. Emerging Pathogens

The challenges posed by novel viruses and mutating variants highlight the need for agile and adaptive vaccine development strategies. Rapid response to emerging pathogens and the development of next-generation vaccines capable of addressing diverse viral strains are crucial to ensure public health security in the face of emerging and evolving threats.

8.7.1. Emerging and Reemerging Viral Diseases

The rapid emergence of novel viruses like the SARS-CoV-2, which causes COVID-19 and the MERS-CoV, which causes Middle East Respiratory Syndrome underscores the urgent need for swift development and deployment of vaccines to counter them at the earliest (Chathappady House *et al.*, 2021). The emergence of novel pathogens often occurs with little caution and remains unnoticed till it takes a dimension of an outbreak. This situation presents significant challenges for the vaccine developers and ultimately affecting the public healthcare system. The process of developers and ultimately affecting the novel viruses involves several stages, which include the identification of the pathogen, designing the appropriate and effective vaccine, preclinical testing, clinical trials and mass production (Singh and Mehta, 2016). Given the fast-paced nature of viral outbreaks, all these stages in the process of vaccine development need to be expedited with uncompromised safety and efficacy.

The experience during the recent pandemic demonstrated that an expeditious vaccine development strategy with uncompromising safety and efficacy parameters is very much practically possible at least for emergency use, and is not just theoretical. For instance, the rapid development of COVID-19 vaccines was unprecedented, with several vaccines being developed and receiving 'emergency use' authorisation within a year of discovery of the virus SARS-CoV-2 (Mohapatra *et al.*, 2024). Such a rapid response could be possible through substantial global investments and working collaborations, and by leveraging the existing cutting-edge technologies, such as the mRNA platforms. Although the vaccine development process could be expedited, however scaling up the production to ensure equitable distribution amidst a global health crisis seemed challenging.

8.7.2. Mutations and Variants

Making the viruses adaptable and amenable for vaccine development through targeted mutations and the emergence of novel variants as the virus evolves through time add another layer of complexity to the design and production of vaccines. Viruses have demonstrated their high ability to mutate and generate new variants as was quite prominent in the case of SARS-CoV-2, and this phenomenon could affect the efficacy of a vaccine (Abulsoud *et al.*, 2023; Mohapatra *et al.*, 2022). Many of these evolving and emerging variants were classified by WHO as variants of concern (VoC; like the Delta and Omicron variants) and variants of interest (VoI). The former classified group has shown increased transmissibility and, also partial resistance to the existing vaccines in certain cases. Such vaccine resistance adaptive behaviour of the virus and its variants that lead to breakthrough infections requires constant monitoring, genome sequencing and adaptive vaccines (such as the next-generation vaccines) for their assured efficacy.

To address these challenges that the mutating viruses present, next-generation vaccines to offer broader protection are being developed adopting the technologically advanced state-of-the-art platforms. These vaccines could target multiple viral epitopes or could incorporate adaptive components that could respond to the altered stimuli by the evolving virus and the emerging variants (Al-Fattah Yahaya *et al.*, 2023). Technological platforms such as the multivalent vaccines and nanoparticle-based carriers are being explored to enhance the ability of vaccines to address various pathogenic strains (Bezbaruah *et al.*, 2022). Further, surveillance systems and genomic sequencing play a critical role in identifying new variants in time and making it available online as updates for vaccine development. Nevertheless, the need to develop vaccines that are constantly adaptable to the evolving viral strains is likely to complicate the design and production process. This would require dedicated ongoing research, development and coordination among the researchers, scientists, manufacturers and the regulatory bodies to ensure that the vaccines remain effective even against the novel emerging variants.

9. Overcoming the Bottlenecks: The New Generation Approach

Advancements in science and technology in general and molecular biology and bioinformatics in particular have paved the way for precision medicine and vaccine designing to the level of an individual's needs. The lessons learnt during mass fatalities due to vaccine-preventable infection diseases as a result of major outbreaks have pushed the scientific community to the wall and forced them to update and integrate their R&D efforts in line with the advanced new generation approach.

9.1. Biological Approach

The mainstay of vaccine research and development is, needless to say, the biological approach. It includes acknowledging an emerging disease, discovering the aetiological agent behind it, identifying the epitope or the antigenic determinant (foreign substance that is responsible for disease manifestation) and the antigen (the protein component that especially binds to the antibody), finding ways-n-measures to counter the pathogenesis by targeting the antigen, developing a vaccine candidate, enhancing the efficacy of the vaccine by formulating with adjuvants and carrier molecules, devising mechanisms to administer the vaccine, and finally, formulating the vaccine for the recipient.

9.1.1. Systems Biology

An effectively designed vaccine is one that mimics the biologically and pathologically active 'entity' in the pathogen as similar as possible to be recognised by the host immune system and thereby induce a cascade of molecular and cellular events between the innate and the adaptive immune system (Buonaguro and Pulendran, 2011). However, the majority of the over-the-counter available vaccines are derived from either live-attenuated or inactivated pathogen particles acting as the active antigen. However, both of these types have their own shortcomings. The live-attenuated vaccine could have light or acute side-effects on the recipient host, while the inactivated vaccines could prove to be less effective thereby requiring a course to be administered in multiple shots/doses. Systems biology utilises the integration of the immune response pathway and computational modelling to improve the efficacy of a vaccine. Systems biology is a promising tool to evaluate vaccine-induced immune responses, identify those specific signatures, assess the response *in silico* and assign a prediction value that is reliably close to the reality.

The early innate immune responses and the gene expression signatures are observed and assessed to predict adaptive immune response (Six *et al.*, 2012; Pezeshki *et al.*, 2019). Systems biology also provides with a hypothesis that is capable of calculating the parameters that control the memory T-cells and antibody production. Systems biology majorly comprises of the following phases:

9.1.1.1. Organise: This includes performing numerous 'omics' assays such as genomics, proteomics, lipidomics, metabolomics, and proteomics. With the use of high-dimensional technologies with a list of *in silico* molecular approaches, the output from these assays are finally organised into pathways and a network of immune responses.

9.1.1.2. Analyse: This phase involves the formulation of strategies to model the methods by understanding the data output from the assay. It also includes the development of a deeper understanding of the antigen-host interactions followed by the analysis of the gene-set, deciphering the biochemical pathways and networks with the help of computational biology (Ng *et al.*, 2006).

9.1.1.3. Utilise to Immunise: The ultimate aim of such in-depth understanding of the obtained dataset, molecular interactions and characterisation of the underlying process is to produce an effective vaccine (Oberg *et al.*, 2011). The information on the factors that can determine what could enhance the performance of the vaccine in the body, such as the antigen dose, type and and category of adjuvants, route of administration, critical epitopes that could be effectively used are gathered using systems biology and bioinformatics. Systems biology is currently being extensively employed in autoimmune diseases infectious diseases, as well as in oncology, and Has recently been increasingly applied in the field of vaccinology.

9.1.2. Reverse Vaccinology

The standard workflow to initiate a systems biology study is identifying the pathogen and the pathogenicity, culturing the organism, and then analysing it through computational biology. This preliminary exercise is done to know about the immunogenicity of the pathogen and the epitope that is responsible in stimulating the desired response. However, this approach has numerous shortcomings. These include identifying and isolating the disease-causing antigens (which is a time-consuming process) and the isolation of antigens from the pathogens that are unculturable (which cannot be grown over media in laboratory conditions). With the advent of the whole-genome sequencing, antigen selection on the basis of their genome has played a major role in vaccine designing as the technique provides a scope to do away with the time-consuming process of culturing the pathogen on media (Chen *et al.*, 2013; Delany *et al.*, 2013). This approach is better described and termed as reverse vaccinology.

Reverse vaccinology is done by initially carrying out the computational analysis to identify the protein antigens that elucidate immunogenicity and thus be a potential vaccine target. After identifying the suitable sequence one could pinpoint the open reading frames (ORFs) that could be the DNA that potentially encode for the exposed proteins outside the surface. Following it, high-throughput screening is carried out to confirm if the antigens are protective, by overexpressing the antigen in the cloning organism (like *Escheria coli*), purification of the antigen to further vaccinate the mice or other model animal, and assessing if the vaccinating animal developed the desired protection against the antigen (Kis *et al.*, 2019; Pizza *et al.*, 2000). The technique of reverse vaccinology was first implemented in the development of the vaccine against *Neisseria meningitis* group B (MenB) (Delany *et al.*, 2013).

A capsular polysaccharide conjugated vaccine was used for the serogroup (a group of bacteria with common antigen) of *Meningococcus* by employing the conventional vaccinology. However, this was not deemed viable for administration to the general public due to the cross-reactivity with several other human antigens. Thus, the first vaccine to provide broader protection against MenB was developed using reverse vaccinology involving three main identified antigens, factor H-binding protein (fHbp), *N. meningitidis* adhesin A (NadA), and Neisserial heparin-binding antigen (NHBA) (McCarthy *et al.*, 2018), and marketed successfully. Reverse vaccinology does not need the antigens to be isolated and be in sufficient quantity, but rather it is dependent on the overexpression of the antigens in the cloning bacteria. However, reverse vaccinology does not facilitate the identification of the protein-carbohydrate milieu that is not encoded by the genome, and their structures.

9.1.3. Synthetic Biology

The field of synthetic biology deals with the modification and optimisation of the existing genes and proteins to improve their performance with an intent to extend the value proposition (Tan *et al.*, 2021). Synthetic biology can be preferably used in developing a sustainable vaccine development model which optimally uses the resources, consumes less time and has little dependency on the experimental data, doing away with the conventional trial-and-error approach. Nucleic acid vaccines produced through synthetic biology would need transportion in kilograms instead of in tonnes (Kitney *et al.*, 2021). mRNA vaccines, developed using codon optimisation and deep learning tools, are often synthetic in nature. Codon optimisation is the process through which a codon is inserted into a specific construct that further optimally translates inside the vaccine recipient, thereby increasing production of the antigen (Pfeifer *et al.*, 2023). mRNA constructs can include nucleic acid modification and polyadenylation as well as inserting a replicase that allows for self-amplification of the mRNA, thus increasing the lifespan of the effect even with a single dose (Pfeifer *et al.*, 2023; Wesselhoeft *et al.*, 2018). Although mRNA platform theoretically seems to be priceless and timeless, specific process optimation and rationalisation of mRNA vaccine constructs to overcome few present limitations like the instability and short lifespan issues may be required.

Synthetic biology approaches in vaccine development could also include setting-up of biofoundries, as in a highly automated facility with robotic work-system that is programmed to perform a specific task, integrated with software that allows simultaneous investigation to observe and act on factors that could optimise the industrial production design (Kitney *et al.*, 2021).

9.2. Management Approach

A vaccine production chain occasionally struggle also to keep up with the market demand and disruptions that could cause unexpected delays. As already mentioned earlier, some of the key underlying reasons could be the shortage of raw materials, lack of a desired well-equipped facility to produce the required huge quantity of vaccine vials especially during a pandemic-like situation, the lack of trained and skilled personnel or the disruptions in the supply cold chain. This overdependence for high-capacity production on a limited manufacturing unit could be a concern. However, it could be resolved by building multi-purpose vaccine production facilities or re-purposing the small vaccine facilities to produce a vaccine in need from time-to-time (Feddema *et al.*, 2023). Veterinary facilities using large and fixed bioreactors could be ramped up for alternate production. Increased flexibility of a manufacturing unit and its working mechanism could further increase the net production.

Maintaining the supply cold chain to maintain the end-to-end integrity of vaccines is necessary, which also is a management bottleneck. Maintaining an uninterrupted cold chain during vaccines transportation over distant places could be full of hassles. Thus, addressing this issue through protocol simplification could be a necessity, such as reducing the geographical distance between the production unit and the end user. This could be achieved through decentralised production. A shortage of raw materials in global vaccine development drive was experienced during the recent COVID-19 pandemic due to the rapid expansion in the production capacity to meet the sudden spike in demand. Thus it was important to maintain the inventory, a stable raw material supply channel, prevention of hoarding, linking the stock suppliers to the manufacturers directly and allocating the resources in a centralised manner through global-level initiatives.

Further, alternative mechanisms of vaccine administration instead of injection could help overcome the shortage of end-use resources like needles (Feddema *et al.*, 2023). Bioprocess development advancements in vaccine production in recent times are appended with modelling of the various production stages (Gernaey *et al.*, 2010). Multidisciplinary modelling of the work station is best suited where mechanistic approach in the initial stage of production with a data-driven approach is involved while developing the vaccine, as well as optimisation and hybrid modelling whilst monitoring the later production stages thereby reducing redundancies (Aars *et al.*, 2021). A flexible vaccine manufacturing set-up with single-use components and through common platform technologies could be adopted at all the stages of vaccine development, from production and processing to fill-and-finish, employed for multiple vaccines and transfer between biologic 'medical countermeasures'. Such flexible set-up could aid in overcoming the specialised manufacturing issues (Sell *et al.*, 2021).

10. Conclusion

The scope in the field of bioprocess technology is on the brink of transformative advancements for vaccine design and scale-up, offering unprecedented opportunities for addressing global health challenges. As vaccines play a critical role in preventing infectious diseases and managing pandemic situations, integrated cutting-edge bioprocess technologies is crucial for their successful development and deployment.

Bioprocess technology encompasses a range of innovative approaches from genetic engineering and advanced cell culture systems to modern bioreactors and continuous manufacturing processes. These advancements have significantly enhanced the ability to design vaccines and efficiently scale-up their production. As a case instance, the mRNA vaccinology platform has revolutionised vaccine development, facilitating rapid responses to contain emerging pathogens. In similar lines, the continuous manufacturing processes promise to improve the production efficiency and reduce the costs, making vaccines more accessible and affordable worldwide.

Despite the numerous promising advancements, several challenges yet remain to be addressed. Ensuring the stability and quality of vaccines, especially against the swiftly spreading novel pathogens and evolving variants, requires continual innovation and rigorous process validation. Cold chain logistics, regulatory harmonisation, and equitable distribution of vaccines are critical intervention facets that need to be addressed to achieve global health equity. Vaccine hesitancy and intellectual property issues further complicate the landscape, necessitating comprehensive strategies to build public trust and delicately balancing the innovative state-of-the-art technologies with accessibility.

Vaccine research in future would focus on enhancing bioprocess technologies to address these challenges. These would include developing next-generation vaccines that could adapt themselves to emerging variants, improving cold chain solutions, and leveraging digital tools for real-time monitoring and quality control. Global investments on infrastructure and global cooperation will be essential to overcome these hurdles. Harmonising the regulatory frameworks across different regions and ensuring that vaccines are affordable and accessible in the low- and middle-income countries (LMIC) will be pivotal in achieving widespread vaccination coverage to effectively combat infectious diseases.

The vaccine development journey from its designing to mass production to equitable global distribution is fraught with numerous challenges. Some of these challenges are technical while some others are mere managerial. However, bioprocess technology promises to offer a pathway to overcome these barriers. Through global sharing of innovations, investments, and collaborations, vaccine development strategies could be fine-tuned which could guarantee the benefits of these life-saving interventions reach the populations worldwide.

References

Abulsoud AI, El-Husseiny HM, El-Husseiny AA, El-Mahdy HA, Ismail A, Elkhawaga SY, Khidr EG, Fathi D, Mady EA, Najda A and Algahtani M, 2023. Mutations in SARS-CoV-2: Insights on structure, variants, vaccines, and biomedical interventions. Biomed. Pharmacother., 157: 113977. doi: 10.1016/j.biopha.2022.113977

Al-Fattah Yahaya AA, Khalid K, Lim HX and Poh CL, 2023. Development of next generation vaccines against SARS-CoV-2 and variants of concern. Viruses, 15(3): 624. doi: 10.3390/v15030624

Bezbaruah R, Chavda VP, Nongrang L, Alom S, Deka K, Kalita T, Ali F, Bhattacharjee B and Vora L, 2022. Nanoparticle-based delivery systems for vaccines. Vaccines, 10(11): 1946. doi: 10.3390/vaccines10111946

Brennan FR, Shaw L, Wing MG and Robinson C, 2004. Preclinical safety testing of biotechnology-derived pharmaceuticals: understanding the issues and addressing the challenges. Mol. Biotechnol., 27: 59–74. doi: 10.1385/MB:27:1:59

Buckland B, Sanyal G, Ranheim T, Pollard D, Searles JA, Behrens S, Pluschkell S, Josefsberg J and Roberts CJ, 2024. Vaccine process technology—A decade of progress. Biotechnol. Bioeng., 121(9): 2604–2635. doi: 10.1002/bit.28703

Busse C, Biechele P, de Vries I, Reardon KF, Solle D and Scheper T, 2017. Sensors for disposable bioreactors. Eng. Life Sci., 17(8): 940–952. doi: 10.1002/elsc.201700049

Chehelgerdi M and Chehelgerdi M, 2023. The use of RNA-based treatments in the field of cancer immunotherapy. Mol. Cancer, 22(1): 106. 10.1186/s12943-023-01807-w

Cid R and Bolívar J, 2021. Platforms for production of protein-based vaccines: from classical to next-generation strategies. Biomolecules, 11(8): 1072. doi: 10.3390/biom11081072

Cross S, Rho Y, Reddy H, Pepperrell T, Rodgers F, Osborne R, Eni-Olotu A, Banerjee R, Wimmer S and Keestra S, 2021. Who funded the research behind the Oxford–AstraZeneca COVID-19 vaccine?. BMJ Global Health, 6(12): e007321. doi: :10.1136/bmjgh-2021-007321

Dash R, Sahoo RN, Pattnaik G, Sarangi AK, Kandi V, Mishra S, Verma S and Mohapatra RK, 2024. An open call for nano-based therapy to address COVID-19 and oncological clinical conditions. Int. J. Surg., 110(4):2430-2. DOI: 10.1097/JS9.0000000000000071

Delany I, Rappuoli R and Seib KL, 2013. Vaccines, reverse vaccinology, and bacterial pathogenesis. Cold Spring Harb. Perspect. Med., 3(5), p.a012476. doi: 10.1101/cshperspect.a012476

Deng S, Liang H, Chen P, Li Y, Li Z, Fan S, Wu K, Li X, Chen W, Qin Y and Yi L, 2022. Viral vector vaccine development and application during the COVID-19 pandemic. Microorganisms, 10(7): 1450. doi: 10.3390/microorganisms10071450

EMA, 2016. Guideline on process validation for the manufacture of biotechnology-derived active substances and data to be provided in the regulatory submission. London, U.K. EMA/CHMP/BWP/187338/2014

Farlow A, Torreele E, Gray G, Ruxrungtham K, Rees H, Prasad S, Gomez C, Sall A, Magalhães J, Olliaro P and Terblanche P, 2023. The future of epidemic and pandemic vaccines to serve global public health needs. Vaccines, 11(3): 690. doi: 10.3390/vaccines11030690

FDA, 2004. Guidance for industry, PAT-A framework for innovative pharmaceutical development, manufacturing and quality assurance. Rockville, USA. http://www. fda. gov/cder/guidance/published. html.

Feddema JJ, Fernald KD, Schikan HG and van de Burgwal LH, 2023. Upscaling vaccine manufacturing capacity-key bottlenecks and lessons learned. Vaccine, 41(30): 4359–4368. doi: 10.1016/j.vaccine.2023.05.027

Garenne D, Haines MC, Romantseva EF, Freemont P, Strychalski EA and Noireaux V, 2021. Cell-free gene expression. Nat. Rev. Methods Primers, 1(1): 49. doi: 10.1038/s43586-021-00046-x

Galagali PM, Kinikar AA and Kumar VS, 2022. Vaccine hesitancy: obstacles and challenges. Curr. Pediatr. Rep., 10(4): 241–248. doi: 10.1007/s40124-022-00278-9

Gernaey KV, Lantz AE, Tufvesson P, Woodley JM and Sin G, 2010. Application of mechanistic models to fermentation and biocatalysis for next-generation processes. Trends Biotechnol., 28(7): 346–354. doi: 10.1016/j.tibtech.2010.03.006

Gerzon G, Sheng Y and Kirkitadze M, 2022. Process analytical technologies–advances in bioprocess integration and future perspectives. J. Pharm. Biomed. Anal., 207: 114379. doi: 10.1016/j.jpba.2021.114379

Gomez PL, Robinson JM and Rogalewicz JA, 2013. Vaccine manufacturing. Vaccines, 44–57. doi: 10.1016/B978-1-4557-0090-5.00019-7

Hajiaghapour Asr M, Dayani F, Saedi Segherloo F, Kamedi A, Neill AO, MacLoughlin R and Doroudian M, 2023. Lipid nanoparticles as promising carriers for mRNA vaccines for viral lung infections. Pharmaceutics, 15(4): 1127. doi: 10.3390/pharmaceutics15041127

Hedley-Whyte J and Milamed DR, 2021. Measles: Progress and failure. Ulst Med. J., 90(2): 107–111.

Hilleman MR, 1987. Yeast recombinant hepatitis B vaccine. Infection, 15(1): 3–7.

Hong MS, Severson KA, Jiang M, Lu AE, Love JC and Braatz RD, 2018. Challenges and opportunities in biopharmaceutical manufacturing control. Comput. Chem. Eng., 110: 106–114. doi: 10.1016/j.compchemeng.2017.12.007

Iqbal M, Tao Y, Xie S, Zhu Y, Chen D, Wang X, Huang L, Peng D, Sattar A, Shabbir MAB and Hussain HI, 2016. Aqueous two-phase system (ATPS): an overview and advances in its applications. Biol. Proced. Online, 18: 1–18. doi: 10.1186/s12575-016-0048-8

James ER, 2021. Disrupting vaccine logistics. International health, 13(3): 211–214. doi: 10.1093/inthealth/ihab010

Kallerup RS and Foged C, 2014. Classification of vaccines. In C Foged, T Rades, Y Perrie, S Hook (Eds) Subunit Vaccine Delivery, Springer, New York: 15–29, doi: 10.1007/978-1-4939-1417-3_2

Karbalaei M, Rezaee SA and Farsiani H, 2020. Pichia pastoris: A highly successful expression system for optimal synthesis of heterologous proteins. J. Cell. Physiol., 235(9): 5867–5881. doi: 10.1002/jcp.29583

Kilbourne ED, 1973. The molecular epidemiology of influenza. J. Infect. Dis., 127(4): 478–487.

Kis Z, Shattock R, Shah N and Kontoravdi C, 2019. Emerging technologies for low-cost, rapid vaccine manufacture. Biotechnol. J., 14(1): 1800376. doi: 10.1002/biot.201800376

Kitney RI, Bell J and Philp J, 2021. Build a sustainable vaccines industry with synthetic biology. Trends Biotechnol., 39(9): 866–874. doi: 10.1016/j.tibtech.2020.12.006

Kiros TG, Levast B, Auray G, Strom S, van Kessel J and Gerdts V, 2012. The importance of animal models in the development of vaccines. In: Baschieri, S. (Eds) Innovation in Vaccinology: from design, through to delivery and testing, Springer, Dordrecht: 251–264. doi: 10.1007/978-94-007-4543-8_11

Kumar R and Kumar P, 2019. Yeast-based vaccines: New perspective in vaccine development and application. FEMS Yeast Res., 19(2): foz007. doi: 10.1093/femsyr/foz007

Kumraj G, Pathak S, Shah S, Majumder P, Jain J, Bhati D, Hanif S, Mukherjee S and Ahmed S, 2022. Capacity building for vaccine manufacturing across developing countries: the way forward. Hum. Vaccin. Immunother., 18(1): 2020529. doi: 10.1080/21645515.2021.2020529

Lee JH and Ko K, 2017. Production of recombinant anti-cancer vaccines in plants. Biomol. Ther., 25(4): 345–353. doi: 10.4062/biomolther.2016.126

Leitner WW, Ying H and Restifo NP, 1999. DNA and RNA-based vaccines: principles, progress and prospects. Vaccine, 18(9–10): 765–777. doi: 10.1016/S0264-410X(99)00271-6

Lembong J, Kirian R, Takacs JD, Olsen TR, Lock LT, Rowley JA and Ahsan T, 2020. Bioreactor parameters for microcarrier-based human MSC expansion under xeno-free conditions in a vertical-wheel system. Bioengineering, 7(3): 73. doi: 10.3390/bioengineering7030073

Lip A, Pateman M, Fullerton MM, Chen HM, Bailey L, Houle S, Davidson S and Constantinescu C, 2023. Vaccine hesitancy educational tools for healthcare providers and trainees: a scoping review. Vaccine, 41(1): 23–35. doi: 10.1016/j.vaccine.2022.09.093

Liu F, Wu X, Li L, Liu Z and Wang Z, 2013. Use of baculovirus expression system for generation of virus-like particles: successes and challenges. Protein Expr. Purif., 90(2): 104–116. doi: 10.1016/j.pep.2013.05.009

Liu S and Schulz BL, 2021. Biopharmaceutical quality control with mass spectrometry. Bioanalysis, 13(16): 1275–1291. doi: 10.4155/bio-2021-0123

Li Y, Wang M, Peng X, Yang Y, Chen Q, Liu J, She Q, Tan J, Lou C, Liao Z and Li X, 2023. mRNA vaccine in cancer therapy: Current advance and future outlook. Clin. Transl. Med., 13(8): e1384. doi: 10.1002/ctm2.1384

Mandenius CF and Brundin A, 2008. Bioprocess optimization using design of experiments methodology. Biotechnol. Prog., 24(6): 1191–1203. doi: 10.1002/btpr.67

Marcuzzi A and Maximova N, 2023. Advances in stem cell therapy: new applications and innovative therapeutic approaches. Front. Med., 10: 1225551. doi: 10.3389/fmed.2023.1225551

McCarthy PC, Sharyan A and Sheikhi Moghaddam L, 2018. Meningococcal vaccines: current status and emerging strategies. Vaccines, 6(1): 12. doi: 10.3390/vaccines6010012

McLemore MR, 2006. Gardasil: Introducing the new human papillomavirus vaccine. Clin. J. Oncol. Nurs., 10(5): 559–560.

Mohapatra RK, El-Shall NA, Tiwari R, Nainu F, Kandi V, Sarangi AK, Mohammed TA, Desingu PA, Chakraborty C and Dhama K, 2022. Need of booster vaccine doses to counteract the emergence of SARS-CoV-2 variants in the context of the Omicron variant and increasing COVID-19 cases: An update. Hum. Vaccin. Immunother., 18(5):2065824. https://doi.org/10.1080/21645515.2022.2065824

Mohapatra RK, Kandi V, Gaidhane AM, Zahiruddin QS, Rustagi S, Satapathy P, Mishra S and Tuglo LS, 2024. Global domination of the recently VoI-classified'JN. 1′ outcompeting other variants–Comparing the vaccines' efficacy. Clinical Infection in Practice, 22:100358. https://doi.org/10.1016/j.clinpr.2024.100358

Mohapatra RK, Mishra S, Kandi V, Branda F, Ansari A, Rabaan AA and Kudrat-E-Zahan M, 2023. Analyzing the emerging patterns of SARS-CoV-2 Omicron subvariants for the development of next-gen vaccine: An observational study. Health Sci. Rep., 6(10):e1596. doi: 10.1002/hsr2.1596

Mohapatra RK, Pintilie L, Kandi V, Sarangi AK, Das D, Sahu R and Perekhoda L, 2020. The recent challenges of highly contagious COVID-19, causing respiratory infections: Symptoms, diagnosis, transmission, possible vaccines, animal models, and immunotherapy. Chem. Biol. Drug Des., 96(5):1187-208. doi: 10.1111/cbdd.13761

Mukherjee P, Roy S, Ghosh D and Nandi SK, 2022. Role of animal models in biomedical research: a review. Lab. Anim. Res., 38(1): 18. doi: 10.1186/s42826-022-00128-1

Ng A, Bursteinas B, Gao Q, Mollison E and Zvelebil M, 2006. Resources for integrative systems biology: from data through databases to networks and dynamic system models. Brief. Bioinformatics, 7(4): 318–330. doi: 10.1093/bib/bbl036

Nadeem AY, Shehzad A, Islam SU, Al-Suhaimi EA and Lee YS, 2022. Mosquirix™ RTS, S/AS01 vaccine development, immunogenicity, and efficacy. Vaccines, 10(5): 713. doi: 10.3390/vaccines10050713

Oberg AL, Kennedy RB, Li P, Ovsyannikova IG and Poland GA, 2011. Systems biology approaches to new vaccine development. Curr. Opin. Immunol., 23(3): 436–443. doi: 10.1016/j.coi.2011.04.005

Olawade DB, Teke J, Fapohunda O, Weerasinghe K, Usman SO, Ige AO and David-Olawade AC, 2024. Leveraging artificial intelligence in vaccine development: A narrative review. J. Microbiol. Methods, 224: 106998. doi: 10.1016/j.mimet.2024.106998

Pambudi NA, Sarifudin A, Gandidi IM and Romadhon R, 2022. Vaccine cold chain management and cold storage technology to address the challenges of vaccination programs. Energy Rep., 8: 955–972. doi: 10.1016/j.egyr.2021.12.039

Panda S, Singh PK, Mishra S, Mitra S, Pattnaik P, Adhikary SD and Mohapatra RK, 2022. Indian biosimilars and vaccines at crossroads–replicating the success of pharmagenerics. Vaccines, 11(1): 110. doi: 10.3390/vaccines11010110

Pavia CS and Wormser GP, 2021. Passive immunization and its rebirth in the era of the COVID-19 pandemic. Int. J. Antimicrob. Agents, 57(3): 106275. doi: 10.1016/j.ijantimicag.2020.106275

Pezeshki A, Ovsyannikova IG, McKinney BA, Poland GA and Kennedy RB, 2019. The role of systems biology approaches in determining molecular signatures for the development of more effective vaccines. Expert Rev. Vaccines, 18(3): 253–267. doi: 10.1080/14760584.2019.1575208

Pfeifer BA, Beitelshees M, Hill A, Bassett J and Jones CH, 2023. Harnessing synthetic biology for advancing RNA therapeutics and vaccine design. NPJ Syst. Biol. Appl., 9(1): 60. doi: 10.1038/s41540-023-00323-3

Pichichero ME, 2013. Protein carriers of conjugate vaccines: characteristics, development, and clinical trials. Hum. Vaccin. Immunother., 9(12): 2505–2523. doi: 0.4161/hv.26109

Pizza M, Scarlato V, Masignani V, Giuliani MM, Arico B, Comanducci M, Jennings GT, Baldi L, Bartolini E, Capecchi B and Galeotti CL, 2000. Identification of vaccine candidates against serogroup B meningococcus by whole-genome sequencing. Science, 287(5459): 1816–1820. doi: 10.1126/science.287.5459.1816

Plotkin S, Robinson JM, Cunningham G, Iqbal R and Larsen S, 2017. The complexity and cost of vaccine manufacturing–an overview. Vaccine, 35(33): 4064–4071. doi: 10.1016/j.vaccine.2017.06.003

Poland GA, Kennedy RB, Ovsyannikova IG, Palacios R, Ho PL and Kalil J, 2018. Development of vaccines against Zika virus. Lancet Infect. Dis., 18(7): e211–e219. doi: 10.1016/S1473-3099(18)30063-X

Pollard DJ and Pralong A, 2018. Single-use technology implementation for biologics and vaccines production. In: G Jagschies, E Lindskog, K Łącki, P Galliher (Eds) Biopharmaceutical Processing, Elsevier:721–740. doi: 10.1016/B978-0-08-100623-8.00035-9

Pramod K, Tahir MA, Charoo NA, Ansari SH and Ali J, 2016. Pharmaceutical product development: A quality by design approach. Int. J. Pharm. Investing., 6(3): 129. doi: 10.4103/2230-973X.187350

Rathore AS, Agarwal H, Sharma AK, Pathak M and Muthukumar SJPB, 2015. Continuous processing for production of biopharmaceuticals. Prep. Biochem. Biotechnol., 45(8): 836–849. doi: 10.1080/10826068.2014.985834

Rosa SS, Prazeres DM, Azevedo AM and Marques MP, 2021. mRNA vaccines manufacturing: Challenges and bottlenecks. Vaccine, 39(16): 2190–2200. 10.1016/j.vaccine.2021.03.038

Ruiz-Palacios, G.M., Pérez-Schael, I., Velázquez, F.R., Abate, H., Breuer, T., Clemens, S.C., Cheuvart, B., Espinoza, F., Gillard, P., Innis, B.L. and Cervantes, Y., 2006. Safety and efficacy of an attenuated vaccine against severe rotavirus gastroenteritis. N. Engl. J. Med., 354(1): 11–22. doi: 10.1056/NEJMoa052434

Sahin U, Karikó K and Türeçi Ö, 2014. mRNA-based therapeutics—developing a new class of drugs. Nat. Rev. Drug Discov., 13(10): 759–780. doi: 10.1038/nrd4278

Salalli R, Dange JR, Dhiman S and Sharma T, 2023. Vaccines development in India: advances, regulation, and challenges. Clin. Exp. Vaccine Res., 12(3): 193–208. doi: 10.7774/cevr.2023.12.3.193

Salian VS, Wright JA, Vedell PT, Nair S, Li C, Kandimalla M, Tang X, Carmona Porquera EM, Kalari KR and Kandimalla KK, 2021. COVID-19 transmission, current treatment, and future therapeutic strategies. Mol. Pharm., 18(3): 754–771. doi: 10.1021/acs.molpharmaceut.0c00608

Salk JE, 1956. Poliomyelitis vaccine in the fall of 1955. Am. J. Public Health Nations Health, 46(1): 1–14.

Sarangi AK, Salem MA, Younus MD, El-Haroun H, Mahal A, Tripathy L, Mishra R, Shabil M, Alhumaydhi FA, Khatib MN and Bushi G, 2024. Advanced biomaterials for regenerative medicine and their possible therapeutic significance in treating COVID-19: a critical overview. Int. J. Surg., 110(12):7508-27. doi: 10.1097/JS9.0000000000002110

Satapathy BS, Pattnaik G, Sahoo RN, Pattanaik S, Sarangi AK, Kandi V, Mishra S, Rabaan AA, Mohanty A, Sah R and Mohapatra RK, 2023. COVID-19 vaccines and their underbelly: Are we going the right way?. Health Sci. Rep., 6(9):e1540. doi: 10.1002/hsr2.1540

Sell TK, Gastfriend D, Watson M, Watson C, Richardson L, Cicero A, Inglesby T and Connell N, 2021. Building the global vaccine manufacturing capacity needed to respond to pandemics. Vaccine, 39(12): 1667–1669. doi: 10.1016/j.vaccine.2021.02.017

Sharma R, Harrison ST and Tai SL, 2022. Advances in bioreactor systems for the production of biologicals in mammalian cells. ChemBioEng Rev., 9(1): 42–62. doi: 10.1002/cben.202100022

Singh K and Mehta S, 2016. The clinical development process for a novel preventive vaccine: An overview. J. Postgrad. Med., 62(1), 4–11. doi: 10.4103/0022-3859.173187

Sinuraya RK, Nuwarda RF, Postma MJ and Suwantika AA, 2024. Vaccine hesitancy and equity: lessons learned from the past and how they affect the COVID-19 countermeasure in Indonesia. Glob. Health, 20(1): 11. doi: 10.1186/s12992-023-00987-w

Six A, Bellier B, Thomas-Vaslin V and Klatzmann D, 2012. Systems biology in vaccine design. Microb. Biotechnol., 5(2): 295–304. doi: 10.1111/j.1751-7915.2011.00321.x

Smanski MJ, Aristidou A, Carruth R, Erickson J, Gordon M, Kedia SB, Lee KH, Prather D, Schiel JE, Schultheisz H and Treynor TP, 2022. Bioindustrial manufacturing readiness levels (BioMRLs) as a shared framework for measuring and communicating the maturity of bioproduct manufacturing processes. J. Ind. Microbiol. Biotechnol., 49(5): kuac022. doi: 10.1093/jimb/kuac022

Smith KA, 2011. Edward Jenner and the small pox vaccine. Front. Immunol., 2: 21. doi: 10.3389/fimmu.2011.00021

Soler E and Houdebine LM, 2007. Preparation of recombinant vaccines. Biotechnol. Annu. Rev., 13: 65–94. doi: 10.1016/S1387-2656(07)13004-0

Sung M, Huang Y, Duan Y, Liu F, Jin Y and Zheng Z, 2021. Pharmaceutical industry's engagement in the global equitable distribution of COVID-19 vaccines: Corporate social responsibility of EUL vaccine developers. Vaccines, 9(10): 1183. doi: 10.3390/vaccines9101183

Sunita, Sajid A, Singh Y. and Shukla P, 2020. Computational tools for modern vaccine development. Hum. Vaccin. Immunother., 16(3): 723–735. doi: 10.1080/21645515.2019.1670035

Szczypka M, Splan D, Woolls H and Brandwein H, 2014. Single-use bioreactors and microcarriers. Bioprocess Int, 12: 54–64.

Takao ITO, Wang H, Hwang SH, Wang B, Wang L and Somasundaram G, 2023. Risk assessment for biopharmaceutical single-use manufacturing: A case study of upstream continuous processing. Biologicals, 84: 101713. doi: 10.1016/j.biologicals.2023.101713

Tan E, Chin CSH, Lim ZFS and Ng SK, 2021a. HEK293 cell line as a platform to produce recombinant proteins and viral vectors. Front. Bioeng. Biotechnol., 9: 796991. doi: 10.3389/fbioe.2021.796991

Tan X, Letendre JH, Collins JJ and Wong WW, 2021. Synthetic biology in the clinic: engineering vaccines, diagnostics, and therapeutics. Cell, 184(4): 881–898. doi: 10.1016/j.cell.2021.01.017

Tavakoli K, Pour-Aboughadareh A, Kianersi F, Poczai P, Etminan A and Shooshtari L, 2021. Applications of CRISPR-Cas9 as an advanced genome editing system in life sciences. BioTech, 10(3): 14. doi: 10.3390/biotech10030014

Thomas SJ and Yoon IK, 2019. A review of Dengvaxia®: development to deployment. Hum. Vaccin. Immunother., 15(10): 2295–2314. doi: 10.1080/21645515.2019.1658503

Tihanyi B and Nyitray L, 2020. Recent advances in CHO cell line development for recombinant protein production. Drug Discov. Today: Technologies, 38: 25–34. doi: 10.1016/j.ddtec.2021.02.003

Uddin MN and Roni MA, 2021. Challenges of storage and stability of mRNA-based COVID-19 vaccines. Vaccines, 9(9): 1033. doi: 10.3390/vaccines9091033

Ulmer JB, Valley U and Rappuoli R, 2006. Vaccine manufacturing: challenges and solutions. Nat. Biotechnol., 24(11): 1377–1383. doi: 10.1038/nbt1261

Urias E and Ramani SV, 2020. Access to medicines after TRIPS: Is compulsory licensing an effective mechanism to lower drug prices? A review of the existing evidence. J. Int. Bus. Policy, 3(4): 367–384. doi: 10.1057/s42214-020-00068-4

USFDA, 2011. Guidance for Industry Process Validation: General Principles and Practices. US Department of Health and Human Services. Rockville, USA. https://www.fda.gov/vaccines-blood-biologics/guidance-compliance-regulatory-information-biologics/biologics-guidances.

van der Burg D, Josefsson L, Emmer Å and Sänger–van de Griend CE, 2023. Recent capillary electrophoresis applications for upstream and downstream biopharmaceutical process monitoring. TrAC Trends Analyt. Chem., 160: 116975. doi: 10.1016/j.trac.2023.116975

Wang R, Hozumi Y, Zheng YH, Yin C and Wei GW, 2020. Host immune response driving SARS-CoV-2 evolution. Viruses, 12(10): 1095. doi: 10.3390/v12101095

Wang YS, Kumari M, Chen GH, Hong MH, Yuan JPY, Tsai JL and Wu HC, 2023. mRNA-based vaccines and therapeutics: An in-depth survey of current and upcoming clinical applications. J. Biomed. Sci., 30(1): 84. doi: 10.1186/s12929-023-00977-5

Wesselhoeft RA, Kowalski PS and Anderson DG, 2018. Engineering circular RNA for potent and stable translation in eukaryotic cells. Nat. Commun., 9(1): 2629. doi: 10.1038/s41467-018-05096-6

Wolf MW and Reichl U, 2011. Downstream processing of cell culture-derived virus particles. Expert Rev. Vaccines, 10(10): 1451–1475. doi: 10.1586/erv.11.111

Xie N, Shen G, Gao W, Huang Z, Huang C and Fu L, 2023. Neoantigens: promising targets for cancer therapy. Signal Transduct. Target Ther., 8(1): 9. doi: 10.1038/s41392-022-01270-x

Yadav DK, Yadav N and Khurana SMP, 2020. Vaccines: present status and applications. In AS Verma and A Singh (Eds) Animal biotechnology, Academic Press: 523–542. doi: 10.1016/B978-0-12-811710-1.00024-0

Yarlagadda H, Patel MA, Gupta V, Bansal T, Upadhyay S, Shaheen N and Jain R, 2022. COVID-19 vaccine challenges in developing and developed countries. Cureus, 14(4): e23951. doi: 10.7759/cureus.23951

Zhang L, Wang W and Wang S, 2015. Effect of vaccine administration modality on immunogenicity and efficacy. Expert Rev. Vaccines, 14(11): 1509–1523. doi: 10.1586/14760584.2015.1081067

Aars OK, Clark M and Schwalbe N, 2021. Increasing efficiency in vaccine Production: A primer for change. Vaccine: X, 8: 100104. doi: 10.1016/j.jvacx.2021.100104

Al Fayez N, Nassar MS, Alshehri AA, Alnefaie MK, Almughem FA, Alshehri BY, Alawad AO and Tawfik EA, 2023. Recent advancement in mRNA vaccine development and applications. Pharmaceutics, 15(7): 1972. doi: 10.3390/pharmaceutics15071972

Ayon NJ, 2023. High-throughput screening of natural product and synthetic molecule libraries for antibacterial drug discovery. Metabolites, 13(5): 625. doi: 10.3390/metabo13050625

Bondi Jr RW and Drennen III JK, 2011. Quality by Design and the Importance of PAT in QbD. In S Ahuja, S Scypinski (Eds.) Separation Science and Technology, Academic Press, 10: 195–224. doi: 10.1016/B978-0-12-375680-0.00005-X

Buonaguro L and Pulendran B, 2011. Immunogenomics and systems biology of vaccines. Immunol. Rev., 239(1): 197–208. doi: 10.1111/j.1600-065X.2010.00971.x

Chathappady House NN, Palissery S and Sebastian H, 2021. Corona viruses: a review on SARS, MERS and COVID-19. Microbiol. Insights, 14: 11786361211002481. doi: 10.1177/11786361211002481

Chen VL, Avci FY and Kasper DL, 2013. A maternal vaccine against group B Streptococcus: past, present, and future. Vaccine, 31: D13–D19. doi: 10.1016/j.vaccine.2012.12.080

5

Designing and Developing Covid 19 Nex-Gen Vaccine: AI as A Potential Tool

Aurobinda Rout[1], Shuvajyoti Kar[2], Snehasish Mishra[3*] and Chandana Mohanty[1*]

[1]School of Applied Sciences, Kalinga Institute of Industrial Technology (Deemed to be University), Bhubaneswar, Odisha, India
[2]School of Computer Sciences Engineering, Kalinga Institute of Industrial Technology (Deemed to be University), Bhubaneswar, Odisha, India
[3]School of Biotechnology, Kalinga Institute of Industrial Technology (Deemed to be University), Bhubaneswar, Odisha, India

Abstract

The severe acute respiratory syndrome coronavirus 2 (SARS-CoV-2) that caused the global COVID-19 (coronavirus disease 2019) pandemic has claimed a considerable number of lives worldwide. The unanticipated global spread of SARS-CoV-2 has resulted in serious issues within the medical systems and healthcare facilities. Creating efficient vaccines against the virus, even after all of efforts, has been on high priority and is time-taking due to the frequent mutations. A critical stage in vaccine development is figuring out the potential antigen. As a ground-breaking technique introduced in 2000, Reverse vaccinology (RV) reduces the required time considerably from 5–15 years to 1–2 years in identifying antigens. Various RV tools are powered by big-data analytics, artificial intelligence (AI) and machine learning (ML) techniques. AI and ML models have demonstrated their potentials in expediting the identification and refinement of novel antivirals or potent vaccination candidates. By utilising datasets available through several dedicated databases, it is more beneficial in identifying current medications that inhibit the human Coronavirus and next-gen healthcare possibilities.

***Keywords*:** SARS, Coronavirus, COVID-19, Pandemic, Mutation, Artificial intelligence, Machine learning, Vaccination

1. Introduction

COVID-19, a deadly disease was identified in Wuhan city of China in December 2019 which spread recklessly that grappled the entire world in no time (Mohapatra *et al.*, 2020; Sah *et al.*, 2021). It attacked particularly human respiratory system making the respiratory organs dysfunctional (Mohapatra *et al.*, 2023[a]). It has affected sixty crores globally since the onset of the pandemic, with about seven million deaths.

COVID-19 pandemic gradually became a serious threat to human community (Mohapatra *et al.*, 2021). Vaccination prevents from critical life-threatening illnesses, restricting the need for hospitalisation (Panda *et al.*, 2022; Mohapatra *et al.*, 2022). Vaccination drives as preventives against smallpox, polio, hepatitis, etc. have been mandatory. Vaccines against COVID-19 were developed in record time in similar lines to protect against the disease, and simultaneously to limit the spread of COVID-19 among the close contacts like family, friends and co-workers (Mohapatra *et al.*, 2023[b]; Satapathy *et al.*, 2023; Sarangi *et al.*, 2024). A vaccine empowers the immune system to create interferons and antibodies for the protection against a disease. It assists in fighting against the disease, often providing a lifelong protection (Mohapatra *et al.*, 2024).

1.1. Vaccine Development - A Brief History

Although vaccination practices started over 500 years ago, the term 'vaccine' was first used by Edward Jenner in the 18th century. The term originates from the Latin word 'Vacca', meaning cow. The inoculation of Jenner's cowpox formulation in 1796 immunised against smallpox. Later, a live-attenuated vaccine against human rabies was successfully developed by Louis Pasteur. 'Germ theory' in the 19th century led to the development of first-generation vaccines against diphtheria and tetanus. Scaling-up of vaccine production process allowing virus cultivation methods beyond the lab advanced during the 1930s, and vaccines against influenza and yellow fever could be developed. The golden period of vaccine development began in the mid-20th century with the cell-culture based polio vaccine synthesis. Vaccines against mumps, varicella, rubella and measles also developed in this era. Whole-genome sequencing and the introduction of recombinant DNA later over the last century facilitated the development of new-age vaccines against numerous pathogens, marking a significant milestone in vaccine development. The rapid emerging COVID-19 in terms of infectivity and transmissibility that the world experienced during the recent pandemic led to the development of the fastest-ever vaccine against a virus in the history of vaccinology. Further, the pandemic witnessed medically sensitive situations like the breakthrough infections, and the emergence and re-emergence of variants, subvariants and sub-lineages.

1.2. The Persisting Pandemic as a Non-ending Malady – The New Normal

The COVID-19 pandemic has exposed the vulnerability of even the most advanced medical systems worldwide, highlighting their inability to manage high influx of critically ill patients. Healthcare infrastructure suspended non-urgent medical care and transformed regular wards into intensive care units (ICUs) or sub-ICUs in response to such emergencies. Accessing the characteristics of novel and imminent variants that might emerge generating an uphill task for the human healthcare set-up is certainly unpredictable. Efforts at the global scale significantly accelerated the development of defenses against SARS-CoV-2 in face of the pandemic's challenges. Until herd immunity developed, sustained public healthcare measures like hand-sanitising, using face-masks and avoiding public gatherings needed to be ensured.

1.3. AI-based Vaccine Development in the Post-Pandemic 'New Normal'

Apart from other societal aspects, managing the healthcare systems and addressing health emergencies is essential. Brought about by John McCarthy in 1956, AI empowers a computer system to perform routine task and reproduce human intelligence. Rapid AI evolution aimed at generating machines that could perform tasks that otherwise depended on the human stimuli. AI algorithms during an ongoing outbreak like COVID-19 could be implemented to overcome difficulties related to production, storage, transportation, and the safety and efficacy of the various vaccine candidates. It is also essential to analyse the clinical data-set bulk during such crises to facilitate prompt response of healthcare authority. AI could expeditiously analyse medical laboratory findings, therapies and case records, accelerate the decision-making process and enrich the patient management measures.

Blue Dot, a Toronto-based start-up utilised AI-enhanced surveillance system to predict pandemic outbreak early immediately after the initial detection before even the COVID-19 Wuhan emergency was declared (Allam *et al.*, 2020). Another AI-based company Metabiota employed similar strategy using big data analytics to monitor information about immigrants and emigrants on-flight, enabling to accurately predict potential outbreak several days in advance in nations like South Korea, Taiwan, Thailand and Japan even without officially-released documents (Sodhi *et al.*, 2022).

2. Fallouts of the COVID-19 Outbreak

COVID-19 brought on by coronavirus SARS-CoV-2 was declared a worldwide pandemic by WHO that affected millions of people and devastated the world. Being infectious in nature, Governments and health organisations imposed numerous measures like social distancing and lockdowns as immediate measures. This global health crisis significantly impacted public health, economies and the daily life. The outbreak promoted extensive research, vaccination campaigns and ongoing efforts to mitigate the adverse effects too.

2.1. The Global-Scale Multiple Waves and the Uncontrolled Deaths – The Reasons Behind

The COVID-19 pandemic death toll has been over 6.3 million worldwide (WHO, 2021). The reported global count of the cases has exceeded half a billion with millions unreported owing to various factors like inadequate testing, asymptomatic infections and challenges in seamless reporting. Due to the emerging and reemerging infections leading to pandemic waves all around with small lull periods, the war against COVID-19 remained quite intricate even with massive and aggressive preventive measures and vaccination drives that were followed.

Without good understandings about the viral epidemiology and biology initially, accurate monitoring of COVID-19 and evaluating its transmissibility were very difficulties. Having appropriate diagnostic kits to detect the virus was one of the initial significant obstacles. Some countries were forced to adopt existing platforms and technologies for mass testing to tackle this highly transmissive, infective and mutating virus, while others lacked the capacity. Erroneous assessments of the spread and the impact of the pandemic was the other challenge in developing global standards to certify COVID-19 as fatal. Excess mortality is the disparity in the number of deaths during a crisis and the number anticipated under normal situation (Msemburi *et al.*, 2023), which includes deaths linked to an aetiological agent and those that are the consequence of indirect effects like interrupted vital health service or mass migration. Thorough assessment of the overall effects of the COVID-19 pandemic associated deaths could be ensured by estimating the excess mortality.

2.2. The Transmission and Infection Patterns of SARS-COV-2

SARS-CoV-2 demonstrated high pathogenicity and broader host base as it infected numerous mammalian species including farmed mink and white-tailed deer (Bashor *et al.*, 2021). SARS-CoV-2 showed limited adaptation and phenotypic changes in humans in the initial months of its evolution that evolved further. Novel SARS-CoV-2 variants with high mutation rates, especially in the spike protein, emerged by October 2020. The variants like Omicron exhibited distinct phenotypes like altered transmissibility and antigenicity. It became evident later that SARS-CoV-2 utilised various mammalian angiotensin-converting enzyme 2 (ACE2) membrane proteins to adopt, evolve and invade the cell and infect wider array of mammals (MacLean *et al.*, 2021). An important factor in higher transmission of SARS-CoV-2 in humans is the FCS (furin cleavage site). Furin-mediated cleavage at the FCS allowed SARS-CoV-2 to penetrate the lungs cells and promote membrane fusion. Original Omicron variant was replaced with evolving variants like JN.1 and HV.1.1, linked to fresh waves (Fan *et al.*, 2024). With undetected recombinations till it surfaces, these variants with intrinsic biology and associated unique antigenic characteristics, these were significantly high on transmission that empowered the pandemic to spread to 'virgin' areas.

2.3. The Globally Encountered Strains, Variants and Subvariants

Coronavirus (CoVs) is the key contributor to common flu since the 60s. Seven of its strains infect humans that include human coronavirus (HCoV-HKU1, HCoV-OC43, HCoV-NL63 and HCoV-229E), severe acute respiratory syndrome coronavirus (SARS-CoV), Middle East respiratory syndrome coronavirus (MERS-CoV) and the coronavirus (2019-nCoV) witnessed recently. Of these, four CoVs strains, HCoV-HKU1, HCoV-OC43, HCoV-NL63 and HCoV-229E cause severe infections. HCoV-229E, isolated from the nasal secretions of healthcare professionals, is the earliest one to be discovered. Contributing to about 30% of all flus, it causes mild upper respiratory tract infection. Serum examination of the subjects revealed that HCoV-229E, HCoV-NL63 and HCoV-OC43 were common in children and HCoV-HKU1 among the adults. Viral RNA of HCoV-229E and HCoV-OC43 are also detected in the brain cells of certain patients, causing severe infection in the central nervous system (CNS). SARS-CoV and MERS-CoV, in contrast, are more lethal causing severe pneumonia, organ failure and even death among the infected.

SARS-CoV started re-spreading through human-human contact in 2002 in Guandong, China and Palm civets were found as the intermediate host, which continued till august 2003. As the Chinese horseshoe bat was identified as the natural source of SARS-CoV in Yunnan, China, a potential resumption of the viral infection was suspected. A decade later, the first MERS-CoV patient was identified in Saudi Arabia in June 2012, and Dromedary camels were the host. There were 2495 confirmed cases of the same by 26 December 2019, with 858 deaths (Tai *et al.*, 2017). MERS-CoV infection kept on increasing with restricted contact spread, yet there was no trace of SARS-CoV infection between 2004 and 2019. SARS-CoV-2 novel coronavirus, allegedly originating from Wuhan, China, sparked an outbreak in December 2019 that spread globally. Similar to SARS-CoV, it spread person to person although researchers are investigating for intermediate hosts (Zhou *et al.*, 2020).

3. SARS-COV-2 and Its Pathogenic Variants

International Committee on Taxonomy of Virus (ICTV) classified Corona Viruses (CoVs) in the subfamily Orthocoronavirinae which is a part of Coronaviridae family and comes under order Nidovirales in the 10th report on viruses (Lefkowitz *et al.*, 2018). The four genera under Orthocoronavirinae affect different organisms. *a* and *b* CoVs affect mammals (human, bat, pig and mice), and γ and δ CoVs usually target birds although some cases of mammals being infected are reported (Wang *et al.*, 2020; Woo *et al.*, 2012; Woo *et al.*, 2014). The WHO declared Lambda (C.37), Mu (B.1.621), Epsilon (B.1.427, B.1.429), Kappa (B.1.617.1), Eta (B.1.525), Lota (B.1.526) and Zeta (P2) strains as variants of interest (VoI), apart from variants of concern (VoCs) (Souza *et al.*, 2022).

3.1. Structure of SARS-CoV-2

Metagenome sequencing detected that the genome of novel SARS-CoV-2 virus was about 79% similar with SARS-CoV and about 51.8% with MERS-CoV (Abulsoud *et al.*, 2023). The about 9–12 nm crown-like projections of the virus justify its name Coronavirus (crown-like projections), seen microscopically (Fig. 1).

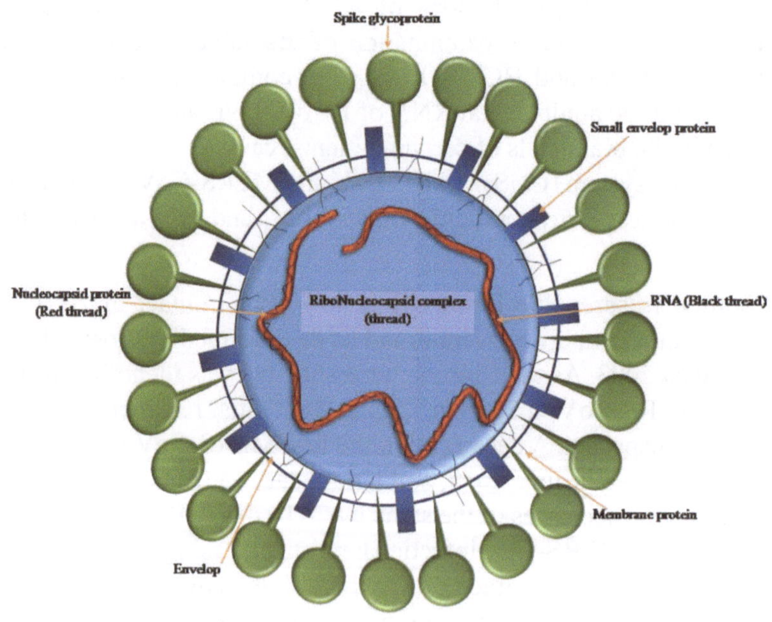

Fig. 1: Detailed structure with ssRNA, structural and non-structural and accessory proteins of the SARS CoV-2 virus

3.1.1. Organisation of the Nucleus

The largest (30 kb) RNA genome with positive-sense RNA strand and approximately 30% adenine, 18% cytosine, 20% guanine and 32% thymine are enveloped by the nucleocapsid of the virion (Zehra *et al.*, 2020). A 5' end and a 3' end encompass the genome with 11 Open reading frames (ORFs) encoding 27 proteins functioning as mRNA to translate replicase polyproteins. The major ORF1/ab constitutes approximately 70% of the genome from the 5' end coding for the replicase complex polyproteins like pp1a having 4405 amino acids or pp1ab with 7096 amino acids, depending on occurring ribosomal frameshifts (Abulsoud *et al.*, 2023). The 5' end has an untranslated region (UTR) and a leader sequence containing multiple stem-loop structures crucial for replication and transcription. The 3' UTR also has RNA structures required for viral RNA replication and synthesis. The organisation of the Coronavirus genome follows the pattern of 5'-leader-UTR-replicase-S (Spike)-E (Envelope)-M (Membrane)-N (Nucleocapsid)-3'UTR poly(A) tail, with accessory genes interspersed within structural genes at the 3' end (Khadse *et al.*, 2020). Additionally, ORFs 3a, 6, 7a, 7b, 8 and 10 encode the accessory and structural (membrane, nucleocapsid, spike and envelope) proteins (Abulsoud *et al.*, 2023).

3.1.2. Structural Protein

Structural proteins of SARS-COV-2 include nucleocapsid, spike, envelope and membrane proteins, which give the virus its pathogenic teeth.

3.1.2.1. Nucleocapsid Protein

Nucleocapsid forms ribonucleoprotein (RNP) in Coronavirus, a long helical nucleocapsid (Zhao *et al.*, 2009). The proteins help release viral genome to the ER-Golgi intermediate compartment (ERGIC) wherein these mature into virion with other structural proteins. The RNP complex maintains the stability of RNA confirmation that is necessary in the viral genome transcription, regulates cytoskeleton reorganisation and host cell apoptosis. Due to their immunogenic phosphoprotein, these also induce protective immune responses (McBride *et al.*, 2014).

3.1.2.2. Spike Protein

The crucial viral entry step depends on the presence of the largest trans-membrane spike protein mainly with three parts i) ectodomain (ED) region, ii) transmembrane (TM) region and iii) intracellular (IC) domain, comprising the intracellular tail region (Duquerroy *et al.*, 2005). The spike protein possesses two domains, S1 and S2 trimeric stalks, both being the main cause of viral infection. S1 with receptor binding domain (RBD) initiates the primary phase of infection by binding to the host cell receptor and S2 helps in the fusion of cellular and viral membranes. The cellular protease Furin activates the S-protein by cleaving S1 and S2 domains that finally enters the lungs cell (Du *et al.*, 2009). The spike protein mediates the infection process that neutralises antibody and the T-cell response (Prajapat *et al.*, 2020).

3.1.2.3. Envelope Protein

Envelope protein is the smallest membrane protein where the transmembrane hydrophobic domain tilts to the membrane. Amphipathic charged cytoplasmic tail moves freely around. Envelop protein found near the host's ERGIC primarily deforms membranes and facilitates viral budding (Kuzmin *et al.*, 2022). The proteins act as ion channel (Vivoporin) by forming pentamers useful in protein trafficking (Schoeman *et al.*, 2019).

3.1.2.4. Membrane Protein

Viral membrane spans thrice with three transmembrane helices, TMH1, TMH2 and TMH3 along with a N-terminal ectodomain and a C-terminal endodomain (Mahtarin *et al.*, 2020). It is the most abundant viral protein to maintain host homeostasis (Wang and Liu, 2016). The membrane protein dimer has a role in genome packaging, viral assembly and morphogenesis (Zhang *et al.*, 2022).

3.1.3. Non-structural Protein

The replicase encodes 16 non-structural proteins (nsps) distributed between two polyproteins pp1 and pp1ab. Chymotrypsin-like cysteine protease (3CLpro) and Papain-like protease (Plpro) are the two cysteine proteases that act on the polyproteins to release 16 nsps by respectively slicing the N-terminal and the C-terminal (Islam *et al.*, 2023).

3.1.4. Accessory Proteins

The accessory proteins include nsp13, nsp12, nsp14, nsp15, nsp16, nsp10, haemagglutin esterase (HE) and transmembrane protease serine 2 (TMPRSS 2) (Zehra *et al.*, 2020).

3.2. The Aetiology of the Infection

SARS-CoV-2 primarily spreads through respiratory droplets infecting the nasal tract initially and progresses to the lungs. It shows symptoms ranging from mild respiratory complications to pneumonia. The virus reaches the lungs using the pulmonary ACE2 receptor to invade the lung epithelium when immune response is inadequate. Other than the pulmonary cells, the ACE2 receptor is found in various other cells like cardiac, renal, intestinal, pancreatic and endothelial cells, which creates critical conditions in case of comorbidities (Dai and Gao, 2021).

The ACE2 receptor on the surface of SARS-CoV-2 spike protein is bound specifically to S1 subunit receptor binding domain (RBD). The S2 transmembrane domain comprising repeated heptapeptide regions and fusion peptides undergoes conformational rearrangement by the host cell's serine protease TMPRSS2, which initiates viral fusion with host cell membrane. The process is facilitated by the host cysteine proteases B (CatB) and L (CatL) cathepsins. Furin at the boundary of S1–S2 cleaves and triggers the infection. SARS-CoV-2 finally invades host cell by endocytosis and fuse at low pH by S cleavage of endosomal proteins.

The N protein of SARS-CoV-2 entering the host cell dissociates from the positive (+) RNA strand and initiates viral gene replication and expression (Fig. 2). Antiviral immune defence and RNA interference (RNAi) of the host is inhibited by the N protein that prevents the viral genome recognition and cleavage. After protease cleavage, ORF1a and ORF1b translate from the positive (+) RNA strand to polyproteins and produce non-structural proteins. The non-structural protein (NSP)-1 shuts down the host translation, NSP2-11 modulates intracellular environment and the core enzymes of NSP12-16 participate in transcription. The viral replication-transcriptional complex (RTC) containing the NSP2-16 and N protein forms replicating organelles and attach to ER. The positive (+) RNA strand is encapsulated by the N protein and assembles with structural proteins S, M and E within the ERGIC. The viral RNA replicates in double-membrane vesicles (DMVs). Ultimately, either the lysosomal transport or exocytosis releases new virions. The N protein alters the interaction, host cell cycle and cell death, and is pivotal in integrating viral RNA (Wu *et al.*, 2023).

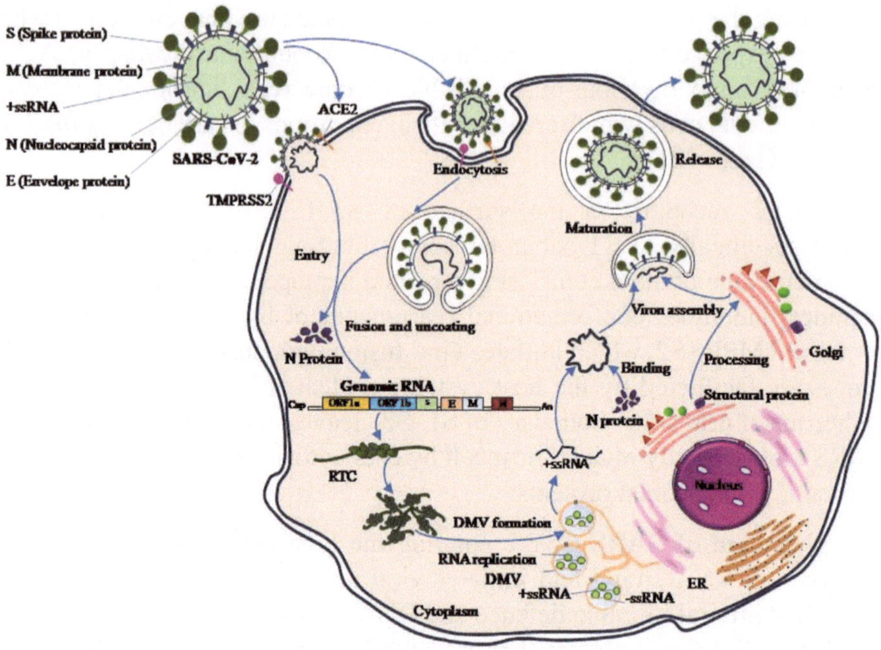

Fig. 2: Life cycle of the SARS-CoV-2 virus within the cell of a human host

3.3. Viral Strains (Involving Variants and Sub-Variants) with Increasing Virulence

The COVID pandemic created the greatest health emergency since the WW-II and constantly affects the mankind with its vigorously mutating strains and variants which almost has left no place on earth without infections. SARS-CoV-2 evolved in to variant strains with increased transmissibility and infectivity. Although numerous viral strains are discovered till date, the prominent pandemic-causing strains as recognised by the WHO are the Alpha (B.1.1.7), Beta (B.1.351), Gamma (P.1), Delta (B.1.617.2) and Omicron (B.1.1.529) strains and their mutating variants (Telenti *et al.*, 2022). The major infectious forms till October 2020 were the alpha, beta and gamma strains, the gamma strain having better fusion ability to host, which were replaced by delta strain. The reason for this is the mutated P681R spike protein of delta strain. It was declared as the variant of concern (VoC) on 11 May 2021 by the WHO (Pal and Yadav 2022). Soon, it was replaced by a new Omicron variant as confirmed by the WHO on 24 November 2021. This strain was more pathogenic, had better immune escape mechanism and induced asymptomatic/ mild infection that made transmission control ever more challenging. It was declared as the variant of concern (VoC) just two days after it was detected in South Africa (Jansen *et al.*, 2021).

Even after mass vaccination drives, infections of COVID-19 and its variants and sub-variants still linger. The most dominating variants were H.V1, JN.1 and EG.5 by December 2023 with respectively 29.6%, 21.4% and 8.8% registered cases. Mutated subvariants EG.5, XBB.1.16.6 and XBB.1.16.11 of the original Omicron strain currently circulate globally (Gong *et al.*, 2023).

3.4. SARS-COV-2 Mutation and The Evolving Strains – the Molecular Differentiation

The primary reason behind such large genome variations in the coronavirus (COVs) is the frequent mutation of the various protein coding genes, mostly the spike proteins responsible to cause infection. It was discovered lately that SARS-CoV-2 infection was similar to the seasonal flu but outbreaks for longer duration accumulated mutations of viral genome with immunological significance (Sehra *et al.*, 2020).

SD614G mutation stabilises and densifies the S-protein through close interaction between S1 and S2 subunits and decreases S1 shedding, which increases the infectivity and transmissivity (Plante *et al.*, 2020).

3.4.1. The Alpha Strain

The evolved Alpha strain has 17 mutations with eight spike mutations and two deletions in the S-protein at N-terminal domain (NTD) region with low viral load and short exposure. The deletion includes 69-70 del (6 bases coding for His and Val) and 144 del (coding for Tyr), both of which induce host immunity escape. The former increases S-protein affinity for AEC2 receptor and the latter alters the NDT-loop that reduce the neutralisation capacity of NDT specific neutralising antibodies (Rees-Spear *et al.*, 2021; Hu *et al.*, 2021).

Substituting asparagine to tyrosine at 501st position of the viral S gene, a N501Y mutation forms a portion of the binding loop at the hACE2 region. It also stabilises K353, a viral binding hotspot residue in the hACE2 region that reduces neutralisation by antibodies. This mutation is seen in Beta and Gamma strains too (Kannan *et al.*, 2021).

Mutations like T7161, S982A and D118H, and the replacement of Alanine by Aspartate at 570 also are found in the Alpha variant whose function is ambiguous. The replacement of Proline by Arginine enhances the furin protease activity (Meng *et al.*, 2021)

3.4.2. The Beta Strain

The Beta lineage strains like K417N, E484K and N501Y have evolved through critically mutated receptor binding domain (RBD). E484 position is an important immunodominant residue and triggers the immune response but an uncommon E484K mutation helps the virus escape antibodies in covalent plasma, as also escaping two monoclonal antibodies REGN10989 and REGN10934 (Weisblum *et al.*, 2020). K417N and N501Y mutations alter antibody binding and reduce the binding phase of the S protein with ACE2 receptor (Baum *et al.*, 2020). The three mutations, if happened together, could reduce neutralisation process by two to three-folds and increase the fitness of Beta strain (Wang *et al.*, 2021). Non-synonymous mutations like D614G, A701Y, D215G, L18F, R246I and D80A in the spike proteins are also present along with two deletions at the NDT region (Gupta *et al.*, 2020).

3.4.3. The Gamma Strain

Due to a total of 37 mutations (including 10 synonymous, 22 missense, one frameshift and three intergenic) in this evolved variant, the Gamma strain is highly virulent even against a vaccinated individual. The mutations exclusively found in the Gamma strain are T20N, P26S, D138Y, R190S, H655Y, H655Y and T1027I. The T20N, P26S, D138Y and R190S mutations are of NDT-supersite region targeted by the antibodies with higher neutralising power. The T20N mutation is formed at N (glycosylation) site which safeguards against antibodies (Du *et al.*, 2021). H655Y mutation is nearer to the furin site and T1027I mutation occurs between HR1 and HR2 sites. These apart, K417, E48K and N501Y mutations are commonly encountered in Alpha, Beta and Gamma strains (Nonaka *et al.*, 2021).

3.4.4. The Delta Strain

Popular as the Indian strain, mutation in the delta strain is at its NDT region that processes the S protein cleavage before contacting the host cell. This increases its infectivity and helps escape the host immunity. Its RBD-region mutation enhances the binding stability. The major development in the Delta strain is the P681R mutation adjacent to the cleavage site that enhances the infection rate three-folds compared to other variants (Callaway *et al.*, 2021[a]). Also, the Delta strain lacks the N501Y that reduces the affinity of RBD to the ACE receptor to certain extent. Rather it has L452R and T478K mutation that allow escaping monoclonal antibodies without reducing the affinity towards RBD receptors (Barnes *et al.*, 2020). Anti-NDT neutralising antibodies target several mutations in the NDT region covering the NDT supersite, including

T19R, T95I, delE156-, delF157-, V70F, R158G, A222V, G142D and W258L (Garcia-Beltran *et al.*, 2021). Non-synonymous mutations in the NDT supersite, like T19R at the N1 site, V70F at the N2 area, G142D and delE156 at the N3 region, and A222V and W258L at the N5 region, alter the structure and reduce the neutralising effect of anti-NDT antibodies.

3.4.5. The Omicron Strain

This variant originated with over fifty mutations of which thirty are on the spike protein only. It developed a completely new spike protein with one insertion at 214 positions at the NDT region acquired from the infected host and three deletions. Mutations like del211, substitution of L212I and ins214EPF at the NDT region helped the variant to easily escape host immunity (McCarthy *et al.*, 2021). The E484A overtook the E484K mutation which helped the virus to escape the 2B04 and 1B07 monoclonal antibodies (Callaway *et al.*, 2021[b]). RBD mutations involved N440K, G446S, S477N, T478K, E484A and Q498R, through which it escaped the anti-RBD neutralising antibodies. Q4 substitution and Q493R/K mutation helped the variant to resist monoclonal antibodies like REGN10989/10934, LY-CoV555 and LY-CoV016 (Starr *et al.*, 2021). These apart, S477N, N501Y, P681H and N679K mutations encouraged high transmissibility of the variant.

4. Strategies to Develop Novel Nest-gen COVID-19 Vaccines

With the power of mutation, SARS-COV-2 exhibited its pathogenicity with the most lethal pandemic that the world had ever witnessed in its spread, intensity and duration. Although vaccines against only the known variants in the current scenario have been developed for emergency use only, the need for a multi-utility next-gen vaccine to counter the mutating and ever-evolving viral form is felt to completely eradicate the malady (Fig. 3).

4.1. Whole Virus Cell as a Candidate for Vaccine Development (The Covaxine Approach)

Inactivated vaccines are conventionally used to protect against deadly diseases like smallpox, polio, rabies, etc. by eliciting greater immunological response. Inactivated vaccines provide substantial epitope coverage reducing the susceptibility to invasion by the emerging variants. Bharat Biotech, India developed BBV152 (Covaxin), the whole virion inactivated Corona virus antigen, indigenously to counter the pandemic (Ahmed *et al.*, 2022). Alhydroxiquim-II was used as a vaccine adjuvant in conjunction to boost the immune response and its shelf-life, with 81% efficacy (Darbar *et al.*, 2021). The experience gained from the formalin-inactivated whole influenza vaccine development helped to develop the whole-cell vaccine against the SARS-CoV-2 on war-footing, within the stipulated time. Two-step inactivation process that used formaldehyde and ultraviolet radiation applications sequentially was used to develop the attenuated virus confirmed the safety of the residual virus for vaccine development.

A Felin Coronavirus used as a vaccine to induce antibodies in the infected opened the way to develop the same for SARS-CoV-2. FIPV (feline infectious peritonitis viruses) inhibitors like Dyphillin, Chloroquine, Hydroxychloroquine, Mefloquine, Itraconazole, GS-441524 and GC376 restricted the growth of SARS CoV-2 (Delaplace *et al.*, 2021) which could be used in vaccine development.

4.2. Potential Target Proteins in Vaccine Development

Approaches like recombinant proteins, DNA and RNA-based vaccinations, vaccines vectored by viruses, inactivated viruses, and particles that resemble viruses are adopted (Soraci *et al.*, 2022). Proteins encoded by S, M, and N genes along with the S-protein by mRNA-1273 and BNT162 are used to develop nucleotide-based vaccines. While S protein induces T-cell response, N protein is targeted for humoral response to secrete antibodies, and the E and M protein induce T-CD_4^+ epitopes (Baghban *et al.*, 2023). The subunit vaccine used spike glycoproteins (S), membrane protein (M) and nucleoproteins (N) as the target. Attenuated vaccines used non-structural proteins (nsp) produced by deleting some essential (S, N and E) genes. Vectored vaccines, protein-based vaccines and mRNA vaccines have all demonstrated significant effectiveness in protecting against COVID-19 (Pandey *et al.*, 2020).

4.3. Antigen Designing for mRNA-based COVID Vaccine (the Covishield Approach)

Being a foreign particle to human body, antigen could be used as a vaccine target. On this principle, the Oxford University collaborated with the British-Swedish-based AstraZeneca to develop the AZD1222 Coronavirus (Covishield) vaccine, with 76% efficacy. They used a modified chimp adenovirus variant ChAdOx1 (Folegatti *et al.*, 2020) that entered the cells but did not multiply there, which stored genetic information in double-stranded instead of single-stranded RNA. While stored, strong adenovirus protein coat protected the genetic material. The genetic material of the non-replicable adenovirus is pushed into the host's nucleus after it invades the host cell, reads the Coronavirus spike protein gene and copies it into the mRNA, which takes over the control machinery of the host cell and generates spike protein. The spike protein fragments were picked up by antigen-presenting cells (APCs) as the infected cell ruptured, and generated humoral response (Patil *et al.*, 2023).

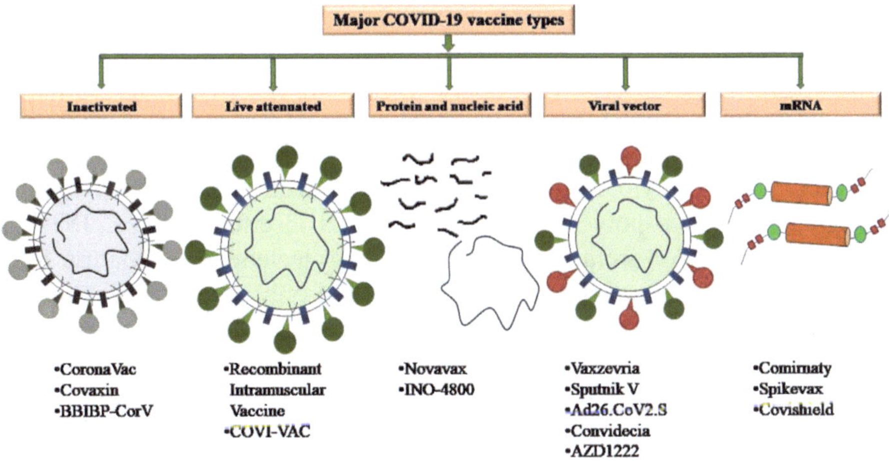

Fig. 3: Illustration of the various strategies to develop COVID-19 vaccines

4.4. mRNA Structure, the Nucleotide Modification and the Nanocarrier-Delivery

With basic and cost-effective production, gradual degradation in the target cell and its safety advantages over DNA therapeutics, mRNA is in use for vaccine production since 1990. It is safe against insertional mutagenesis, as mRNA does not integrate into the human genome like the DNA, and translates into cytoplasmic proteins with ease (Karam *et al.*, 2022). Liposome-encased mRNA vaccine based on nucleoprotein using *in vitro* transcription was generated to successfully induce both cytotoxic T-cells and antibodies *in vivo* to treat influenza (Hoerr *et al.*, 2000). RNA-based vaccines primarily altered the immune cell function by orchestrating ribosomal translation, ultimately triggering the immune response.

As the benefits of first-generation mRNA vaccines unfolded, mRNA-based technology is gaining increasing popularity at the global scale. Clinical research on mRNA vaccines against the infectious diseases dramatically increased consequently. Experts opine that the mRNA platforms shall increasingly be sought for a range of therapeutic purposes. Pfizer-BioNTech vaccine used lipid nanoparticle-encapsulated nucleoside-modified mRNAs. Two proline mutations encoding the SARS-CoV-2 spike protein are added to the mRNA to keep it steady in the prefusion configuration (Walsh *et al.*, 2020). Novel vaccines to augment its stability and translational efficacy due to the intrinsic instability of RNA have been designed.

4.5. mRNA Vaccine-Induced Cellular and Humoral Immune Responses

Human body triggers cellular and humoral immune responses against foreign substances for sustenance. Proteins produced within the body as the injected transcribed mRNA expresses generate the immune responses. It is the fundamental basis of mRNA vaccine development. The generation of the immune response follows usually involve four steps: The antigen is encoded in the DNA format and the host machinery transcribes and translates to generate the protein in the cytoplasm → The transcribed mRNA stabilises through 5'-capping and a 3'-poly-A tailing → 5' cap is inserted to the COVID-19 BNT162b1 mRNA vaccine through 'clean cap' technique → Mature RNA is protected from degradation by 5' cap, and the poly-A tail ensures mRNA stability, translation and transport (Jeeva *et al.*, 2021). Overstimulated immune system triggers allergic reactions and anaphylactic shock. The third step above is consolidated and the nucleobase is modified to avoid it. N1-methylpseudouridin, a modified nucleobase, increases the protein yield and decreases TLR3 activation. Modification by RIG-1 also decreases signal differentiation capacity of mRNAs (Nance and Meier, 2021). A multilamellar vesicular lipid nanoparticle (homogenous nano core-shell for mRNA delivery) structure as a carrier enhances vaccine stability and targeting (Schoenmaker *et al.*, 2021).

4.6. Other Vaccine Development Approaches (Gene Silencing by Moderna)

The WHO granted mRNA-1273 (Moderna COVID-19 vaccine) for emergency use. It is a liquid nanoparticle encapsulated mRNA vaccine having mRNA core encoding for the spike protein. The liquid nanoparticle helps intra-muscular invasion of mRNA which subsequently enters the cytosol. The translation process within the ribosome generates the S-protein to which the host immune system reacts and develops the immunity. This mRNA-1273 vaccine reportedly exhibited 94.1% efficacy (Shabu and Nishtala, 2023).

Most vaccines like that of Pfizer-BioNTech and AstraZeneca utilised RNA and DNA-based viral vectors taking advantage of the next-gen platforms. Sinopharm vaccine, in contrast, used conventional technology, employing an inactivated virus. The attenuation involved the mixing of β-propionolactone using the extracted viral solution. The final vaccine formulation used aluminum hydroxide as an adjuvant (Imrie *et al.*, 2018). Table 1 lists the major COVID-19 vaccines developed around the world.

Table 1: A list of the various vaccines developed against COVID-19 throughout the globe

Vaccine name	Country of origin	Year approved	The viral component
Covovax	Serum Institute of India Pvt Ltd, India	2021	Recombinant spike protein (rS) with nanoparticle
SKYCovione	SK Bioscience Co., Ltd., Republic of Korea	2023	Recombinant protein subunit
Nuvaxovid	Novavax CZ a.s.	2021	Recombinant spike protein (rS) with adjuvant
Spikevax	Spain	2021	Nucleoside modified
Comirnaty Original/Omicron	Pfizer BioNTech Manufacturing GmbH, Germany	2020	mRNA
Convidecia	CanSino Biologics Inc., People's Republic of China	2022	Non-replicating viral vector
Vaxzevria	AstraZeneca AB, Sweden	2021	Non-replicating viral vector
Jcovden	Janssen–Cilag International NV, Belgium	2021	Non-replicating viral vector
Covishield	Serum Institute of India Pvt. Ltd, India	2021	Non-replicating viral vector
Covaxin	Bharat Biotech International Ltd, India	2021	Inactivated virus
Covilo	Sinopharm (Beijing), People's Republic of China	2021	Inactivated virus
CoronaVac	Sinovac Life Sciences Co., Ltd., People's Republic of China	2021	Inactivated virus
Corbevax	Biological E. Ltd, India	2024	Protein subunit
ZyCoV-D	Cadila Healthcare Limited, India	2021	Plasmid DNA with gene for S-protein
GEMCOVAC-19	Gennova Biopharmaceuticals Limited, India	2023	RNA
Spikevax	Moderna	2021	mRNA
iNCOVACC	Bharat Biotech	2022	Non-replicating viral vector
Sputnik V	Gamaleya	2020	Non-replicating viral vector
Sputnik Light	Gamaleya	2021	Non-replicating viral vector
HGCO19	Gennova Biopharmaceuticals Limited	2021	RNA
Noora vaccine	Bagheiat-allah University of Medical Sciences	2022	Protein subunit
Ad26.COV2.S	Janssen Pharmaceutical Companies and Johnson & Johnson	2021	Recombinant spike (rS) protein
BBIBP-CorV	Sinopharm, People's Republic of China	2021	Inactivated, produced in vero cells

5. Application of AI in Vaccine Development

AI has the capacity to optimise and hasten the process of vaccine development and its distribution at an unparalleled speed and accuracy. It enhances and automatises large subsections of the vaccine development processes simultaneously, that primarily include assisted data gathering to identify the target, optimising the clinical trials and integrating the real-world data by utilising enhanced data analysis, predictive modelling and bioinformatics. AI could predict antigenic epitopes during vaccine development itself, and optimise the overall vaccine design. AI accelerates the process by rapidly analysing the large datasets, assisting in identifying the promising target and expediting the overall vaccine development timeline.

5.1. AI-assisted Data Gathering Through Social Media

The traditional vaccine development approach largely relied on manually collecting and the analysing the data, which has numerous limitations. Also, it is often very expensive, time-consuming and laborious, where millions of small-scale repetitive data-gathering techniques are used that has larger propensity to generate mistakes and anomalies that ultimately affects the overall development of an effective vaccine, resulting in time overrun of several years to develop a particular strain-specific vaccine. It could drag vaccine development significantly. A particular advantage that AI-assisted data gathering with minimal human interference provides is data quality. Machine learning (ML) technique was employed to analyse the data during the initial COVID-19 vaccine development and the results were obtained in 22 hours (Basheeruddin Asdaq *et al.*, 2022). Demonstrating their dexterity, versatility and reliability in giving valuable insights that contribute to improving health policy and management, the use of predictive computing tools is rising. AI researchers employ advanced ML techniques (like deep learning) to gather data from social media conversations of individuals discussing their fever and respiratory distress symptoms. AI algorithms can effectively combine the data by harmonising the data from social media platforms, public health organisations and electronic health records. It allows identify subtle signs of the spread of the disease and facilitates its tracking (Bobdey and Ray 2020).

Electronic media and online platforms like Facebook, Twitter, YouTube and Instagram could be extremely important in distributing pandemic-related information. Despite variations in quality and sources, information from these platforms and the internet is readily accessible in less time. Collection and processing of these data allow an in-depth analysis. As a potent tool to handle extensive data, AI is used to enhance the understanding of social network dynamics and help address the situational difficulties during COVID-19 (Ganasegeran and Abdulrahman 2020). So, incorporating AI-assistance in gathering data across social media platforms as a predictive tool to analyse the trends to target and predict the spread of a pandemic like COVID-19 remains a largely unexplored domain that the mankind may benefit from.

5.2. Predicting the Pandemic Waves

AI-based algorithms increasingly demonstrate growing trends in predicting the outcome better using the available health data. It progressively contributes to enhanced anticipation of disease outbreaks. Research trend in this increased tremendously during the pandemic as noticed through a spike in the PubMed query keywords like 'artificial intelligence', 'machine learning', 'deep learning' and 'disease surveillance'. Computational techniques to forecast the connection between the human immune system and the vaccine enhances the accuracy of the developed vaccine. AI-propelled biosensors could detect biological substances to address COVID-19 issues.

Multiple major developed economies deployed mobile and web-server-based applications that relied heavily on predictive analysis techniques and collaborative data sharing with external data servers to provide real-time data on the pandemic that included information like COVID-19 risk assessment tests, COVID-19 symptoms, Government initiatives or directives, nearby COVID-19 suspect or quarantine zone, nearest available ICU, high risk and low-risk areas based on pandemic proliferation, efficient slot booking at the nearest vaccination centre with comprehensive display of availability of particular vaccines and provisions for effective vaccination, certificate distribution and sharing. Diverse tools like audio and video messages and chatbots were deployed within such applications to monitor the infected individuals. COVID Safe in Australia, Aarogyasetu in India and COVIDALERT in Canada are a few such smart-phone applications. Patients with COVID-19 symptoms in Taiwan were made more comfortable by redirecting from packed rooms to quarantine tents through the Smart-phone Quarantine Station and the AI trio (Liu *et al.*, 2020).

COVID-19 era witnessed increased number of AI-based software-as-a-service companies that targeted bioinformatics in healthcare system. One such software-as-a-service company is BlueDot which uses its flagship product Insights, a SAAS Product to map the transmission of contagious illnesses. It is developed as a tool to model transport networks that is expanded to incorporate open-source intelligence and clustering tools to identify the potential hotspots of infectious disease outbreaks. The company allegedly was the first to send alerts to customers through the usage of data on airline tickets to precisely forecast the spread of the virus across four major cities (Bangkok, Seoul, Taipei and Tokyo). Accessible on payment bases, it employs both AI and human moderation supporting multi-languages using closed-source government and client data (MacIntyre *et al.*, 2023). BlueDot was able to identify eight out of the first ten cities to import novel Coronavirus by analysing the international flight tickets and predicted the occurrence in those places months ahead of time. BlueDot identified Brazil and India as possible epicentres in its regular focus reports. Receiving significant coverage during COVID-19 through collaborations with multiple governments to access closed data for public safety it was the first to release a COVID-19 scientific publication (Goldust *et al.*, 2023).

Metabiota, a risk analytic software start-up company, contributed significantly to data mapping. The publicly accessible the Metabiota epidemic tracker shows a heat map showing the epidemics epicentres for 208 diseases. The serviced extends beyond the effects of illness by generating diverse Pathogen Sentiment Indices important for travel agencies and insurance firms. Metabiota uses big data and cloud computing to provide a legitimate library through peer-review process with a variety of disease models and a sizable number of simulated events for risk analysis and informed planning (Goldust *et al.*, 2023). EPIWATCH, an AI-driven open-source data analysis platform, analyses the information from various sources to detect patterns and trends indicating emerging health threats. It serves as an early warning system to facilitate early responses and interventions regarding potential epidemics (Goldust *et al.*, 2023). Apart from these, ProMED-mail, HealthMap, Epidemic Intelligence from Open Sources (EIOS), Global Biosurveillance Portal (GBSP) and Epitweetr are other significant IT-enabled intelligence systems active in the healthcare sector for similar data mapping purposes (Goldust *et al.*, 2023).

5.3. Recent Trends in AI-based Data Interpretation

Along with traditional wet-lab methods, network-based computational model simulation is a prominent approach to unravel the complex virus–host interactions (Messina *et al.*, 2020). Recent application of AI in addressing the obstacles in COVID-19 is a multifaceted approach, focusing primarily on virtual screening for vaccine development and drug repurposing. The major intent of drug repurposing and vaccine development using AI is to predict quickly and use the interconnected biological pathways of existing medications with their known safety profiles to optimise fresh clinical trials.

AI-based approaches interpret existing medications, screen targets for vaccines and identify suitable vaccine adjuvants, thus, enabling vaccine discovery against novel variants (Ghosh *et al.*, 2023). PolypharmDB by Cyclica is an outstanding case of collective power of AI in exploring and discovering drugs. This cutting-edge software is a deep learning-based resource that acts as a platform, offering details about established medications and their expected bindings to targets for drug repurposing, and also assisting vaccine development by identifying the target. Pfizer is transitioning to AI-incorporation to deduce purposeful information from the millions of datasets (Basheeruddin Asdaq *et al.*, 2022).

5.4. AI-driven Epitope/Target Prediction

AI-based genome analysis identifies potential vaccine targets (antigens) more efficiently than the conventional manual approach. It helps researchers to prioritise the candidates that are most promising to investigate further. Epitopes recognised by the host immune system could play a significant role in designing specific vaccine target. Numerous AI-based techniques have been used since the emergence of the first Coronavirus to anticipate possible epitopes to formulate vaccine (Ton *et al.*, 2020). Fast *et al.*, (2020) used two supervised neural network-driven methods, MARIA (Guan *et al.*, 2020) and NetMHCPan4 (Jurtz *et al.*, 2017) to find possible SARS-CoV2 T-cell epitopes nearer to the 2019-nCoV spike receptor-binding domain (RBD).

Long Short-Term Memory (LSTM) network has also shown encouraging outcomes. Spike protein epitopes are predicted using the Recurrent Neural Network (RNN). Similarly, deep-learning RNN is used to generate spike protein simulation sequences and pinpoint possible targets to develop vaccines. The sequences produced by RNN having high sequence identity to BLAST could be a protein candidate of interest. iNeo tool is a unique method to create a vaccine that has T-cell and B-cell epitopes. The discovered 17 vaccine peptides targeting both the immune cells in multi-peptide vaccine uniquely protects against SARS-CoV-2 (Rangan *et al.*, 2020). Nsp3 is the largest non-structural protein of the coronavirus family that was found to be the most attractive target candidate for vaccine development, after the spike protein. Vaxign-RV selects non-structural proteins as targets for SARS-CoV-2 vaccine (Ong *et al.*, 2020). Malone *et al.* (2020) analysed the whole SARS-CoV-2 proteome thoroughly beyond the spike to provide a comprehensive guide to develop vaccines. They used the NEC Immune Profiler, Immune Epitope Database (IEDB) and BepiPred tools to construct an epitope map for various HLA alleles.

Deep Learning (DL)-based virtual screening of primary protease of SARS-CoV-2 is a notable example of the role of AI in combating COVID-19 pandemic. These efforts included sharing the newly predicted chemical structures transparently, reflecting a collaborative and open approach to address the pandemic (Bung *et al.*, 2021; Zhang *et al.*, 2020). Structural analysis using AI-powered tools to predict the 3D structure of proteins and their interactions with the immune system enabled researchers to design vaccines that targeted the weaknesses of the pathogen. Machine Learning (ML)-based molecular docking has emerged as a pivotal and versatile virtual screening approach.

The intricate high-powered computerised process involved a comprehensive dataset comprising of approved molecules, a molecular docking program, homology model or crystal structure of the target (Pagadala *et al.*, 2017). The viral replication and infection targets include a multitude of molecules with potential functions that span to numerous SARS-CoV-2 proteins, like PLpro, RdRP, spike protein and ACE2 receptor in the host, and TMPRSS2 protease in the virus (Choudhary *et al.*, 2020; Kong *et al.*, 2020). Deep Docking (DD) network technology approach identifies thousands of potential protease inhibitors. It is crucial to highlight that the model training involved applying Quantitative Structure-Activity Relationship (QSAR) without novel docking. While the approach demonstrated substantial progress, it lacked unique docking score (Ton *et al.*, 2020). Following are some approaches in Artificial Neural Network (ANN)-based viral host prediction:

- k1 time-steps of certain viral sequence are processed using truncated back propagation through time (TBPTT) algorithm that reduces error in the expected output for a given input.
- Recurrent Neural Networks (RNNs): Viral host traits are predicted by repeatedly training the RNNs. While building the neural network, nearest neighbours are obtained.
- Convolutional Neural Networks (CNNs): The predicted viral mutation is analysed using CNNs. It can also be used to analyse the course of an outbreak (Kannan *et al.*, 2020).

5.5. Machine-learning and Clinical Trial Optimisation

Machine Learning (ML) is a set of tools that identifies the data patterns. Powered by AI, ML tools excel at recognising patterns in an ocean of data, being faster and having the ability to improve as they encounter fresh sets of information. It is much different from the traditional pattern identification techniques, exploring and applying in combating COVID-19 (Verma, 2023). These techniques could predict, detect and manage infectious diseases, examining its use at various stages of an epidemic, dissecting the problems and potential challenges in combating COVID-19-like pandemics. Machine learning (ML) is increasingly applied in healthcare especially since the SARS-CoV-2 pandemic. It is applied to evaluate and carry out public health initiatives to manage epidemiological curve. Such systematic analysis aims to evaluate the efficacy of AI and ML in public health initiatives to curb the spread of SARS-CoV-2 (Combi *et al.*, 2023).

ML-based Patient selection, based on AI algorithms can be a pivotal step in healthcare. Analysing medical history to identify individuals who are likely to respond well to the vaccine with minimal risks, ML Models can provide predictive analysis of the demographics to facilitate vaccine development and delivery methods as well. Through AI, automated data collection during clinical trials like electronic health records, wearable sensors could analyse it in real-time, allowing for faster identification of trends and potential safety concerns. Also, Predictive modelling using AI models can predict vaccine efficacy based on collected data, helping researchers to optimise trial design and resource allocation.

AI has recently witnessed notable progress in data analysis importantly after the pandemic, as the deep learning and transfer learning advanced (Fig. 4). Mostly through tools like Google Translator and reverse image searching these have transformed the day-to-day life, and have significantly enhanced clinical diagnosis (Verma, 2023). AI algorithms may replace or significantly assist trained radiology professionals too. Despite its large potentials, new challenges posed by the recent breakthroughs need to be addressed.

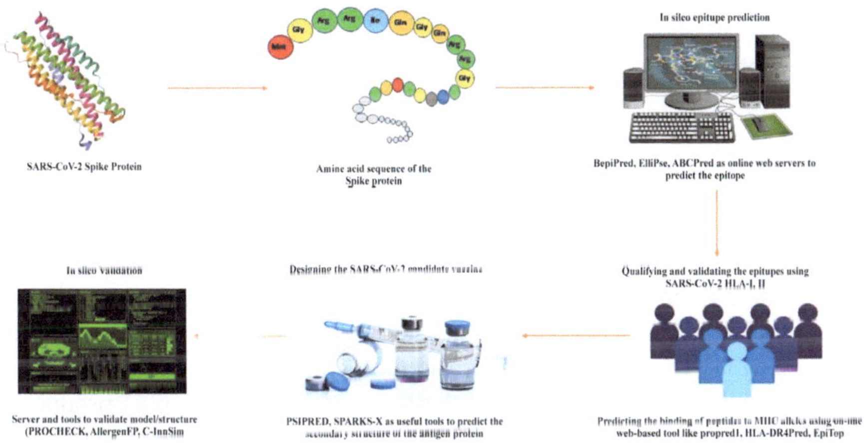

Fig. 4: Flow-chart of next-gen COVID-19 vaccine development using immunoinformatics: Spike protein as a case example; it shows the several instruments, database and servers and software tools used in vaccine invention and innovation

5.6. Information Filtration and Virtual Designing from Scratch

Using computer models that are adept at filtering data and producing dependable treatments could greatly accelerate vaccine development. Application of supervised learning techniques and artificial neural networks has shown to be revolutionary particularly in virtual filtering and *de novo* designing. Selecting the most pertinent targets with access to a sizable training dataset is necessary to attain optimal performance through such approaches. The most often selected targets for vaccine development and treatment with great potential are proteases and the viral spike proteins. 'CoronaDBAI' was developed as a dataset collection to address the issues associated with obtaining the training data and extract meaningful information. It shall eventually enhance the research and development results, benefitting bioinformaticians and computer scientists equally (Keshavarzi *et al.*, 2020).

5.7. Molecular Model Prediction/Protein Interaction

Natural language processing models and methods are vital in developing COVID-19 vaccine. Protein interactions are predicted using pre-trained transformers and simulate molecular reactions in carbohydrate chemistry, offering valuable insights in to vaccine development. Model application of an LSTM-based seq-2-seq predicted the secondary configuration of several SARS-COV-2 proteins (Tong *et al.*, 2024). This can potentially generate simulated sequences guiding the COVID-19 vaccine research further and would potentially address the emerging zoonosis. AI-assisted computer image technology could potentially analyse and monitor vaccine production facilities to ensure quality production with minimal alterations.

5.8. Surveillance Through AI: A Paradigm Shift in Data Acquisition and Analysis

While developing and approving vaccines for the global population is itself a herculean task, monitoring its safety and tracking its efficacy are two extremely important follow-ups. AI can ably analyse the humongous datasets including that of post-vaccination reports to identify rare or subtle safety errands that might go unnoticed by traditional methods. AI analyses the data on disease-spread propensity and hospitalisation, and track vaccine efficacy in the real-world settings to guide public healthcare interventions. The vaccine safety and efficiency while in transit is a critical challenge which requires post-production strategies. It allows the detection of long-term adverse effects by examining the population more extensively.

Surveillance was primarily reliant on human analysis and passive reporting systems before AI revolution, which had limitations on comprehending and monitoring the real-time data. Advanced algorithms efficiently analyse both structured and unstructured data (Sekaran *et al.*, 2023). AI system recognises patterns, trends and possible negative occurrences automatically, making it easier to quickly notice and evaluate the results, and finally improve patient care. Real-time dataset monitoring and an early alert system could help identify potential adversity due to vaccination thereby reducing human biases and increasing accuracy. AI algorithms could easily quantify patient-specific variables like determining vaccine coverage, identify high-risk population and evaluating potential confounding factors. Prioritising safety signals during post-marketing vaccine surveillance is crucial. AI algorithms excel in prioritising signals by considering factors like clinical relevance, statistical significance and the magnitude (Ghosh *et al.*, 2023). This guarantees a more effective use of resources to deal with possible unfavourable situations such as a pandemic. Using comprehensive population analysis-level data and AI algorithms, vaccine efficacy and safety profiles could be assessed. Decision and policy makers get a thorough grasp of the advantages and possible hazards associated with vaccinations or immunisation through this thorough analysis. AI software could be deployed in the form of smart-phone applications, thereby further increasing their reach, effectiveness and utility in the collection and analysis of data to understand the prominent trends and do informed prediction.

6. Limitations and Challenges in Implementing Ai in Vaccine Development

While AI could revolutionise vaccine development, many challenges are currently restricting the manoeuvrability and flexibility of deploying AI-assisted software. Broadly, the significant challenges hindering the integration of AI in healthcare are the absence of prospective validated studies and the difficulty in enhanced algorithms. The following are the possible outcomes regarding this.

6.1. Data Scarcity

The COVID 19 pandemic put forward the challenge of data insufficiency for AI models to precisely diagnose and predict COVID-19. AI-generated hypotheses required validation. The suitability of training data directly impacts the quality of an AI model in the real-world settings. Training the AI models on diverse and representative datasets is paramount to avoid biases (Enughwure and Febaide, 2020).

While it is worth noting that global databases exist that deal with the information on pathogen and protein, like the National Centre for Biotechnology Information (NCBI; GenBank), Virus Pathogen Resource (ViPR), UniProt and IMG/VR (Camargo *et al.*, 2023), and databases that deal with immune responses like IEDB (Vita *et al.*, 2015), Comprehensive T-cell receptor database (TCRdb) and BCIDE (Chen *et al.*, 2021), and Cyber Cell Database (CCDB) (Chew and Karr, 2021), there is a need to develop enhanced unified database along the lines of Next-Generation Immunogenome Project (NGIP), Global Microbial Identifier (GMI) with interactive open-access for active contribution to enhance the existing dataset.

6.2. Global Challenges in AI-based COVID-19 Vaccine Development

As SARS-CoV-2 is yet a novel virus and its research is still in its infancy, the information available to help with the creation of vaccines is scanty. To overcome this limitation, one approach could be to employ transfer learning, using the knowledge acquired from earlier studies. Deep learning plays a crucial role in developing strategies against SARS-CoV-2, providing prompt and precise answer in spite of the minimal data to accelerate the SARS-CoV-2 vaccine development and efficient therapeutics (Theobald, 2020).

6.3. Risk in M-protein Manipulation

It is understood that a more rigid outer shell made of M-protein enhances the contagiousness of the virus by increasing its resistance to antimicrobial enzymes in body and improving its viability outside the body. Considering M-protein to manipulation and attenuate the virus might be threatening, by increasing the probability of the spread of virus (or its mutated form) through the vaccine. However, before drawing any conclusion on such possibility, a deeper comprehension of the associated risks with increasing disorders is needed, with sound idea about the pathogenesis of the viruses with a manipulated outer shell (Goh *et al.*, 2020).

6.4. Ethical Concerns on Developing AI-based Vaccines

While AI is useful in creating vaccines, understanding its limitations and continuing to rely on large-scale clinical trials is necessary to assess vaccine efficacy and safety. Ethical concerns on the data privacy, prejudice, accountability, transparency and potential societal ramifications are there while employing AI in vaccine research. AI algorithms are majorly dependent on extensive datasets, potentially with genetic information and health records of the affected subjects. Prioritising the adequate protection of data and securing the subject's consent for appropriate data usage is crucial (Gerke *et al.*, 2020).

AI-based software developers are concerned about biasness ensuring algorithmic justice and fairness across AI models, e.g., in distributing vaccine across heterogeneous population. Transparency is an essential parameter in vaccine development to build public confidence. Even though certain AI models are considered 'black boxes', working on creating explainable algorithms is important so that researchers are able to comprehend the decision-making. The responsibilities and roles of AI-related researchers, developers and regulatory authorities while handling adversities must be clear through stringent regulatory frameworks, clear accountability and liability. Fair access to all AI resources is necessary to encourage ethical use of AI in vaccine research, enabling the marginalised communities to benefit from the advanced technologies and minimising the global health inequalities.

However, relying exclusively on AI algorithms for crucial decisions would grossly neglect the essential human ethical judgment, particularly in critical ethically dilemmatic situations concerning, say, vaccine development. Thus, ethical norms, rules and ethical regulations to apply AI in vaccine development are crucial to establish to uphold the safety principles, rights of the individuals and public confidence in the healthcare systems. It needs cooperation from regulatory authorities, researchers and software developers. Timely revision of rules, ethical assessments and routine monitoring of the performance shall guarantee ethically sound AI system based vaccine development in line with social and ethical values (Gerke *et al.*, 2020).

7. AI-based Analyses of After-effects, re-and Breakthrough Infections and Potential Risks of COVID-19 Vaccine

Observations on T-cell and IgG responses against SARS-CoV-2 up to a year after COVID-19 showed no additional benefits from booster dose vaccination in individuals infected earlier. The heterogeneity in the durability of humoral and cellular immunity was identified, emphasising the importance of T-cell assessments. Severe COVID-19 cases without effective T-cell response showed prolonged lungs inflammation. Alpha and Beta variants partially evaded humoral but could not interfere with the T-cell responses. The Delta variant showed lower titre of neutralising antibodies after vaccination but facilitated T-cell responses. The unique attempt to assess the responses a year after the infection revealed sustained T-cell and antibody responses in the recovered subject, effectively boosted by single vaccination (Reynolds *et al.*, 2021).

Machine learning (ML) approach offers a fresh perspective to aid policymakers in effectively responding to potentially pandemic infectious outbreaks in future (Lalmuanawma *et al.*, 2020; Vaishya *et al.*, 2020; Pal *et al.*, 2022).

Implementing effective ML in vaccination strategies is crucial to mitigate the impact of the persisting viral variants, especially owing to the uncertainty posed. The innovative ML method shows how immunisation campaigns significantly reduced the negative impact of the COVID-19 pandemic with a notable drop in death rate (Magazzino *et al.*, 2022).

While this approach prevents future outbreaks by COVID-19 variants and similar infectious diseases, it also offers valuable insights to policymakers enabling them to formulate effective vaccination strategies and set realistic goals to address existing infectious diseases. Vaccine development strategies need to consider the intricate relationship between immunisation campaigns and the evolving pandemic with impending variations due to factors beyond even the clinical parameters. It could enhance the preparedness for future pandemics with least additional burden on the existing healthcare infrastructure, and mitigate their adverse effects on public health, the economy and the society in general. Yet, the accuracy of AI predictions to detect epitopes of mutants and developing targeted vaccines and body's response against it remains to be tested every time.

Low toxicity, good stability, ease of manufacturing and storage are several benefits of DNA vaccines. Still, there are questions about their safety and immunogenicity to be answered. Rhesus macaque model revealed that the AstraZeneca vaccine had a detectable viral burden in every 5 out of 6 cases, while the Sinopharm vaccine showed no detectable viral load (Hatmal *et al.*, 2021). However, both Sinopharm and AstraZeneca vaccines provided good protection by preventing viral interstitial pneumonia.

8. Suggested AI Interventions and Future Directions

While COVID-19 drug discovery and vaccine development benefited from AI, accuracy of AI predictions throughout the vaccine development is unknown. Although research suggest possible COVID-19 vaccine targets, mass immunisation campaigns to offset the fast mutating virus and promote long-term herd immunity is needed. Few AI-based strategies to combat such infections are discussed below.

8.1. Personalised Vaccine

Tailored vaccine is capable of boosting efficacy and efficiency against a specific ailment by accounting for the unique genetic, immunological and environmental features of each individual, thus reducing the side-effects. Sophisticated algorithms and machine learning powers of AI essentially evaluate large, complicated datasets and determine which vaccine candidate fits best (Zeng *et al.*, 2020), an exercise that is humanly unattainable and seemed impractical even during the advanced pre-AI IT era.

8.2. AI-enabled Immunogenomics

Immunoinformatics strategies for COVID-19 vaccine development are in the rise due to a pressing global need to design vaccines swiftly (Ishack and Lipner 2021). Easy access to genomic sequences in the GenBank using bioinformatics (immunoinformatics) approach opens up a plethora of gene-level information to identify antigenic epitopes. Immunoinformatics and bioinformatics are pivotal in developing next-gen COVID-19 vaccines.

There are immediate challenges in developing vaccines using immunoinformatics though. Firstly, there is a need for advanced algorithms for fast and accurate calculations without any computational error. Secondly, there is a need for *in vitro* and *in vivo* data validation of the algorithms illustrating the post-vaccination adaptive and innate immunity scenario. Thirdly, no epitope-based vaccine has successfully combated diseases like HIV and malaria yet despite the advancements (Chakraborty *et al.*, 2021). Fourthly, considering the various factors associated with the efficacy of constructed multi-epitope vaccines is essential. It is mandatory to combine peptide linkers and epitopes (linker peptides) to keep the vaccine candidate stable.

8.3. Cost-effective and flexible Vaccines

Progress in AI methodologies in healthcare has extended prospects to identify the genomes of COVID-19 and VoC (variant of concern). AI is the key in swiftly creating advanced vaccine, to address and manage pandemics like the COVID-19. AI offers advantages like flexibility and cost-effectiveness (Basu *et al.*, 2020). However, its extensive application is hampered due to issues like data collection, external and internal validation, the duration of clinical studies, evaluation of therapeutic impact and the associated ethical issues.

8.4. Deep Learning Models

Concerns regarding next-gen vaccine development necessitate enhanced comprehension of the deep learning (DL) models. An advanced system AlphaFold introduced by Google DeepMind specialises in predicting 3D structures of proteins based on the genetic sequences, which was tested during COVID-19. AlphaFold predictions were crucial to accurately predict the structure of spike protein. DeepMind published structural predictions for various proteins associated with SARS-CoV-2. The University of Texas, Austin and the National Institutes of Health utilised a conventional biological approach to create the first 3D atomic map of a spike protein component of the virus responsible in human cell binding.

8.5. Nex-gen vaccine Development

Developed based purely on nucleotide or protein sequences and predictive modelling, next-gen vaccines are significantly advantageous. Coding sequences of viral proteins are crucial to protect against infectious diseases. These are included in viral antigen construct and vaccine development without relying completely on the viral culture. Such cutting-edge adaptability makes the platform highly versatile and significantly accelerates vaccine development. The majority of the COVID-19 vaccines with ongoing clinical trials have used next-gen platforms considering these advantages. Artificial antigen-presenting cells (aAPC) vaccine and LV-SMENP-DC vaccine are some vaccines that are developed based on such new approaches.

aAPC vaccine uses dendritic cells (DCs) that are highly proficient in activating the T-cells. The options of *in situ* delivery of cargo to DCs is advantageous in developing easily scalable, stable and humoral immune response inducing (rather than cell-mediated immune response) more effective next-gen vaccine (Rezaei and Nazari, 2022). As the isolation of specific DCs is expensive and labour-intensive, the process has limitations. An essential and conserved SARS-CoV-2 protein antigen is used to develop lentiviral synthetic minigene vaccine. The method involves expressing SARS-CoV-2 minigene (SMENP) on DCs using lentivirus. LV-DC expression for the desired antigen is subsequently stimulated to produce antigen-specific cytotoxic T-lymphocytes (Rezaei and Nazari, 2022).

9. Conclusion: AI tools in Combating Such Pandemics That Occur Over and Over Again

Human race has seemingly overcome the deadliest COVID-19 pandemic that created havoc over the last three years. Although the most deadly phase of the pandemic is seemingly over attributable to the widespread healthcare initiatives, yet the world needs to learn from the painful experiences and remain vigilant and prepared for the future as the COVID-19 variants still emerge and reemerge. The increasing breakthrough infection cases are also worrisome.

This calls for foolproof analyses on the possible extended applications of the AI in managing COVID-19, the discovery of the new-age healthcare interventions, vaccine research, case detection and contact-tracing, and predicting the outcomes. AI training using large datasets emulates human thinking, like learning and problem-solving. Rapid real-time gathering and global accessibility of data has generated fresh prospects for advanced AI to create adaptable surveillance platforms. Machine learning (ML) subset of AI is also promising to address problems using the knowledge by carefully choosing the data. Numerous publications during the COVID-19 pandemic pointed at how well AI approaches could prioritise, deliver, monitor and supply preventives and therapeutics (Arora *et al.*, 2021). To build trust among the public with varying mindsets in the use of AI systems, it needs to work seamlessly in altered critical situations and should be understandable to a layman. Such analyses to explore the benefits of AI, how it helps in real-time monitoring of public opinions during such pandemics and the acceptability of its use in healthcare sectors is grossly necessary.

References

Abulsoud AI, El-Husseiny HM, El-Husseiny AA, El-Mahdy HA, Ismail A, Elkhawaga SY, Khidr EG, Fathi D, Mady EA, Najda A and Algahtani M, 2023. Mutations in SARS-CoV-2: Insights on structure, variants, vaccines, and biomedical interventions. Biomed. Pharmacother., 157: 113977. doi: 10.1016/j.biopha.2022.113977

Ahmed TI, Rishi S, Irshad S, Aggarwal J, Happa K and Mansoor S, 2022. Inactivated vaccine Covaxin/BBV152: A systematic review. Front. Immunol., 13: 863162. doi: 10.3389/fimmu.2022.863162

Allam Z, Dey G and Jones DS, 2020. Artificial intelligence (AI) provided early detection of the coronavirus (COVID-19) in China and will influence future Urban health policy internationally. Ai, 1(2): 156–165. doi: 10.3390/ai1020009

Barnes CO, Jette CA, Abernathy ME, Dam KMA, Esswein SR, Gristick HB, Malyutin AG, Sharaf NG, Huey-Tubman KE, Lee YE and Robbiani DF, 2020. SARS-CoV-2 neutralizing antibody structures inform therapeutic strategies. Nature, 588(7839): 682–687. doi: 10.1038/s41586-020-2852-1

Basu S, Mitra S and Saha N, 2020. December. Deep learning for screening covid-19 using chest x-ray images. In: Symposium series on computational intelligence (SSCI). 01 December 2029, IEEE, ISBN 978-1-7281-2548-0: 2521–2527. doi: 10.1109/SSCI47803.2020.9308571

Bung N, Krishnan SR, Bulusu G and Roy A, 2021. De novo design of new chemical entities for SARS-CoV-2 using artificial intelligence. Future Med. Chem., 13(06): 575–585. doi: 10.4155/fmc-2020-0262

Camargo AP, Nayfach S, Chen IMA, Palaniappan K, Ratner A, Chu K, Ritter SJ, Reddy TBK, Mukherjee S, Schulz F and Call L, 2023. IMG/VR v4: an expanded database of uncultivated virus genomes within a framework of extensive functional, taxonomic, and ecological metadata. Nucleic Acids Res., 51(D1): D733–D743. doi: 10.1093/nar/gkac1037

Chen SY, Yue T, Lei Q and Guo AY, 2021. TCRdb: a comprehensive database for T-cell receptor sequences with powerful search function. Nucleic Acids Res., 49(D1): D468–D474. doi: 10.1093/nar/gkaa796

Chew YH and Karr JR, 2021. Centralizing data to unlock whole-cell models. Curr. Opin. Syst. Biol., 27: 100353. doi: 10.1016/j.coisb.2021.06.004

Combi C, Facelli JC, Haddawy P, Holmes JH, Koch S, Liu H, Meyer J, Peleg M, Pozzi G, Stiglic G and Veltri P, 2023. The IHI Rochester Report 2022 on Healthcare Informatics Research: Resuming After the CoViD-19. J. Healthc. Inform. Res., 7(2): 169–202. doi: 10.1007/s41666-023-00126-5

Dai L and Gao GF, 2021. Viral targets for vaccines against COVID-19. Nat. Rev. Immunol., 21(2): 73–82. doi: 10.1038/s41577-020-00480-0

Du L, Yang Y and Zhang X, 2021. Neutralizing antibodies for the prevention and treatment of COVID-19. Cell. Mol. Immunol., 18(10): 2293–2306. doi: 10.1038/s41423-021-00752-2

Duquerroy S, Vigouroux A, Rottier PJ, Rey FA and Bosch BJ, 2005. Central ions and lateral asparagine/glutamine zippers stabilize the post-fusion hairpin conformation of the SARS coronavirus spike glycoprotein. Virology, 335(2): 276–285. doi: 10.1016/j.virol.2005.02.022

Delaplace M, Huet H, Gambino A and Le Poder S, 2021. Feline coronavirus antivirals: A review. Pathogens, 10(9): 1150. doi: 10.3390/pathogens10091150

Du L, He Y, Zhou Y, Liu S, Zheng BJ and Jiang S, 2009. The spike protein of SARS-CoV—a target for vaccine and therapeutic development. Nat. Rev. Microbiol., 7(3): 226–236. doi: 10.1038/nrmicro2090

Enughwure AA and Febaide IC, 2020. Applications of artificial intelligence in combating Covid-19: a systematic review. Open Access Libr., 7(8): 1–12. doi: 10.4236/oalib.1106628

Fan H, Qin S and Cui Y, 2024. Emergence and Characterization of the SARS-CoV-2 JN. 1 Variant: Global Prevalence and Implications for Public Health. Zoonoses, 4(1): 994. doi: 10.15212/ZOONOSES-2023-0061

Ganasegeran K and Abdulrahman SA 2020. Artificial Intelligence Applications in Tracking Health Behaviors During Disease Epidemics. In: Hemanth D (eds) Human Behaviour Analysis Using Intelligent Systems. Learning and Analytics in Intelligent Systems, Cham, Springer: 141–155. doi: 10.1007/978-3-030-35139-7_7.

Ghosh A, Larrondo-Petrie MM and Pavlovic M, 2023. Revolutionizing Vaccine Development for COVID-19: A Review of AI-Based Approaches. Information, 14(12): 665. doi: 10.3390/info14120665

Gong W, Parkkila S, Wu X and Aspatwar A, 2023. SARS-CoV-2 variants and COVID-19 vaccines: Current challenges and future strategies. Int. Rev. Immunol., 42(6): 393–414. doi: 10.1080/08830185.2022.2079642

Guan WJ, Ni ZY, Hu Y, Liang WH, Ou CQ, He JX, Liu L, Shan H, Lei CL, Hui DS and Du B, 2020. Clinical characteristics of coronavirus disease 2019 in China. N. Engl. J. Med., 382(18): 1708–1720. doi: 10.1056/NEJMoa2002032

Gupta AM, Chakrabarti J and Mandal S, 2020. Non-synonymous mutations of SARS-CoV-2 leads epitope loss and segregates its variants. Microbes Infect., 22(10): 598-607. doi: 10.1016/j.micinf.2020.10.004

Goldust Y, Sameem F, Mearaj S, Gupta A, Patil A and Goldust M, 2023. COVID-19 and artificial intelligence: Experts and dermatologists perspective. J. Cosmet. Dermatol., 22(1): 11–15. doi: 10.1111/jocd.15310

Hatmal MMM, Al-Hatamleh MA, Olaimat AN, Hatmal M, Alhaj-Qasem DM, Olaimat TM and Mohamud R, 2021. Side effects and perceptions following COVID-19 vaccination in Jordan: a randomized, cross-sectional study implementing machine learning for predicting severity of side effects. Vaccines, 9(6): 556. doi: 10.3390/vaccines9060556

Hoerr I, Obst R, Rammensee HG and Jung G, 2000. In vivo application of RNA leads to induction of specific cytotoxic T lymphocytes and antibodies. Eur. J. Immunol., 30(1): 1–7. doi: 10.1002/1521-4141(200001)30:1<1::AID-IMMU1>3.0.CO;2-%23

Hu J, Peng P, Wang K, Fang L, Luo FY, Jin AS, Liu BZ, Tang N and Huang AL, 2021. Emerging SARS-CoV-2 variants reduce neutralization sensitivity to convalescent sera and monoclonal antibodies. Cell. Mol. Immunol., 18(4): 1061–1063. doi: 10.1038/s41423-021-00648-1

Imrie F, Bradley AR, van der Schaar M and Deane CM, 2018. Protein family-specific models using deep neural networks and transfer learning improve virtual screening and highlight the need for more data. J. Chem. Inf. Model., 58(11): 2319–2330. doi: 10.1021/acs.jcim.8b00350

Ishack S and Lipner SR, 2021. Bioinformatics and immunoinformatics to support COVID-19 vaccine development. J. Med. Virol., 93(9): 5209–5211. doi: 10.1002/jmv.27017

Islam MJ, Islam NN, Alom MS, Kabir M and Halim MA, 2023. A review on structural, non-structural, and accessory proteins of SARS-CoV-2: Highlighting drug target sites. Immunobiology, 228(1): 152302. doi: 10.1016/j.imbio.2022.152302

Jansen L, Tegomoh B, Lange K, Showalter K, Figliomeni J, Abdalhamid B, Iwen PC, Fauver J, Buss B and Donahue M, 2021. Investigation of a SARS-CoV-2 B. 1.1. 529 (omicron) variant cluster—Nebraska, November–December 2021. Morbidity and Mortality Weekly Report, 70: 1782.

Jeeva S, Kim KH, Shin CH, Wang BZ and Kang SM, 2021. An update on mRNA-based viral vaccines. Vaccines, 9(9): 965. doi: 10.3390/vaccines9090965

Jurtz VI, Johansen AR, Nielsen M, Almagro Armenteros JJ, Nielsen H, Sønderby CK, Winther O and Sønderby SK, 2017. An introduction to deep learning on biological sequence data: examples and solutions. Bioinformatics, 33(22): 3685–3690. doi: 10.1093/bioinformatics/btx531

Kannan S, Subbaram K, Ali S and Kannan H, 2020. The role of artificial intelligence and machine learning techniques: Race for covid-19 vaccine. Arch. Clin. Infect. Dis., 15(2): e103232. doi: 10.5812/archcid.103232

Kannan S, Ali PSS and Sheeza A, 2021. Evolving biothreat of variant SARS-CoV-2-molecular properties, virulence and epidemiology. Eur. Rev. Med. Pharmacol. Sci., 25(12): 4405–4412.

Karam M and Daoud G, 2022. mRNA vaccines: Past, present, future. Asian J. Pharm. 17(4): 491–522. doi: 10.1016/j.ajps.2022.05.003

Keshavarzi Arshadi A, Webb J, Salem M, Cruz E, Calad-Thomson S, Ghadirian N, Collins J, Diez-Cecilia E, Kelly B, Goodarzi H and Yuan JS, 2020. Artificial intelligence for COVID-19 drug discovery and vaccine development. Front. Artif. Intell., 3: 65. doi: 10.3389/frai.2020.00065

Khadse NA, Wankhade AM, Patil SR and Kathale SV, 2020. A review on corona virus disease. European J. Biomed. Pharm. Sci., 7(4): 1–8.

Kong R, Yang G, Xue R, Liu M, Wang F, Hu J, Guo X and Chang S, 2020. COVID-19 Docking Server: A meta server for docking small molecules, peptides and antibodies against potential targets of COVID-19. Bioinformatics, 36(20): 5109–5111. doi: 10.1093/bioinformatics/btaa645

Kuzmin A, Orekhov P, Astashkin R, Gordeliy V and Gushchin I, 2022. Structure and dynamics of the SARS-CoV-2 envelope protein monomer. Proteins: Structure, Function, and Bioinformatics, 90(5): 1102–1114. doi: 10.1002/prot.26317

Lalmuanawma S, Hussain J and Chhakchhuak L, 2020. Applications of machine learning and artificial intelligence for Covid-19 (SARS-CoV-2) pandemic: A review. Chaos, Solitons & Fractals, 139: 110059. doi: 10.1016/j.chaos.2020.110059

Lefkowitz EJ, Dempsey DM, Hendrickson RC, Orton RJ, Siddell SG and Smith DB, 2018. Virus taxonomy: the database of the International Committee on Taxonomy of Viruses (ICTV). Nucleic Acids Res., 46(D1): D708–D717. doi: 10.1093/nar/gkx932

Liu PY, Tsai YS, Chen PL, Tsai HP, Hsu LW, Wang CS, Lee NY, Huang MS, Wu YC, Ko WC and Yang YC, 2020. Application of an artificial intelligence trilogy to accelerate processing of suspected patients with SARS-CoV-2 at a smart quarantine station: Observational study. J. Med. Internet Res., 22(10): e19878. doi: 10.2196/19878

MacIntyre CR, Chen X, Kunasekaran M, Quigley A, Lim S, Stone H, Paik HY, Yao L, Heslop D, Wei W and Sarmiento I, 2023. Artificial intelligence in public health: the potential of epidemic early warning systems. J. Int. Med. Res., 51(3), p.03000605231159335. doi: 10.1177/03000605231159335

MacLean OA, Lytras S, Weaver S, Singer JB, Boni MF, Lemey P, Kosakovsky Pond SL and Robertson DL, 2021. Natural selection in the evolution of SARS-CoV-2 in bats created a generalist virus and highly capable human pathogen. PLoS biology, 19(3): e3001115. doi: 10.1371/journal.pbio.3001115

Magazzino C, Mele M and Coccia M, 2022. A machine learning algorithm to analyse the effects of vaccination on COVID-19 mortality. Epidemiol. Infect., 150: e168. doi: 10.1017/S0950268822001418

Mahtarin R, Islam S, Islam MJ, Ullah MO, Ali MA and Halim MA, 2022. Structure and dynamics of membrane protein in SARS-CoV-2. J. Biomol. Struct. Dyn., 40(10): 4725–4738. doi: 10.1080/07391102.2020.1861983

Malone B, Simovski B, Moliné C, Cheng J, Gheorghe M, Fontenelle H, Vardaxis I, Tennøe S, Malmberg JA, Stratford R and Clancy T, 2020. Artificial intelligence predicts the immunogenic landscape of SARS-CoV-2 leading to universal blueprints for vaccine designs. Scientific reports, 10(1): 22375. doi: 10.1038/s41598-020-78758-5

McBride R, Van Zyl M and Fielding BC, 2014. The coronavirus nucleocapsid is a multifunctional protein. Viruses, 6(8): 2991–3018. doi: 10.3390/v6082991

McCarthy KR, Rennick LJ, Nambulli S, Robinson-McCarthy LR, Bain WG, Haidar G and Duprex WP, 2021. Recurrent deletions in the SARS-CoV-2 spike glycoprotein drive antibody escape. Science, 371(6534): 1139–1142. doi: 10.1126/science.abf6950

Meng B, Kemp SA, Papa G, Datir R, Ferreira IA, Marelli S, Harvey WT, Lytras S, Mohamed A, Gallo G and Thakur N, 2021. Recurrent emergence of SARS-CoV-2 spike deletion H69/V70 and its role in the Alpha variant B. 1.1. 7. Cell Rep., 35(13): 109292. doi: 10.1016/j.celrep.2021.109292

Messina G, Polito R, Monda V, Cipolloni L, Di Nunno N, Di Mizio G, Murabito P, Carotenuto M, Messina A, Pisanelli D and Valenzano A, 2020. Functional role of dietary intervention to improve the outcome of COVID-19: a hypothesis of work. Int. J. Mol. Sci., 21(9): 3104. doi: 10.3390/ijms21093104

Mohapatra RK, Das PK and Kandi V, 2020. Challenges in controlling COVID-19 in migrants in Odisha, India. Diabetes Metab. Syndr., 14(6):1593-9. doi: 10.1016/j.dsx.2020.08.024

Mohapatra RK, El-Shall NA, Tiwari R, Nainu F, Kandi V, Sarangi AK, Mohammed TA, Desingu PA, Chakraborty C and Dhama K, 2022. Need of booster vaccine doses to counteract the emergence of SARS-CoV-2 variants in the context of the Omicron variant and increasing COVID-19 cases: An update. Hum. Vaccin. Immunother., 18(5):2065824. https://doi.org/10.1080/21645515.2022.2065824

Arora G, Joshi J, Mandal RS, Shrivastava N, Virmani R and Sethi T, 2021. Artificial intelligence in surveillance, diagnosis, drug discovery and vaccine development against COVID-19. Pathogens, 10(8): 1048. doi: 10.3390/pathogens10081048

Baghban R, Ghasemian A and Mahmoodi S, 2023. Nucleic acid-based vaccine platforms against the coronavirus disease 19 (COVID-19). Archives of Microbiology, 205(4): 150. doi: 10.1007/s00203-023-03480-5

Basheeruddin Asdaq SM, Jomah S, Rabbani SI, Alamri AM, Salem Alshammari SK, Duwaidi BS, Alshammari MS, Alamri AS, Alsanie WF, Alhomrani M and Sreeharsha N, 2022. Insight into the advances in clinical trials of SARS-CoV-2 vaccines. Can J Infect Dis Med Microbiol, 2022(1): 6913772. doi: 10.1155/2022/6913772

Bashor L, Gagne RB, Bosco-Lauth AM, Bowen RA, Stenglein M and VandeWoude S, 2021. SARS-CoV-2 evolution in animals suggests mechanisms for rapid variant selection. PNAS, 118(44): e2105253118. doi: 10.1073/pnas.2105253118

Baum A, Fulton BO, Wloga E, Copin R, Pascal KE, Russo V, Giordano S, Lanza K, Negron N, Ni M and Wei Y, 2020. Antibody cocktail to SARS-CoV-2 spike protein prevents rapid mutational escape seen with individual antibodies. Science, 369(6506): 1014–1018. doi: 10.1126/science.abd0831

Bobdey S and Ray S, 2020. Going viral-Covid-19 impact assessment: A perspective beyond clinical practice. J. Mar. Med. Soc., 22(1): 9–12. doi: 10.4103/jmms.jmms_12_20

Callaway E, 2021a. The mutation that helps Delta spread like wildfire. Nature, 596(7873): 472–473. doi: 10.1038/d41586-021-02275-2

Callaway E, 2021b. Heavily mutated Omicron variant puts scientists on alert. Nature, 600(7887): 21. doi: 10.1038/d41586-021-03552-w

Chakraborty C, Sharma AR, Bhattacharya M and Lee SS, 2021. Lessons learned from cutting-edge immunoinformatics on next-generation COVID-19 vaccine research. Int J Pept Res Ther, 27: 2303–2311. doi: 10.1007/s10989-021-10254-4

Choudhary S, Malik YS and Tomar S, 2020. Identification of SARS-CoV-2 cell entry inhibitors by drug repurposing using in silico structure-based virtual screening approach. Front. Immunol., 11: 1664. doi: 10.3389/fimmu.2020.01664

Darbar S, Agarwal S and Saha S, 2021. COVID19 vaccine: COVAXIN®-India's first indigenous effective weapon to fight against coronavirus (A Review). Parana J. Sci. Educ., 7(3): 1–9.

Fast E, Altman RB and Chen B, 2020. Potential T-cell and B-cell epitopes of 2019-nCoV. BioRxiv, 2020–02. doi: 10.1101/2020.02.19.955484

Folegatti PM, Ewer KJ, Aley PK, Angus B, Becker S, Belij-Rammerstorfer S, Bellamy D, Bibi S, Bittaye M, Clutterbuck EA and Dold C, 2020. Safety and immunogenicity of the ChAdOx1 nCoV-19 vaccine against SARS-CoV-2: a preliminary report of a phase 1/2, single-blind, randomised controlled trial. The Lancet, 396(10249): 467–478. doi: 10.1016/S0140-6736(20)31604-4

Garcia-Beltran WF, Lam EC, Denis KS, Nitido AD, Garcia ZH, Hauser BM, Feldman J, Pavlovic MN, Gregory DJ, Poznansky MC and Sigal A, 2021. Multiple SARS-CoV-2 variants escape neutralization by vaccine-induced humoral immunity. Cell, 184(9): 2372–2383. doi: 10.1016/j.cell.2021.03.013

Gerke S, Minssen T and Cohen G, 2020. Ethical and legal challenges of artificial intelligence-driven healthcare. In A Bohr and K Memarzadeh (Eds) Artificial intelligence in healthcare, Academic Press: 295–336. doi: 10.1016/B978-0-12-818438-7.00012-5

Goh GKM, Dunker AK, Foster JA and Uversky VN, 2020. A novel strategy for the development of vaccines for SARS-CoV-2 (COVID-19) and other viruses using AI and viral shell disorder. J. Proteome Res., 19(11): 4355–4363. doi: 10.1021/acs.jproteome.0c00672

Mohapatra RK, Kandi V, Gaidhane AM, Zahiruddin QS, Rustagi S, Satapathy P, Mishra S and Tuglo LS, 2024. Global domination of the recently VoI-classified'JN. 1′ outcompeting other variants–Comparing the vaccines' efficacy. Clinical Infection in Practice, 22:100358. https://doi.org/10.1016/j.clinpr.2024.100358

Mohapatra RK, Mishra S, Azam M and Dhama K, 2021. COVID-19, WHO guidelines, pedagogy, and respite. Open Med., 16(1):491-3. doi: 10.1515/med-2021-0266

Mohapatra RK, Mishra S, Kandi V, Branda F, Ansari A, Rabaan AA and Kudrat-E-Zahan M, 2023a. Analyzing the emerging patterns of SARS-CoV-2 Omicron subvariants for the development of next-gen vaccine: An observational study. Health Sci. Rep., 6(10):e1596. doi: 10.1002/hsr2.1596

Mohapatra RK, Verma S, Kandi V, Sarangi AK, Seidel V, Das SN, Behera A, Tuli HS, Sharma AK and Dhama K, 2023b. The SARS-CoV-2 Omicron variant and its multiple sub-lineages: transmissibility, vaccine development, antiviral drugs, monoclonal antibodies, and strategies for infection control–a review. ChemistrySelect., 8(9):e202201380. https://doi.org/10.1002/slct.202201380

Msemburi W, Karlinsky A, Knutson V, Aleshin-Guendel S, Chatterji S and Wakefield J, 2023. The WHO estimates of excess mortality associated with the COVID-19 pandemic. Nature, 613(7942): 130–137. doi: 10.1038/s41586-022-05522-2

Nance KD and Meier JL, 2021. Modifications in an emergency: the role of N1-methylpseudouridine in COVID-19 vaccines. ACS Cent. Sci., 7(5): 748–756. doi: 10.1021/acscentsci.1c00197

Nonaka CK, Franco MM, Gräf T, de Lorenzo Barcia CA, de Ávila Mendonça RN, De Sousa KAF, Neiva LM, Fosenca V, Mendes AV, De Aguiar RS and Giovanetti M, 2021. Genomic evidence of SARS-CoV-2 reinfection involving E484K spike mutation, Brazil. Emerging Infect. Dis., 27(5): 1522–1524. doi: 10.3201/eid2705.210191

Ong E, Wong MU, Huffman A and He Y, 2020. COVID-19 coronavirus vaccine design using reverse vaccinology and machine learning. Front. Immunol., 11: 1581. doi: 10.3389/fimmu.2020.01581

Pagadala NS, Syed K and Tuszynski J, 2017. Software for molecular docking: a review. Biophysical Rev., 9: 91–102. doi: 10.1007/s12551-016-0247-1

Pal M, Parija S, Mohapatra RK, Mishra S, Rabaan AA, Al Mutair A, Alhumaid S, Al-Tawfiq JA and Dhama K, 2022. Symptom-Based COVID-19 Prognosis through AI-Based IoT: A Bioinformatics Approach. BioMed Research International. 2022(1):3113119.

Pal R and Yadav U, 2022. Resurgence of COVID-19 in India: time for introspection. Postgraduate Med. J., 98(e2): e86–e87. doi: 10.1136/postgradmedj-2021-140410

Panda S, Singh PK, Mishra S, Mitra S, Pattnaik P, Adhikary SD and Mohapatra RK, 2022. Indian biosimilars and vaccines at crossroads–replicating the success of pharmagenerics. Vaccines, 11(1): 110. doi: 10.3390/vaccines11010110

Pandey SC, Pande V, Sati D, Upreti S and Samant M, 2020. Vaccination strategies to combat novel corona virus SARS-CoV-2. Life Sci., 256: 117956. doi: 10.1016/j.lfs.2020.117956

Patil PB, Patil DM, Khan ZG, Patel SA and Patel JK, 2023. Review on CoviShield and Covaxin Vaccine against Covid-19. Health, 2: 50-56.

Plante JA, Liu Y, Liu J, Xia H, Johnson BA, Lokugamage KG, Zhang X, Muruato AE, Zou J, Fontes-Garfias CR and Mirchandani D, 2021. Spike mutation D614G alters SARS-CoV-2 fitness. Nature, 592(7852): 116–121. doi: 10.1038/s41586-020-2895-3

Prajapat M, Sarma P, Shekhar N, Avti P, Sinha S, Kaur H, Kumar S, Bhattacharyya A, Kumar H, Bansal S and Medhi B, 2020. Drug targets for corona virus: A systematic review. Indian J. Pharmacol., 52(1): 56–65. doi: 10.4103/ijp.IJP_115_20

Rangan R, Zheludev IN, Hagey RJ, Pham EA, Wayment-Steele HK, Glenn JS and Das R, 2020. RNA genome conservation and secondary structure in SARS-CoV-2 and SARS-related viruses: a first look. Rna, 26(8): 937–959. doi: 10.1261/rna.076141.120.

Rees-Spear C, Muir L, Griffith SA, Heaney J, Aldon Y, Snitselaar JL, Thomas P, Graham C, Seow J, Lee N and Rosa A, 2021. The effect of spike mutations on SARS-CoV-2 neutralization. Cell reports, 34(12): 108890. doi: 10.1016/j.celrep.2021.108890

Reynolds CJ, Pade C, Gibbons JM, Butler DK, Otter AD, Menacho K, Fontana M, Smit A, Sackville-West JE, Cutino-Moguel T and Maini MK, 2021. Prior SARS-CoV-2 infection rescues B and T cell responses to variants after first vaccine dose. Science, 372(6549): 1418–1423. doi: 10.1126/science.abh1282

Rezaei M and Nazari M, 2022. New generation vaccines for COVID-19 based on peptide, viral vector, artificial antigen presenting cell, DNA or mRNA. Avicenna J. Med. Biotechnol., 14(1): 30–36. doi: 10.18502/ajmb.v14i1.8167

Sah R, Khatiwada AP, Shrestha S, Bhuvan KC, Tiwari R, Mohapatra RK, Dhama K and Rodriguez-Morales AJ, 2021. COVID-19 vaccination campaign in Nepal, emerging UK variant and futuristic vaccination strategies to combat the ongoing pandemic. Travel Med. Infect. Dis., 41:102037. doi: 10.1016/j.tmaid.2021.102037

Sarangi AK, Salem MA, Younus MD, El-Haroun H, Mahal A, Tripathy L, Mishra R, Shabil M, Alhumaydhi FA, Khatib MN and Bushi G, 2024. Advanced biomaterials for regenerative medicine and their possible therapeutic significance in treating COVID-19: a critical overview. Int. J. Surg., 110(12):7508-27. doi: 10.1097/JS9.0000000000002110

Satapathy BS, Pattnaik G, Sahoo RN, Pattanaik S, Sarangi AK, Kandi V, Mishra S, Rabaan AA, Mohanty A, Sah R and Mohapatra RK, 2023. COVID-19 vaccines and their underbelly: Are we going the right way?. Health Sci. Rep., 6(9):e1540. doi: 10.1002/hsr2.1540

Schoeman D and Fielding BC, 2019. Coronavirus envelope protein: current knowledge. Virol. J., 16(1): 1–22. doi: 10.1186/s12985-019-1182-0

Schoenmaker L, Witzigmann D, Kulkarni JA, Verbeke R, Kersten G, Jiskoot W and Crommelin DJ, 2021. mRNA-lipid nanoparticle COVID-19 vaccines: Structure and stability. Int. J. Pharm., 601: 120586. doi: 10.1016/j.ijpharm.2021.120586

Sehra ST, Salciccioli JD, Wiebe DJ, Fundin S and Baker JF, 2020. Maximum daily temperature, precipitation, ultraviolet light, and rates of transmission of severe acute respiratory syndrome coronavirus 2 in the United States. Clin. Infect. Dis., 71(9): 2482–2487. doi: 10.1093/cid/ciaa681

Sekaran K, Gnanasambandan R, Thirunavukarasu R, Iyyadurai R, Karthick G and Doss CGP, 2023. A systematic review of artificial intelligence-based COVID-19 modeling on multimodal genetic information. Prog. Biophys. Mol. Biol., 179: 1–9. doi: 10.1016/j.pbiomolbio.2023.02.003

Shabu A and Nishtala PS, 2023. Safety outcomes associated with the Moderna COVID-19 vaccine (mRNA-1273): a literature review. Expert Rev. Vaccines, 22(1): 393–409. doi: 10.1080/14760584.2023.2209177

Sodhi GK, Kaur S, Gaba GS, Kansal L, Sharma A and Dhiman G, 2022. COVID-19: role of robotics, artificial intelligence and machine learning during the pandemic. Curr. Med. Imaging, 18(2): 124–134. doi: 10.2174/1573405617666210224115722

Soraci L, Lattanzio F, Soraci G, Gambuzza ME, Pulvirenti C, Cozza A, Corsonello A, Luciani F and Rezza G, 2022. COVID-19 vaccines: current and future perspectives. Vaccines, 10(4): 608. doi: 10.3390/vaccines10040608

Souza PF, Mesquita FP, Amaral JL, Landim PG, Lima KR, Costa MB, Farias IR, Belém MO, Pinto YO, Moreira HH and Magalhaes IC, 2022. The spike glycoprotein of SARS-

CoV-2: A review of how mutations of spike glycoproteins have driven the emergence of variants with high transmissibility and immune escape. Int. J. Biol. Macromol., 208: 105–125. doi: 10.1016/j.ijbiomac.2022.03.058

Starr TN, Greaney AJ, Dingens AS and Bloom JD, 2021. Complete map of SARS-CoV-2 RBD mutations that escape the monoclonal antibody LY-CoV555 and its cocktail with LY-CoV016. Cell Rep. Med., 2(4): 100255 doi: 10.1016/j.xcrm.2021.100255

Tai W, Wang Y, Fett CA, Zhao G, Li F, Perlman S, Jiang S, Zhou Y and Du L, 2017. Recombinant receptor-binding domains of multiple Middle East respiratory syndrome coronaviruses (MERS-CoVs) induce cross-neutralizing antibodies against divergent human and camel MERS-CoVs and antibody escape mutants. J. Virol., 91(1): e01651. doi: 10.1128/jvi.01651-16

Telenti A, Hodcroft EB and Robertson DL, 2022. The evolution and biology of SARS-CoV-2 variants. Cold Spring Harb. Perspect. Med., 12(5): a041390. doi: 10.1101/cshperspect.a041390

Theobald N, 2020. Emerging vaccine delivery systems for COVID-19: Functionalised silica nanoparticles offer a potentially safe and effective alternative delivery system for DNA/RNA vaccines and may be useful in the hunt for a COVID-19 vaccine. Drug Discov. Today, 25(9): 1556–1558. doi: 10.1016/j.drudis.2020.06.020

Ton AT, Gentile F, Hsing M, Ban F and Cherkasov A, 2020. Rapid identification of potential inhibitors of SARS-CoV-2 main protease by deep docking of 1.3 billion compounds. Mol. Inform., 39(8): 2000028. doi: 10.1002/minf.202000028

Tong J, Gao P, Xu H and Liu Y, 2024. Improved SAR and QSAR models of SARS-CoV-2 Mpro inhibitors based on machine learning. J. Mol. Liq., 394: 123708. doi: 10.1016/j.molliq.2023.123708

Vaishya R, Javaid M, Khan IH and Haleem A, 2020. Artificial Intelligence (AI) applications for COVID-19 pandemic. Diabetes Metab. Syndr., 14(4): 337–339. doi: 10.1016/j.dsx.2020.04.012

Verma R, 2023. Development of machine learning model for vaccination simulation tool using artificial intelligence. In: IoT in Social, Mobile, Analytics and Cloud (I-SMAC). 7th Intl. Conf., 11 October 2023, IEEE, ISBN 979-8-3503-4149-2: 450-455. doi: 10.1109/I-SMAC58438.2023.10290601

Vita R, Overton JA, Greenbaum JA, Ponomarenko J, Clark JD, Cantrell JR, Wheeler DK, Gabbard JL, Hix D, Sette A and Peters B, 2015. The immune epitope database (IEDB) 3.0. Nucleic Acids Res., 43(D1): D405–D412. doi: 10.1093/nar/gku938

Walsh EE, Frenck Jr RW, Falsey AR, Kitchin N, Absalon J, Gurtman A, Lockhart S, Neuzil K, Mulligan MJ, Bailey R and Swanson KA, 2020. Safety and immunogenicity of two RNA-based Covid-19 vaccine candidates. N. Eng. J. Med., 383(25): 2439–2450. doi: 10.1056/NEJMoa2027906

Wang N, Shang J, Jiang S and Du L, 2020. Subunit vaccines against emerging pathogenic human coronaviruses. Front. Microbiol., 11: 298. doi: 10.3389/fmicb.2020.00298

Woo, P.C., Lau, S.K., Lam, C.S., Tsang, A.K., Hui, S.W., Fan, R.Y., Martelli, P. and Yuen, K.Y., 2014. Discovery of a novel bottlenose dolphin coronavirus reveals a distinct species of marine mammal coronavirus in Gammacoronavirus. J. Virol., 88(2): 1318–1331. doi: 10.1128/jvi.02351-13

Woo PC, Lau SK, Lam CS, Lau CC, Tsang AK, Lau JH, Bai R, Teng JL, Tsang CC, Wang M and Zheng BJ, 2012. Discovery of seven novel Mammalian and avian coronaviruses in the genus deltacoronavirus supports bat coronaviruses as the gene source of alphacoronavirus and betacoronavirus and avian coronaviruses as the gene source of gammacoronavirus and deltacoronavirus. J. Virol., 86(7): 3995–4008. doi: 10.1128/jvi.06540-11

World Health Organization, 2021. COVID-19 weekly epidemiological update, 9 March 2021.

Zehra Z, Luthra M, Siddiqui SM, Shamsi A, Gaur NA and Islam A, 2020. Corona virus versus existence of human on the earth: A computational and biophysical approach. Int. J. Biol. Macromol., 161: 271–281. doi: 10.1016/j.ijbiomac.2020.06.007

Zhao C, Lou Z, Guo Y, Ma M, Chen Y, Liang S, Zhang L, Chen S, Li X, Liu Y and Bartlam M, 2009. Nucleoside monophosphate complex structures of the endonuclease domain from the influenza virus polymerase PA subunit reveal the substrate binding site inside the catalytic center. J. Virol., 83(18): 9024–9030. doi: 10.1128/jvi.00911-09

Zhou P, Yang XL, Wang XG, Hu B, Zhang L, Zhang W, Si HR, Zhu Y, Li B, Huang CL and Chen HD, 2020. A pneumonia outbreak associated with a new coronavirus of probable bat origin. Nature, 579(7798): 270–273. doi: 10.1038/s41586-020-2012-7

Wang Y and Liu L, 2016. The membrane protein of severe acute respiratory syndrome coronavirus functions as a novel cytosolic pathogen-associated molecular pattern to promote beta interferon induction via a toll-like-receptor-related TRAF3-independent mechanism. MBio, 7(1): e01872. doi: 10.1128/mbio.01872-15

Wang Z, Schmidt F, Weisblum Y, Muecksch F, Barnes CO, Finkin S, Schaefer-Babajew D, Cipolla M, Gaebler C, Lieberman JA and Oliveira TY, 2021. mRNA vaccine-elicited antibodies to SARS-CoV-2 and circulating variants. Nature, 592(7855): 616–622. doi: 10.1038/s41586-021-03324-6

Weisblum Y, Schmidt F, Zhang F, DaSilva J, Poston D, Lorenzi JC, Muecksch F, Rutkowska, M, Hoffmann HH, Michailidis E and Gaebler C, 2020. Escape from neutralizing antibodies by SARS-CoV-2 spike protein variants. elife, 9: e61312. doi: 10.7554/eLife.61312

Wu W, Cheng Y, Zhou H, Sun C and Zhang S, 2023. The SARS-CoV-2 nucleocapsid protein: its role in the viral life cycle, structure and functions, and use as a potential target in the development of vaccines and diagnostics. Virol. J., 20(1): 6. doi: 10.1186/s12985-023-01968-6

Zeng L, Li Y, Liu J, Guo L, Wang Z, Xu X, Song S, Hao C, Liu L, Xin M and Xu C, 2020. Rapid, ultrasensitive and highly specific biosensor for the diagnosis of SARS-CoV-2 in clinical blood samples. Mater. Chem. Front., 4(7): 2000–2005. doi: 10.1039/D0QM00294A

Zhang H, Penninger JM, Li Y, Zhong N and Slutsky AS, 2020. Angiotensin-converting enzyme 2 (ACE2) as a SARS-CoV-2 receptor: molecular mechanisms and potential therapeutic target. Intensive Care Med., 46: 586–590. doi: 10.1007/s00134-020-05985-9

Zhang Z, Nomura N, Muramoto Y, Ekimoto T, Uemura T, Liu K, Yui M, Kono N, Aoki J, Ikeguchi M and Noda T, 2022. Structure of SARS-CoV-2 membrane protein essential for virus assembly. Nat. Commun., 13(1): 4399. doi: 10.1038/s41467-022-32019-3

6

The Biological, Commercial and Economic Impacts of Vaccine Boosters

Ranjan K. Mohapatra[1], Snehasish Mishra[2,*], Puneet Kumar Singh[2] and Venkataramana Kandi[3]

[1]*Department of Chemistry, Government College of Engineering Keonjhar-758 002, Odisha, India;*
[2]*School of Biotechnology, Campus-11, KIIT Deemed-to-be-University Bhubaneswar-751 024, Odisha, India*
[3]*Department of Microbiology, Prathima Institute of Medical Sciences Karimnagar-505 417, Telangana, India*

Abstract

Recent pandemic (COVID-19) impacted global economy significantly and increased economic disparity. Vaccines are significantly beneficial and cost-effective compared to other public healthcare preventives. Vaccines reduce hospitalisation, treatment costs and associated morbidity and mortality. Although COVID-19 vaccination and natural viral infection protected against reinfection, it waned in part due to emerging novel variants. Waning immunity from vaccine and natural infection are documented, and it was more so in severe hospitalised COVID-19. Many countries developed their own vaccines successfully to counter as COVID-19 became global. Vaccines needed updates to effectively fight COVID-19 as the wild strain constantly mutated. Among the intrinsic, perinatal, extrinsic, environmental, behavioural and nutritional aspects, the host factors included antibiotics usage pattern, sleep habits, physical activities, smoking habit and alcohol intake. Similarly, the external factors influencing vaccine response included childhood vaccination, early-age infections, nutrient supplements soon after birth, and breastfeeding pattern. Vaccination time also affected the efficacy. Forenoon vaccination developed less breakthrough infection compared to afternoon or evening vaccination due to varying immunological responses like immune cell functions, recruitment and transport, owing to circadian rhythm. Although vaccination side-effects are there, almost all vaccines are reportedly safe, effective *and prevented serious illness, hospitalisation and death. Vaccine usually takes two weeks to manifest, and it prevented 14·4–19.8 million pandemic fatalities globally in 185 nations in a single year during December 2020 and December 2021. It was necessary that the boosters alongside vaccines enhanced immunological effects and provided extended protection. Thus, vaccine and booster design and development, dosing, targeted immunisation, cost-efficacy and vaccine acceptance are challenges to address. Government, not-for-profit organisations, health agencies and researchers may systematically analyse, justify and validate vaccine R&D and vaccinations economics. This chapter comprehends biological, commercial and economic benefits and impacts of booster dose in vaccination drives, and the roadmap ahead.*

***Keywords*:** vaccines, boosters, vaccine hesitancy, vaccination, infectious disease, variants

1. Introduction

Several viral variants emerged and reemerged (especially the variants of Omicron, *a*, *b*, γ and δ) since initial days of reported infective SARS-CoV-2 cases in the Wuhan city which triggered multiple COVID-19 waves. The significance of vaccination as the most significant preventive strategy is well documented and duly acknowledged, more so with the pandemic. Honestly, the health authorities across several countries were initially not very serious about the consequences of the viral spread as SARS-CoV-2 emerged in the Mainland China on 31 December 2019. This was attributed primarily to its symptoms and clinical presentations being similar to the seasonal flu (influenza), which made it difficult for a foolproof diagnosis and differentiation from the usual influenza. This deadly virus spread rapidly globally since then, infected the human population across the globe very fast, challenged the healthcare infrastructure hard and raised serious healthcare concerns worldwide (Mohapatra *et al.*, 2023a). Before anything superior could be ascertained on the diagnostics, therapeutics and preventives about COVID-19, people were advised to stay indoors as a need to self-protect, through the imposed COVID-19 lockdown and shutdown guidelines. The WHO declared COVID-19 as a public health emergency of international concern (PHEIC) on 30 January 2020, and later as a pandemic declared on 11 March 2020 (WHO, 2024a). This viral disease has been recorded as the seventh coronavirus disease. The other two previously reported coronavirus diseases that infected human subjects with serious health concerns were SARS-CoV and MERS-CoV (Mohapatra *et al.*, 2023b; Mohapatra *et al.*, 2023c; Sah *et al.*, 2023), and these emerge and reemerge currently too.

The COVID-19-causing aetiological agent SARS-CoV-2 was genome-sequenced soon after it was pure-isolated (WHO, 2024b). The researchers and the vaccine manufacturers started working collaboratively complementing each other's strengths to develop the COVID-19 vaccines to fight the pandemic. It is beyond doubt that, vaccines are one of the most complex medical products to develop (Panda *et al.*, 2023). Sufficient evidences on the quality, safety and efficacy were needed to be collected to confirm that a vaccine candidate would provide more benefits than risks when administered for 'emergency use' especially during a public health emergency situation. Although regulatory authorities have established the vaccine development and procedural guidelines to maximise vaccine efficacy (WHO, 2024b), the emergency situation that COVID-19 posed needed an expeditious action. Several vaccine vendors had prepared their roadmaps to come up with their perfected vaccines as fast as practicable to counter COVID-19. The USFDA approved Pfizer-BioNTech's vaccine as the first COVID-19 vaccine on December 11, 2020 (USFDA, 2020), marketed under the emergency use approval (EUA) on 23 August 2021 to counter COVID-19 (USFDA, 2021).

With the passage of time, numerous countries had developed their own COVID-19 vaccines to counter this deadly disease. Almost all the COVID-19 vaccines thus developed were safe, effective and prevented serious illnesses, hospitalisation and deaths, although there were some reported post-vaccination side-effects (Satapathy *et al.*, 2023). Usually, a vaccine takes about two weeks to manifest its activity after administration. Staying up-to-date with the vaccines and getting vaccinated in time was the most prudent approach to protect the citizen from deadly diseases like the COVID-19. As per a study, it is estimated that 14·4–19.8 million pandemic deaths could be prevented between 8 December 2020 and 8 December 2021 in 185 countries and territories through COVID-19 vaccinations (Watson *et al.*, 2022). Several emerging and reemerging viral variants were identified since the reported first case of SARS-CoV-2 infection (Mohapatra *et al.*, 2023d). These viral variants, particularly the SARS-CoV-2 VOCs, were responsible for multiple COVID-19 waves across the globe. Five VOCs had been reported till date, namely alpha (B.1.1.7), beta (B.1.351), gamma (P.1), delta (B.1.617.2) and omicron (B.1.1.529). This virus and its numerous variants impacted significantly the global economy and inequalities (Mohapatra *et al.*, 2023e). Also, the vaccines needed to be updated to help fight the disease more effectively as the original virus strain that caused COVID-19 continued to mutate.

2. Vaccination

Vaccinations against the various infectious diseases gained increased attention and approved after the emergence of SARS-CoV-2 causing the pandemic, with emergency use. COVID-19 pandemic had caused the biggest ever global public health catastrophe of the 21st century in documented history that affected billions of people and killing millions of them. Despite the stupendous advancements made in terms of healthcare infrastructure and scientific endeavours, the COVID-19 associated morbidity and mortality remained a cause for concern for the healthcare administrations around the globe. The WHO, the European Medicine Agency (EMA) and the USFDA along with other international drug control agencies in specific countries fast-forwarded the vaccine availability during the pandemic through 'emergency use' approvals of COVID-19 vaccines. It enabled the availability of the potentially efficacious vaccines in the open market for public consumption as also the sponsored vaccination drives even before the completion of Phase III (final stage) clinical trials.

Clinical trial research intended to develop a vaccine usually takes at least a decade to complete. However, the COVID-19 vaccine development was carried out in less than a year. It resulted in the uncertainty about its efficacy and long-term safety, and informed vaccine hesitancy. Moreover, emerging SARS-CoV-2 variants, subvariants and lineages with unique genetic mutations resulted in vaccine resistance and breakthrough infections (Mohapatra *et al.*, 2022a). This called for the development of the nest-generation vaccines that could counter the emerging variants (Mohapatra *et al.*, 2023e). Assessment of the safety and efficacy of the vaccines among various population groups like children, the pregnant etc. was urgently needed (Li *et al.*, 2023).

It was observed that vaccine dosages needed to be standardised, and the protection conferred by a full-dose vaccination was short-term that waned in about a month. It required the adoption of booster shots of the vaccine for increased protection conferred against future infections, especially among the susceptible populations like the elderly (>60 years) and individuals with debilitating conditions and comorbidities. Thus, it is clear that there were several vaccine development and mass vaccination challenges to address, like the manufacturing of sufficient vaccine doses to immunise the global population, cost rationalisation to make it available to people in the LMICs, and the vaccine safety among the population (Yarlagadda *et al.*, 2022; Ansari *et al.*, 2022). Fig. 1 details the biological (parental nutrition, breastfeeding, age, sex, nutrition, internal and external stress, comorbidities, smoking and alcoholism), commercial (vaccine type, safety, efficacy, preservatives, adjuvants and duration of protection) and economic (cost of distribution and equity, import and export, acceptance issues and cost of development and production) factors that affect vaccination drives around the globe against especially the infectious diseases.

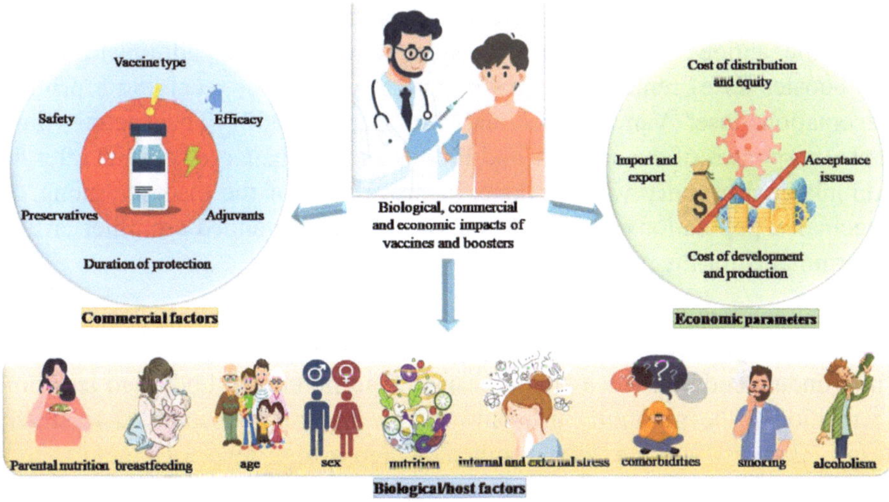

Fig. 1: The biological, commercial and economic factors that affect vaccination drives

3. COVID-19 Vaccine Booster

A booster vaccine dose is the administration of an extra dose of the same (homologolous boosting) or a different (homologolous boosting) vaccine after administering an initial (preliminary) dose. A booster dose after initial vaccination exposes the vaccinee repeatedly to the immunising antigen or immunogen. Booster vaccination helps to increase the immunity against a particular target antigen at protective level (titre) after memory against the antigen waned. For instance, it is recommended to receive booster shots against tetanus are every ten years as the memory cells specific against tetanus tend to undergo programmed cell death or lose their function by this time (van der Heiden *et al.*, 2017).

Notably, Arthus reaction develops if a booster dose is administered in a subject who possesses a high antibody titre. Arthus reaction is a localised hypersensitivity (Type III) induced by high IgG antibody titre that could cause swelling (Leuridan and Van Damme, 2011). Although this swelling or inflammation self-limits in few days but, however it could be thorough avoided with increased duration between primary vaccine dose and the booster dose (Chavda *et al.*, 2022). Thus, whether there is a need for the booster dose after primary vaccination needs to be ascertained. This is done through numerous approaches. One of the approaches is the spatial estimation of the antibody titre specific to a disease after administration of primary dose. Rapid production of antibodies after the vaccination stimuli (anamnestic response) to ascertain the need for a vaccine booster dose is a typical approach. The need for a booster dose is most likely little if an anamnestic response (rapid antibody production the same antigen is subsequently encountered or upon administration of the booster dose) remained high for several years after receiving a primary vaccination dose (Van Damme and Van Herck, 2007). The spatial (time-lapse) responses of the active T and B cells against the target antigen after the administered primary vaccine dose, or prevalence of the disease among the vaccinated populations for which the vaccine was intended are other critical determinants for the purpose.

The factors behind some (like hepatitis A, hepatitis B) vaccines being effective for a lifetime while others (like tetanus) needing boosters are not fully understood yet. It was hypothesised that the human body had less time to memorise the immunity efficiently if the immunity responded relatively faster against a vaccine, as a result of which a high level of memory cells did not persist for a lifetime in humans (Abdulla *et al.*, 2023). As a immunity response, the memory B and T helper cells maintain at a fairly high titre in the germinal centres (with slow to nonexistent cell division rate) after a primary vaccination dosing. While these memory cells live long, they typically don't undergo mitosis. As a result of it, the loss rate of these cells is eventually greater than the gain rate. Thus, the booster dose of a vaccine is needed in such instances to 'boost' the memory T and B cell counts (Natalini *et al.*, 2022). Booster dosing became impending in COVID-19 vaccination process.

The COVID-19 pandemic posed global health concerns of very high order which had resulted 704,753,890 confirmed human infections worldwide with 7,010,681 deaths till 13 April 2024 (Mbonigaba *et al.*, 2024). Although vaccination was carried out almost everywhere across the globe, however inequitable distribution of the vaccines among the developed and developing countries was glaringly noticed which might have been a possible reason for the further viral spread (Sharun and Dhama, 2021; Wouters *et al.*, 2021), and the emergence of numerous variants that were increasingly transmissive and infective. Further, the vaccination drives were also severely affected due to the alleged post-vaccination side-effects as was observed throughout the world resulting in vaccine hesitancy (Troiano and Nardi, 2021; Dhama *et al.*, 2021). The vaccine hesitancy was further witnessed even among the educated and informed community as all the 'emergency use' vaccines had not yet undergone a thorough clinical trial process. The waning vaccine efficacy and the constantly emerging deadly viral variant forms emphasised the need for COVID-19 booster shots (Burki, 2022; Garcia-Beltran *et al.*, 2022). The booster shot of COVID-19 vaccine is an extra dose that was administered when the protection from the original shot gradually became weaker and increasingly ineffective. The booster shot helped the vaccinated subject to maintain the antibody contents and immunity levels in the body appreciably high for longer duration (Mohapatra *et al.*, 2022b).

Numerous countries had administrated booster doses of the vaccines among the citizens through their vaccination drives especially to control the spread of the novel viral variants of SARS-CoV-2. The fully-vaccinated human subjects who received the booster doses reportedly had a ten times lower risk of sicking with COVID-19 as compared with unvaccinated individuals (Khandia *et al.*, 2022). A UK-based study suggested that the booster shots were moderately to highly effective which provided 70–75% extra protection (Antonelli *et al.*, 2023). The study also reported that third dose (second booster dose) of Pfizer-BioNTech induced up to an additional 25-fold increase in the titre of the neutralising antibodies when compared with the titre levels that were elicited after the first booster dose (Hvidt *et al.*, 2022). As per the single blind randomised clinical trial study, it was noticed that the heterologous boosting (booster dose of another vaccine form than the initial) resulted more robust immune response as compared to homologous boosting (Atmar *et al.*, 2022). However, the efficacy and safety of such vaccination strategies (especially of the heterologous boosting) in the face of the numerous constantly emerging and reemerging novel viral variants from time to time was still debatable and needed further scientific investigations and detailed insights.

Substantial evidences on the currently available COVID-19 vaccine's efficacy against the numerous deadly SARS-CoV-2 variants were currently missing. It was also reported that two vaccine shots were insufficient to protect against the most infectious Omicron variant. Keeping this in mind, vaccination drives and booster shots were critical especially in the countries with high virus circulation to reduce the immediate and the long-term health consequences of the disease. As numerous subvariants of the COVID-19 viral variants were currently circulating and the immunity against Omicron was poor without a booster dose, focussed research and deeper insights are still needed to examine the vaccination efficacy in preventing symptomatic and asymptomatic ailments caused by the Omicron variants. The COVID-19 vaccine doses including the boosters administrated country-wise, as per the collated data of 2024 (till 12 August 2024) from the World Health Organisation (WHO) sites, are presented in Fig. 2.

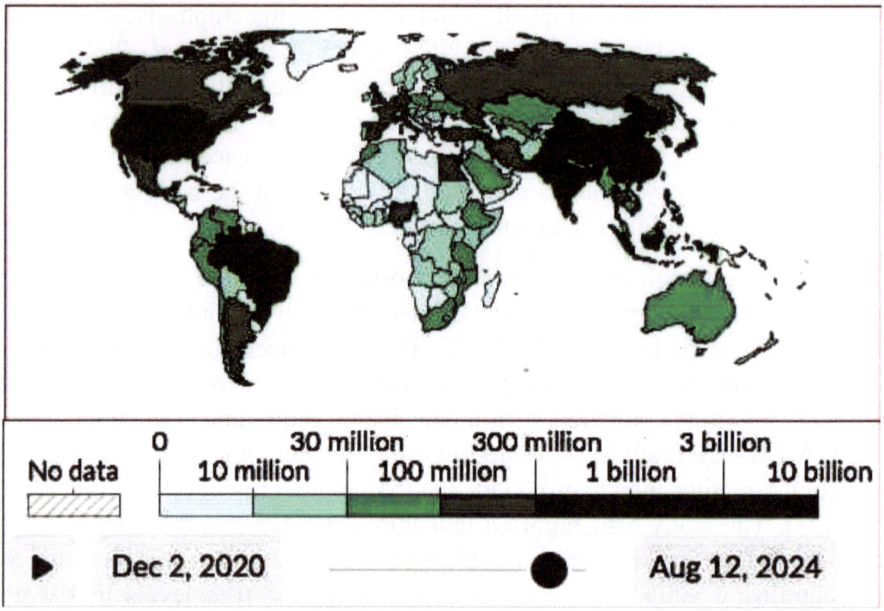

Fig. 2: The country-wise COVID-19 vaccine dosages including the boosters as administrated till 12 August 2024 (Our world in data, 2024)

Based on vaccination history, age and the overall health condition (including comorbidities) of the human subjects, the updated recommendations of the WHO's SAGE on immunisation for vaccination have been outlined in Table 1.

Table 1: Updated SAGE recommendations for vaccination during COVID-19 (WHO, 2023)

Vaccination status	Target recipient	Dose recommendation
Never received a vaccine	• All adults	Single dose
	• Child and adolescent	
	• Healthcare worker	
	• Pregnant woman	
	• Immuno-compromised individual	Multiple (2-3) doses
Has received at least a dose earlier	• Pregnant woman	Single dose during each pregnancy
	• Healthy adult, child and adolescent	Routine revaccination not recommended
	• Healthcare worker	Revaccination after 12 months of the most recent dose
	• Adult with comorbidity	
	• Adult > 50 years	
	• Immuno-compromised individual	Revaccination after 6–12 months of the most recent dose
	• Adult > 50 years with comorbidity	
	• Adult > 75 years	

3.1. Booster Dosing During COVID-19 Vaccination

Despite the low efficacy of the vaccines in protecting from COVID-19 infection, the protection from this deadly disease remained high till six months after the vaccination as of September 2021. Experts from WHO, US FDA and several other healthcare institutions of international repute opined that the available dataset to assess the sustained protection of the booster dose was insufficient as the observed data were only with regard to the short-term protective effects. Their immediate recommendation was to make the existing vaccine stock available to the population worldwide who had not received any vaccination yet to save most lives (Hartzell and Blaylock, 2014).

As the first country, Israel introduced booster dosage of Pfizer–BioNTech mRNA vaccine of COVID-19 in July 2021 for it's citizens who were at a 'high risk' (Yamin *et al.*, 2023), and expanding the option for the rest of its population in August. It was found that, the efficacy of the vaccine against the disease severity was lower among those who were vaccinated during January and April as compared to those who were vaccinated during February and March. Immediately after the booster dosing was approved and was deployed widely during the first three weeks of August 2021, a third shot (relative to the two doses) was suggested for an extended short-term protection (Hartzell and Blaylock, 2014).

The CDC (Centres for Disease Prevention and Control) in the US launched booster shots during 2021 summer for the immuno-compromised individuals, with an original plan to allow an adult to receive a third COVID-19 vaccine dose starting in September 2021. The condition was that an individual would become eligible for the second booster (third) dose eight months after receiving the second dose (Gavish *et al.*, 2022). Later, the CDC allowed receiving the booster shot six months after the second shot after further data about the delta variant and the long-term vaccine efficacy was understood, in late October (Gavish *et al.*, 2022). The vaccinations in the US surged subsequently (Gavish *et al.*, 2022). The JCVI in the UK recommended booster shots, preferably the Pfizer–BioNTech mRNA vaccine, for the 'at-risk' groups and the population over the age of 50 years in September 2021 which meant that a third (second booster) dose was needed to be administered to about 30 million adults (Gavish *et al.*, 2022). Subsequently, the booster-shot rollout was extended in the UK to the population over the age of 40 years in November 2021 (Willis *et al.*, 2024). The Sputnik V COVID-19 vaccine of Russia, that used a similar technology as that of COVID-19 vaccine of AstraZeneca, introduced a COVID-19 booster (Sputnik Light) in November 2021 with a 70% efficacy against the delta variant (as per the GRIEM studies) (Willis *et al.*, 2024). Further, it was opined that Sputnik Light might be potent with the mRNA vaccine combinations than the mRNA boosters (Satapathy *et al.*, 2023).

The National Health Service of the UK recommended to its citizens a waiting period of 28 days after testing COVID-19 positive before getting the booster shots. It was evidenced that a booster dose vaccination after recovering from COVID-19 infection provided additional immunity protection (Gilboa *et al.*, 2022). Thus, booster shots were reportedly useful even after contracting a COVID-19 infection. Below are mentioned some other case instances of the vaccination campaign against numerous other common infectious diseases (cases of polio, hepatitis B, tetanus and whooping cough) wherein a booster dosing became fairly imminent and beneficial for the ailing or the 'at-risk' subject.

3.1.1. COVID-19 Booster Vaccination in the Europe

COVID-19 vaccination drives saved lakhs of lives in the EU by the end of 2021, as per an estimate (Meslé *et al.*, 2021). Additional COVID-19 vaccine booster dosing on annual bases were recommended in the UK and other countries from 2022, particularly for 'at-high-risk' individuals including the elderly and the comorbid individual (with an underlying comorbid medical condition). UK based studies showed that booster dose of the originally formulated vaccine diminished hospitalisation risk against BA.4/BA.5 (Kirsebom *et al.*, 2022) and BA.1 (Nyberg *et al.*, 2022). COVID-19 vaccines were updated in 2022 autumn by including an Omicron strain alongside the original strain. The US used a BA.4/BA.5 bivalent vaccine while the UK used a BA.1 bivalent vaccine (Kirsebom *et al.*, 2023a).

Vaccine efficacy is about estimating the protection level guaranteed through vaccination to a vaccinated individual (Sullivan *et al.*, 2015). Choosing the comparison group to study and interpret the impact of COVID-19 booster shot matters which needs meticulous spadework. Individuals receiving the fourth dose recently were compared with the unvaccinated subjects. And similarly, between the eligible individuals for a fourth dosage who chose not to be vaccinated. However, as almost all vaccine dosages being administered currently were the booster doses, comparing with the nonvaccinated subjects was quite selective with low community health significance.

Multiple healthcare digital records were linked in England to estimate vaccination efficacy against COVID-19 during December 2022 and April 2023. The patients who tested positive for acute respiratory illness were considered as the cases and those with COVID-19 negative test reports were considered as controls that were limited to the persons with only the primary diagnosis codes for the respiratory illness (Kirsebom *et al.*, 2023a). 3881 cases and 187,348 test-negative controls were included in the study, with stratified subvariant analyses. It was found that bivalent COVID-19 vaccines could effectively prevented COVID-19 hospitalisation against BQ.1, CH.1.1 and XBB.1.5 variants, five to nine weeks after the vaccination (Kirsebom *et al.*, 2023b). Booster doses of bivalent vaccine could effectively prevent COVID-19 hospitalisations between the time period 5 September 2022 and 5 February 2023 when the various Omicron subvariants circulated (Kirsebom *et al.*, 2023a). With the evidence that bivalent vaccines protected against the antigenically-distinct Omicron subvariants that circulated then, this observation supported using bivalent vaccines to protect against severe COVID-19 infections.

Data linkage approach adopted by Kirsebom *et al.* (2023b) on multiple digital records was functionally limited. Data linkage could be erroneous where a unique identifier was not available or the linkage was imperfectly executed. In line with the conventional clinical case definition, deriving the cases as well as the non-cases from the digital records of one source population might not be a good proposition. It might complicate the study prospects on the negative tests subjects. Thus, the approach may not be a good approach to study booster dose, especially when the data related to the reason behind hospitalisation was updated after discharging a patient and the testing performed in the hospital was informed later. After the successful formulation of a monovalent vaccine using XBB.1.5 (COVID variant) strain for the northern hemisphere winter during 2023 and 2024, an updated strain was recommended in the UK and elsewhere to use in boosting COVID-19 vaccination. Assessing the sustained protection over a longer period beyond six months was needed to be studied further to provide relevant data related to the booster dosage drives. A sustained monitoring of the COVID-19 booster vaccination was crucial as a regular community healthcare activity.

3.1.2. COVID-19 Booster Vaccination in the US

Understanding the risk mitigation by the various COVID-19 vaccine boosters against the severely manifested COVID-19 across various age-group and immunity levels were needed for public healthcare purpose. Microsimulation models on the surveillance and the seroprevalence data of COVID-19 revealed that booster vaccination frequently in six to twelve month time period among the immunocompromised and the older population effectively reduced the COVID-19 burden in the US. It is learnt that frequent booster vaccination benefitted against severe disease only modestly among the young. The model estimated that annual booster dose administration reduced absolute severe COVID-19 risk by 199 cases in every lakh elderly (above 75 years) compared to booster vaccination only once. While frequent administration of the booster vaccines benefitted the immunocompromised more, it had less benefit on those with prior COVID-19 infection. Frequent dosing of variant-targeted booster vaccines increasingly benefitted against the immune-evading emerging variants. Due consideration of key risk factors about COVID-19 booster vaccination frequency among the public in general and facilitate foolproof annual booster dosing among high-risk population was needed as health guidance and advisory.

Studies have shown that severe COVID-19 infection that led to hospitalisation or even death could be prevented through mild infection and/or vaccination (Bobrovitz *et al.*, 2023; Lin, 2023). While likely infection as also vaccination protected from severe COVID-19, however the protection waned with time partly as novel variants emerged (Menegale *et al.*, 2023; Stein *et al.*, 2023). Despite a prior declining trend, additional booster shots restored the protection levels (Bobrovitz *et al.*, 2023; Lin, 2023). Severe COVID-19 risk was complex and person-specific. While studies on introducing the COVID-19 vaccines on priority were many (Bubar *et al.*, 2021; Matrajt *et al.*, 2021; Giordano *et al.*, 2021; Gozzi *et al.*, 2021; Chapman *et al.*, 2022), evidences for a guided decision on the timing of the booster vaccination to prevent COVID-19 severity were limited. Individual considerations to assess the booster vaccination frequency (like monovalent vaccine targeting a single variant like XBB.1.5 or a bivalent vaccine that targeted the wild strain as well as the Omicron subvariants BA.4/5) included: i) age-correlated baseline risk of infection severity, or an immunocompromised state; ii) the dose number and the time lapse since last vaccination (vaccination history); iii) earlier COVID-19 infection(s) like the duration since the last infection and the variants that were involved; and iv) the overall infection risk by the transmitted SARS-CoV-2 within the community. A comparison of the COVID-19 booster vaccination efficacy based on the frequency may vary based on the numerous critical parameters given the heterogeneous nature of the risk of COVID-19 severity within a population.

The decision on the optimal need of a COVID-19 booster vaccine and its right timing would be dependent on the value judgments, the associated factors considered, evaluating COVID-19 severity on the absolute and the relative scales, and the perspectives of individual and the community level effects. The decision-making on COVID-19 booster vaccination frequency shall more likely be influenced by the emerging novel variants, subvariants and strains, and the formulated novel vaccine.

3.2. Booster Dosing Against Polio

After administering the polio vaccine orally (OPV), the generated B and T memory cells persisted for about six months. This booster dosing was found to be ineffective as the results revealed that the immune response still decreased after every six months. However, the immune response was found to enhance the antibody titre by 39–75% when a booster shot of the IPV was used in the test subject (Deng *et al.*, 2022). OPV is often preferred over the IPV in the developing countries owing to economics and logistics reasons. Further, IPVs were challenging to store in tropical countries primarily attributed to the prevailing climate. Inactivated polio vaccine (IPV) boosting after the primary OPV dose could eradicate the disease in the regions where polio was persistent (Jafari *et al.*, 2014). There is a caution here; the OPV reportedly developed critical illness and paralysed the vaccine recipient although the cases were rare which was about one in every 2.7 million cases. For this, IPV is administered in the USA incrementally in instalments; three in the first year, a half after birth (post-parturition), and a booster dose between four and six years of age (Deng *et al.*, 2022). It is noteworthy that the US insists on the use of only the IPV.

3.3. Booster Dosing Against Hepatitis B

Whether there is the need for a booster dosing of hepatitis B is debated since long. Studies to estimate the memory cell titre in the vaccinated individuals in the early 2000s have revealed that a booster shot was not needed later in life in the fully vaccinated adults who received all the three vaccination rounds as per the prescribed timeline during their infancy. The CDC of the US and the NACI of Canada supported the recommendations and advised against the need for the booster dosing of hepatitis B (Ford-Jones *et al.*, 2016). However, the scenario might differ in case of immuno-compromised individuals who would be advised to assess the immune response, and could receive booster shots of hepatitis B if the B and T cell titres against hepatitis B went below the subminimal levels as per the clinical findings (Ford-Jones *et al.*, 2016).

3.4. Booster Dosing Against Tetanus

There is a requirement of a booster dose every ten years against tetanus disease. It could be administered immediately following tetanus infection in certain circumstances. The recommended booster shot for adults is Td (Tetanus and adult diphtheria, a tetanus and diphtheria combination with a lower diphtheria antigen titre). It differed from primary tetanus vaccine dose (DPT) as the immunisation against pertussis (whooping cough) was not included (Cook *et al.*, 2001). While the USA recommended tetanus booster dosing after every ten years, other countries (like the UK) suggested booster shots twice only in the initial twenty years with no additional booster shots after that (Cook *et al.*, 2001). As neonatal tetanus in case of some women is a concern during pregnancy, the administration of a booster shot against tetanus is recommended to expecting mothers during pregnancy to protect the child in the womb against the disease (Cook *et al.*, 2001).

3.5. Booster Dosing Against Whooping Cough

Whooping cough, also known as pertussis, is an infectious disease that affected the respiratory tract. *Bordetella pertussis*, the causal bacterium, sticks to the cilia (tiny hair-like extensions) in the upper respiratory tract. The disease is particularly fatal for babies who had not yet developed their immune system fully. If unattended, the ailment could result in troubled breathing in the baby or would develop into pneumonia (Rodrigo *et al., 2014)*. Also known as DPT, DTaP (diphtheria, tetanus, pertussis) is the primary vaccine administered typically in five shots before the child attains seven years of age. Tdap is the booster shot against pertussis, and the US advised for its administration every ten years and the expecting mothers during every pregnancy. It is also recommended as a booster dose to be used against tetanus (Hartzell and Blaylock 2014). The pertussis vaccine was administered as inactivated bacterium entirely (whole-cell) when it was invented in the 1950s. The vaccine caused localised reactions and fever in the vaccine recipient. However, the acellular vaccine that was developed in the 1990s which contained only a small fraction of *Bordetella pertussis* with less side-effects, because of which it was recommended in the US. However, as only a small fraction of *B. pertussis* was present, this vaccine was reportedly less effective in eliciting immunological memory responses as the antigen that was presented to the immune system was incomplete (Hartzell and Blaylock 2014). This alternate vaccine was popular due to its high safety levels, however it led to developing the Tdap vaccine as a booster for a sustained immune response as the vaccine was less effective (Hartzell and Blaylock, 2014).

4. Biologicals

Biologicals are the diverse group of third generation pharmaceuticals including vaccines, monoclonal antibodies (mAbs), immune modulators (substance that stimulated immunity), the growth factors (biologically active molecule affecting cellular growth) and the numerous products derived from human fluid connective tissue (Eaglstein and Eaglstein, 2014). Usually, these are purified proteins that are obtained from living systems including human blood. However, other 'small molecule' medicines are synthetically produced or purified from the numerous plant sources. Also considered as biologicals, biological therapeutics are the class of medicines that are grown and then purified from mass culture of bacterial, yeast, plant or animal cells. Due to the inherent differences in their nature, biological therapeutics are tested, regulated and controlled differently than other similar medicines. Each batch of a biological therapeutic product should be tested at various production stages till its patient administration to ensure their safety, quality and efficacy.

5. Biologics

Biologics are designed with the use of living cells/organisms to treat the life-threatening diseases (Halimi *et al.*, 2020). These include a range of products like transplant tissue, blood and blood components, recombinant proteins, gene therapies, insulin therapies, mAbs and stem cell therapies. Biologics may be composed of proteins, sugars, nucleic acids or their complex combinations, and living entities like the cells and tissues (Eaglstein and Eaglstein, 2014). Biologics are isolated from a range of natural (animal, human, microbial) sources. Biologics differ from the conventional drugs in terms of the manufacturing process, the sources of materials, structural complexities and the regulatory requirements (Eaglstein and Eaglstein, 2014). Owing to these reasons, biologics are seemingly highly priced that is obviously a barrier to patient accessibility; everyone could not afford it (Halimi *et al.*, 2020). These are used to treat many severe and seemingly untreatable ailments, like the autoimmune inflammatory conditions (Hsiao et al. 2020). These are a special group of modern third generation pharmaceutical products used to treat a variety of clinical conditions for which no other treatment was available. Numerous USFDA-approved biologics are now being actively employed in the various medical interventions in immunology, oncology, rheumatology, gastroenterology, neurology, diabetes and genetically inherited clinical conditions (Dash *et al.*, 2021).

6. Biosimilars

Biosimilars are another group of third generation pharmaceutical (biopharmaceuticals) products designed particularly to increase the patients' access to biologic medicine treatment. Although technically different, biosimilars are equivalent to biologic medications with no clinically meaningful variations, and possess the same levels of safety and efficacy. These are the medicines that are specifically designed to have similar properties to a similar conventional drug available over the counter. As defined by the USFDA, a biosimilar is a biological product which is similar and has no clinically meaningful difference from the existing FDA-approved reference product in terms of purity, safety and potency (Patil *et al.*, 2024). Due to the streamlined development process adopted, biosimilars are expected be less expensive than the biologics.

7. Biological Aspects Of Vaccines and Vaccination

Vaccine development and success of any vaccination programme is reflected by the conferred protection by the vaccine against infections. An immunised person produces the protective neutralisation antibody after vaccination. But, antibodies have specific lifespan predisposing people to infections after the vaccine's effects diminish (Shahapur *et al.*, 2022). A vaccine booster dose extends the duration of the protection. Vaccine safety and efficacy depends on biological factors like the environment, the host and traits of pathogens. Vaccination results in a unique response. Some people response positively to a vaccine and develop immunity against infections, while some others fail to develop protective immunity thereby being predisposed to infections (Grassly *et al.*, 2015). Such variations in the response to vaccination by different people are not well explained (Plotkin, 2013). However, studies attributed it to the role of genetic traits in influencing the response (Newport *et al.*, 2004). The factors that were found to influence the response include childhood vaccination history, microbial exposure during early age, breastfeeding patterns and nutritional supplementation after birth, etc. (Parker *et al.*, 2014). Among many intrinsic, perinatal, extrinsic, environmental, nutritional and behavioural factors, the host factors influencing vaccine efficacy are antibiotics usage, sleep pattern, physical exercise, smoking and alcohol intake (Zimmermann and Curtis, 2019).

A successful vaccine must elicit both humoral (antibody-mediated) and the cell-mediated immune responses that confer protection against the invading pathogen. Applying advanced technologies like high-throughput evaluation of immunological and related parameters after vaccination in host and role of vaccine adjuvants (high-molecular weight carrier compounds) in increasing vaccine immunogenicity were suggested (Pulendran *et al.*, 2010). Varying immunological response and the protection conferred by vaccines also depends on the mode of vaccine administration. It may be explained by the fact that most infections are acquired through microbial contact to mucus membranes like respiratory epithelium and oropharyngeal mucosal surfaces. The COVID-19 vaccine is administered parenterally, and the Bacillus Calmette Guerin (BCG) vaccine intramuscular. It could impact vaccine efficacy, and the conferred protection. Despite limitations, oral vaccination in infants still seems to be most effective (Liu *et al.*, 2024).

Studies on humans exposed to soil microbiome and the response to pneumococcal vaccine were recently conducted. As evidenced by the raised IFN-gamma level, the results showed that people exposed to soil microbes induced better cellular immune response as against the control group. It was noticed that gut microbiome decreased the levels of proinflammatory cytokines like tissue growth factor (TGF)-*β* plasma (Roslund *et al.*, 2024). The role of intestinal microbiota in influencing the immunological responses to vaccines was verified by a study in paediatrics. It was observed that children born through vaginal delivery had a good balance of beneficial microbes in the intestines compared to those born through caesarean sections. It influenced the vaccination response wherein children born through vaginal delivery demonstrated better immunological responses to vaccination (de Koff *et al.*, 2022).

Varying immunological response based on the geographical regions was investigated recently (van Dorst *et al.*, 2024). It was noted that people in high-income countries developed 100% protection against malaria vaccine compared to only up to 50% protection conferred among people in low-income nations. Similar trends were seen in others, like BCG, rota and yellow fever vaccines. These differences were attributed mainly to the genetic factors and nutritional status (van Dorst *et al.*, 2024). The role of adiponectin, a hormone that participated in the metabolism was noted to influence immunological response to vaccination. The study evaluated the impact of weight on the success of pneumococcal (PCV13) vaccination. High adiponectin activity (-1.15; 95% CI: 2.22–0.072) and overweight (-0.19; 95% CI: 0.24–0.14) correlated with low immunological response (antibody content) (Siegers *et al.*, 2022).

Alternate to the host factors, the vaccine type also influences the immunological responses. The vaccine types include live-attenuated (measles, smallpox, rubella, mumps, rota virus, etc.), killed-whole cell (typhoid, rabies, influenza, Japanese B encephalitis), toxoid (diphtheria, tetanus), sub-unit (anthrax, influenza, typhoid, etc.), virus-like particle (hepatitis B virus, Human papillomavirus), outer membrane vesicle (group B meningococcal), protein-polysaccharide conjugate (*Hemophilus influenzae* type b), viral vector (SARS-CoV-2, Ebola), and nucleic acid based vaccines. Other vaccine types using bacteria as vectors and antigen-presenting cell-based vaccines are at experimental stage. Administering live vaccine among the immunocompromised is cautioned, as attenuated virus may potentially revert back to the original strain after vaccination with the ability to manifest the disease. The killed and other vaccine types would need adjuvants that enhanced immunogenicity in vaccine. The adjuvants used are liposomes, aluminium salts, etc. Vaccines also use preservatives, stabilisers and excepients like polysorbate 80, gelatine, sorbitol, antibiotics, egg, yeast, latex, formaldehyde, glutaraldehyde, and potassium/ sodium salts to ensure longevity and functionality (Pollard and Bijker, 2021).

In a recent observational study among the COVID-19 vaccinated, the time of vaccination was found to influence the efficacy. It was observed that people vaccinated in the forenoon were less likely to develop breakthrough infections as compared to those who were vaccinated in the afternoon and in the evening (HR=0.64, morning vs. evening; 95% CI: 0.43–0.97; P=0.038) (Hazan *et al.*, 2023). It could be due to the varying immunological responses like immune cell functions and their recruitment and transportation are affected by circadian rhythm (Karaboué *et al.*, 2024).

8. Commercial and Economical Aspects Of Vaccines

Developing a vaccine is a complex process, and the associated costs are also high owing to the clinical research and trials carried out throughout the process. While vaccine development and manufacturing costs are high, the scopes for profits are limited as most governments offer vaccines at a discounted price and often free under the free-for-all initiatives. This was the case with COVID-19 vaccines wherein the Indian government distributed the vaccines to the global population free-of-cost. Vaccine production may be profitable if exported to the countries in need. Many developing countries have limited logistics and equipment that necessitate import-related expenses. Vaccine development goes through research and clinical trials to confirm the safety and efficacy for approval by regulatory agencies (Kandi and Vadakedath, 2023; Kandi *et al.*, 2023).

COVID-19 pandemic could grossly be controlled by adopting two molecular-level vaccine development strategies, the rDNA and mRNA vaccine technologies. It is appreciated that although the rDNA technology is comparatively a cost-effective strategy, the mRNA vaccines seemed to be better in terms of the speed of development of such vaccines, the flexibility of the technique to accommodate even the evolving strains and the timely availability in the global market (Davidopoulou *et al.*, 2024). However, the vaccines developed by adopting the latter technology needs a strong cold-chain in logistics as these are highly sensitive to fluctuating high temperatures. Thus, although mRNA and ribonucleoproteins (RNPs) with the lipid nanoparticles as the delivery systems have been explored in vaccine development, efficient vaccines supply systems could be financially demanding which seems to be a major hurdle in acceptance of such vaccines as the most preferred ones (Eftekhari *et al.*, 2024).

Despite the technological advancements in vaccine development strategies, there are numerous infectious (like syphilis caused by *Treponema pallidum*) and non-infectious (like various cancers) diseases for which appropriate vaccines are still lacking. This state-of-affairs could be attributed to several factors that could include but are not limited to vaccine acceptance among the general population (Waugh and Cameron, 2024). Non-acceptance of vaccines (vaccine hesitancy) owing to misinformation and disinformation often make the development and commercialisation of vaccines challenging for the pharmaceutical manufacturing companies and the buyers of the vaccines like the public healthcare administrations, the governments and the non-government organisations.

9. Women Empowerment and Healthcare Equity

Women education and the degree of literacy among them vary considerably across the world. Women empowerment has been seen to have significantly affected vaccination programmes (Rodrigues and Plotkin, 2020). Women could have the autonomy on health-related decisions for themselves and their children. It would also improve childhood immunisation rates. An Indian survey on women empowerment programme conducted in rural Bihar where the participants were largely the women who were educated on health and hygiene reported higher rates of DTP, BCG and measles vaccination in children (Janssens, 2011). This study suggested that the rates of vaccination in children improved with women education and empowerment as compared to the non-participant groups where such education and awareness programmes were not conducted especially among the rural communities.

A public healthcare initiative in the Indian state of Haryana conducted between 2005 and 2012 improved the provision of healthcare resources in the rural belt and access to healthcare provision among the poor, women and children in the society (Gupta *et al.*, 2016). This initiative reduced the maternal and child healthcare inequalities. More children will allegedly survive to adulthood with a healthy life through such initiatives thereby the infant and childhood mortality could be improved. As women spend more time with the children, so women education and empowerment was crucial (Shearley, 1999). It also helped vaccinating the infants against pertussis, tetanus and influenza (Marchant *et al.*, 2017). The strategy of maternal vaccination brings great success at preventing the vaccine-preventable infectious diseases.

Mission Indradhanush envisaged manufacturing life-saving vaccines and making them available to all the pregnant women and children by 2020 in India (Rodrigues and Plotkin, 2020). A significant degree of healthcare infrastructure was required to achieve this, ranging from primary care to public healthcare. Various listed challenges in the process were financial resources, uniform implementation policy, and identifying the eligible children through public health messaging and outreach programmes. Public health personnel could be engaged to promote and broadcast critical messages timely, personal health education related to the hygiene and sanitation and malnutrition-related complications about the vaccine-preventable diseases like malaria and HIV.

The access to vaccines, therapeutics and other wellbeing-related products is still uneven in many regions worldwide. Vaccine equity and the access to medicines is a fundamental component of community healthcare and everyone's right to good health. The lack of equitable distribution especially in the low-and-medium income countries has affected the uniformity and universality of healthcare interventions, causing human miseries. Thus, vaccines and medicines must be produced and made available and accessible to everyone. It shall reduce the impact of several lethal infectious diseases (Assembly, 1985). Poverty, malnutrition, dense population, poor hygiene and sanitation, discriminating approaches, etc. are glaring factors behind vaccine inequity. Other factors that contribute to the worries are the elderly, infants, women and girls, ethnicity or racial minorities, indigenous population, people with physical and mental disabilities, and migrants (George *et al.*, 2015). Improving the access of such population to the vaccines could save millions of precious human lives each year.

EPI program of the WHO strives to ensure that everyone has a fair and timely access to the relevant vaccines. As per the reported of EPI of the WHO, the vaccine coverage in the developing countries increased from 5% to about 80% in the last 15 years (Levine and Robins-Browne, 2009). Further, the global distribution of vaccines particularly among the infants, children, women and low poverty people was affected due to several civil unrests around the world. A study observed that the phased introduction of vaccine for measles in Bangladesh in 1982 in an equitable manner improved the healthcare outcome there (Bishai *et al.*, 2003). The modelling to understand the impact of rotavirus vaccine in India suggested that the vaccine programme could provide direct healthcare benefits and indirect financial benefits to the poor (Verguet *et al.*, 2013). Such economic modelling on vaccines with regard to the healthcare interventions would improve the policy decisions at the governmental level with an eye on the targeted and most vulnerable population in the society (Riumallo-Herl *et al.*, 2018). Implementation of the combined public healthcare initiatives with proper health infrastructure and improved provision of nutrition would provide additional cost-effective benefits and prevent the occurrence of infectious diseases (Gessner *et al.*, 2017).

As vaccines reduce the risks of contracting a vaccine-preventable infectious disease, immunisation drives have saved millions of human lives. Immunisation reportedly currently prevents 3.5-5 million annual deaths from infectious diseases like tetanus, pertussis, diphtheria, influenza and measles (WHO, 2024a). The Austrian government imposed a mandatory COVID-19 vaccination for all its citizens during the COVID-19 pandemic, on Dec 9, 2021 (Desson *et al.*, 2022). Strengthening the healthcare and human rights efforts including the climate crisis, right to a sustainable environment, social media, social injustice, social determinants of health arising from inequity, conflict and displacement were suggested (Rami *et al*, 2023).

10. Conclusion

Compared with other public healthcare interventions, vaccines seem to be preferred, being highly beneficial and cost-effective. A successful vaccine programme would reduce the associated morbidity and mortality, provide protection against target vaccine-preventable infectious diseases, and also lead to reduced healthcare costs on treating the diseases. It is highly recommended that the government agencies, non-governmental organisations, health authorities and line researchers perform systematic economic analyses on vaccines and vaccination programmes that are carried out across the globe to justify the situation further. In such a scenario, vaccine boosters could play a critical and effective role to moderate the situation and provide extended benefits through vaccination programmes.

References

Abdulla ZA, Al-Bashir SM, Alzoubi H, Al-Salih NS, Aldamen AA and Abdulazeez AZ, 2023. The role of immunity in the pathogenesis of SARS-CoV-2 infection and in the protection generated by COVID-19 vaccines in different age groups. Pathogens, 12(2): 329. doi: 10.3390/pathogens12020329

Ansari MH, Aborode AT, Aboufandi Y, Hassan J, Suvvari TK and Kandi V, 2022. Vaccine equity-The need of the hour in the face of emerging SARS-CoV-2 variants. Asian Pac. J. Trop. Med., 15(2): 95–96. doi: 10.4103/1995-7645.338445

Antonelli M, Penfold RS, Canas LDS, Sudre C, Rjoob K, Murray B, Molteni E, Kerfoot E, Cheetham N, Pujol JC and Polidori L, 2023. SARS-CoV-2 infection following booster vaccination: illness and symptom profile in a prospective, observational community-based case-control study. J. Infect., 87(6): 506–515. doi: 10.1016/j.jinf.2023.08.009

Assembly WH, 1985. The expanded programme on immunization: the 1974 resolution by the world health assembly. Assignment child., 69: 87–88.

Atmar RL, Lyke KE, Deming ME, Jackson LA, Branche AR, El Sahly HM, Rostad CA, Martin JM, Johnston C, Rupp RE and Mulligan MJ, 2022. Homologous and heterologous Covid-19 booster vaccinations. N Eng. J. Med., 386(11): 1046–1057. doi: 10.1056/NEJMoa2116414

Bishaia D, Koenig M and Khan MA, 2003. Measles vaccination improves the equity of health outcomes: evidence from Bangladesh. Health Econ., 12(5): 415–419. doi: 10.1002/hec.732

Bobrovitz N, Ware H, Ma X, Li Z, Hosseini R, Cao C, Selemon A, Whelan M, Premji Z, Issa H and Cheng B, 2023. Protective effectiveness of previous SARS-CoV-2 infection and hybrid immunity against the omicron variant and severe disease: a systematic review and meta-regression. Lancet Infect. Dis., 23(5): 556–567. doi: 10.1016/S1473-3099(22)00801-5

Bubar KM, Reinholt K, Kissler SM, Lipsitch M, Cobey S, Grad YH and Larremore DB, 2021. Model-informed COVID-19 vaccine prioritization strategies by age and serostatus. Science, 371(6352): 916–921. doi: 10.1126/science.abe6959

Burki TK, 2022. Omicron variant and booster COVID-19 vaccines. Lancet Respir. Med., 10(2): e17.doi:10.1016/S2213-2600(21)00559-2.

Chapman LA, Shukla P, Rodríguez-Barraquer I, Shete PB, León TM, Bibbins-Domingo K, Rutherford GW, Schechter R and Lo NC, 2022. Risk factor targeting for vaccine prioritization during the COVID-19 pandemic. Sci. Rep., 12(1): 3055. doi: 10.1038/s41598-022-06971-5

Chavda VP, Patel AB, Pandya A, Vora LK, Patravale V, Tambuwala ZM, Aljabali AA, Serrano-Aroca Á, Mishra V and Tambuwala MM, 2022. Co-infection associated with SARS-CoV-2 and their management. Fut. Sci. OA, 8(9): FSO819. doi: 10.2144/fsoa-2022-0011

Cook TM, Protheroe RT and Handel JM, 2001. Tetanus: a review of the literature. Br. J. Anaesth., 87(3): 477–487. doi:10.1093/bja/87.3.477.

Dash P, Mohapatra S, Ghosh S and Nayak B, 2021. A scoping insight on potential prophylactics, vaccines and therapeutic weaponry for the ongoing novel coronavirus (COVID-19) pandemic-a comprehensive review. Front. Pharmacol., 11: 590154. doi: 10.3389/fphar.2020.590154

Davidopoulou C, Kouvelas D and Ouranidis A, 2024. COMPARING vaccine manufacturing technologies recombinant DNA vs in vitro transcribed (IVT) mRNA. Sci. Rep., 14(1): 21742. doi: 10.1038/s41598-024-67797-x.

de Koff EM, van Baarle D, van Houten MA, Reyman M, Berbers GA, van den Ham F, Chu MLJ, Sanders EA, Bogaert D and Fuentes S, 2022. Mode of delivery modulates the intestinal microbiota and impacts the response to vaccination. Nat. Commun., 13(1): 6638. doi: 10.1038/s41467-022-34155-2.

Deng Y, Yi L, Li Y, Zhao Z, Zhong Z, Shi H, Li J, Liang Y and Yang J, 2022. Safety evaluation on concomitant immunization with inactivated poliomyelitis vaccine produced from Sabin strains and other vaccines (from 2015 to 2020). Hum. Vaccin. Immunother., 18(1): 2041944. doi: 10.1080/21645515.2022.2041944

Desson Z, Kauer L, Otten T, Peters JW and Paolucci F, 2022. Finding the way forward: COVID-19 vaccination progress in Germany, Austria and Switzerland. Health Policy Technol., 11(2): 100584. doi: 10.1016/j.hlpt.2021.100584

Dhama K, Sharun K, Tiwari R, Dhawan M, Emran TB, Rabaan AA and Alhumaid S, 2021. COVID-19 vaccine hesitancy–reasons and solutions to achieve a successful global vaccination campaign to tackle the ongoing pandemic. Hum. Vaccin. Immunother., 17(10): 3495–3499. doi:10.1080/21645515.2021.1926183.

Eaglstein WH and Eaglstein WH, 2014. What Are Biologics, Biological Products and Biological Drugs?. The FDA for Doctors, 19–20. doi: 10.1007/978-3-319-08362-9_4

Eftekhari Z, Zohrabi H, Oghalaie A, Ebrahimi T, Shariati FS, Behdani M and Kazemi-Lomedasht F, 2024. Advancements and challenges in mRNA and ribonucleoprotein-based therapies:

From delivery systems to clinical applications. Mol. Ther. Nucleic Acids, 35(3): 102313. doi: 10.1016/j.omtn.2024.102313.

Ford-Jones EL and Calvin S, 2010. Literature Review on Rotavirus: Disease and Vaccine Characteristics: An Advisory Committee Statement (ACS)• National Advisory Committee on Immunization (NACI). Can. Commun. Dis. Rep., 36(ACS-14): 1–31. doi: 10.14745/ccdr.v36i00a14

Garcia-Beltran WF, Denis KJS, Hoelzemer A, Lam EC, Nitido AD, Sheehan ML, Berrios C, Ofoman O, Chang CC, Hauser BM and Feldman J, 2022. mRNA-based COVID-19 vaccine boosters induce neutralizing immunity against SARS-CoV-2 Omicron variant. Cell, 185(3): 457–466. doi: 10.1016/j.cell.2021.12.033

Gavish N, Yaari R, Huppert A and Katriel G, 2022. Population-level implications of the Israeli booster campaign to curtail COVID-19 resurgence. Sci. Transl. Med., 14(647): eabn9836. doi: 10.1126/scitranslmed.abn9836

George U, Thomson MS, Chaze F and Guruge S, 2015. Immigrant mental health, a public health issue: Looking back and moving forward. Int. J. Environ. Res. Public Health, 12(10): 13624–13648. doi: 10.3390/ijerph121013624

Gessner BD, Kaslow D, Louis J, Neuzil K, O'Brien KL, Picot V, Pang T, Parashar UD, Saadatian-Elahi M and Nelson CB, 2017. Estimating the full public health value of vaccination. Vaccine, 35(46): 6255–6263. doi: 10.1016/j.vaccine.2017.09.048

Gilboa M, Regev-Yochay G, Mandelboim M, Indenbaum V, Asraf K, Fluss R, Amit S, Mendelson E, Doolman R, Afek A and Freedman LS, 2022. Durability of immune response after COVID-19 booster vaccination and association with COVID-19 omicron infection. JAMA Net. Open, 5(9): e2231778–e2231778. doi: 10.1001/jamanetworkopen.2022.31778

Giordano G, Colaneri M, Di Filippo A, Blanchini F, Bolzern P, De Nicolao G, Sacchi P, Colaneri P and Bruno R, 2021. Modeling vaccination rollouts, SARS-CoV-2 variants and the requirement for non-pharmaceutical interventions in Italy. Nat. Med., 27(6): 993–998. doi: 10.1038/s41591-021-01334-5

Gozzi N, Bajardi P and Perra N, 2021. The importance of non-pharmaceutical interventions during the COVID-19 vaccine rollout. PLoS Comput. Biol., 17(9): e1009346. doi: 10.1371/journal.pcbi.1009346

Grassly NC, Kang G and Kampmann B, 2015. Biological challenges to effective vaccines in the developing world. Philos. Trans. R. Soc. Lond., B, Biol. Sci., 370(1671): 20140138. doi: 10.1098/rstb.2014.0138.

Gupta M, Angeli F, Bosma H, Rana M, Prinja S, Kumar R and Van Schayck OC, 2016. Effectiveness of multiple-strategy community intervention in reducing geographical, socioeconomic and gender based inequalities in maternal and child health outcomes in Haryana, India. PloS one, 11(3): e0150537. doi: 10.1371/journal.pone.0150537

Halimi V, Daci A, Ancevska Netkovska K, Suturkova L, Babar ZUD and Grozdanova A, 2020. Clinical and regulatory concerns of biosimilars: a review of literature. Int. J. Environ. Res. Public Health, 17(16): 5800. doi: 10.3390/ijerph17165800

Hartzell JD and Blaylock JM, 2014. Whooping cough in 2014 and beyond: an update and review. Chest, 146(1): 205–214. doi:10.1378/chest.13-2942.

Hazan G, Duek OA, Alapi H, Mok H, Ganninger A, Ostendorf E, Gierasch C, Chodick G, Greenberg D and Haspel JA, 2023. Biological rhythms in COVID-19 vaccine effectiveness in an observational cohort study of 1.5 million patients. J. Clin. Invest., 133(11). doi: 10.1172/JCI167339.

Hsiao B, Khan A and Kang I, 2020. Vaccinations and Biologics. Infect. Dis. Clin., 34(2): 425–450. doi: 10.1016/j.idc.2020.02.012.

Hvidt AK, Baerends EA, Søgaard OS, Stærke NB, Raben D, Reekie J, Nielsen H, Johansen IS, Wiese L, Benfield TL and Iversen KK, 2022. Comparison of vaccine-induced antibody neutralization against SARS-CoV-2 variants of concern following primary and booster doses of COVID-19 vaccines. Front. Med., 9: 994160. doi: 10.3389/fmed.2022.994160

Jafari H, Deshpande JM, Sutter RW, Bahl S, Verma H, Ahmad M, Kunwar A, Vishwakarma R, Agarwal A, Jain S and Estivariz C, 2014. Efficacy of inactivated poliovirus vaccine in India. Science, 345(6199): 922–925. doi:10.1126/science.1255006.

Janssens W, 2011. Externalities in program evaluation: the impact of a women's empowerment program on immunization. J. Eur. Econ. Assoc., 9(6), pp.1082-1113. doi: 10.1111/j.1542-4774.2011.01041.x

Kandi V, Vadakedath S, Addanki PS, Godishala V and Pinnelli VB, 2023. Clinical Trials: The Role of Regulatory Agencies, Pharmacovigilance Laws, Guidelines, Risk Management, Patenting, and Publicizing Results. Borneo J. Pharm., 6(1): 93-109. doi: 10.33084/bjop.v6i1.3263

Kandi V and Vadakedath S, 2023. Clinical trials and clinical research: a comprehensive review. Cureus, 15(2). doi: 10.7759/cureus.35077.

Karaboué A, Innominato PF, Wreglesworth NI, Duchemann B, Adam R and Lévi FA, 2024. Why does circadian timing of administration matter for immune checkpoint inhibitors' efficacy?. Br. J. Cancer, 1–14. doi: 10.1038/s41416-024-02704-9.

Khandia R, Singhal S, Alqahtani T, Kamal MA, Nahed A, Nainu F, Desingu PA and Dhama K, 2022. Emergence of SARS-CoV-2 Omicron (B. 1.1. 529) variant, salient features, high global health concerns and strategies to counter it amid ongoing COVID-19 pandemic. Environ. Res., 209: 112816. doi: 10.1016/j.envres.2022.112816

Kirsebom FCM, Andrews N, Stowe J, Groves N, Chand M, Ramsay M and Bernal JL, 2022. Effectiveness of the COVID-19 vaccines against hospitalisation with Omicron sub-lineages BA. 4 and BA. 5 in England. Lancet Reg. Health Eur., 23. doi: 10.1016/j.lanepe.2022.100537

Kirsebom FCM, Andrews N, Stowe J, Ramsay M and Bernal JL, 2023a. Duration of protection of ancestral-strain monovalent vaccines and effectiveness of bivalent BA. 1 boosters against COVID-19 hospitalisation in England: a test-negative case-control study. Lancet Infect. Dis., 23(11): 1235–1243. doi: 10.1016/S1473-3099(23)00365-1

Kirsebom FCM, Harman K, Lunt RJ, Andrews N, Groves N, Aziz NA, Hope R, Stowe J, Chand M, Ramsay M and Dabrera G, 2023b. Vaccine effectiveness against hospitalisation estimated using a test-negative case-control study design, and comparative odds of hospital admission and severe outcomes with COVID-19 sub-lineages BQ. 1, CH. 1.1. and XBB. 1.5 in England. Lancet Reg. Health Eur., 35. doi: 10.1016/j.lanepe.2023.100755

Leuridan E and Van Damme P, 2011. Hepatitis B and the need for a booster dose. Clin. Infect. Dis., 53(1): 68–75. doi:10.1093/cid/cir270.

Levine MM and Robins-Browne R, 2009. Vaccines, global health and social equity. Immunol. Cell Biol., 87(4): 274–278. doi: 10.1038/icb.2009.15

Li HJ, Yang QC, Yao YY, Huang CY, Yin FQ, Xian-Yu CY, Zhang C and Chen SJ, 2023. COVID-19 vaccination effectiveness and safety in vulnerable populations: a meta-analysis of 33 observational studies. Front. Pharmacol., 14: 1144824. doi: 10.3389/fphar.2023.1144824.

Lin DY, 2023. Bivalent Boosters against Severe Omicron Infection. Reply. N Eng. J. Med., 388(18): 1726–1727. doi: 10.1056/nejmc2303753

Liu Y, Lam DMK, Luan M, Zheng W and Ai H, 2024. Recent development of oral vaccines. Exp. Ther. Med., 27(5): 1–12. doi: 10.3892/etm.2024.12511.

Marchant A, Sadarangani M, Garand M, Dauby N, Verhasselt V, Pereira L, Bjornson G, Jones CE, Halperin SA, Edwards KM and Heath P, 2017. Maternal immunisation: collaborating with mother nature. Lancet Infect. Dis., 17(7): e197–e208. doi: 10.1016/S1473-3099(17)30229-3

Matrajt L, Eaton J, Leung T and Brown ER, 2021. Vaccine optimization for COVID-19: Who to vaccinate first?. Sci. Adv., 7(6): eabf1374. doi: 10.1126/sciadv.abf1374

Mbonigaba E, Yu F, Reñosa MDC, Mwikarago IE, Cho FN, Elad PCK, Metzger W, Muhindo R, Chen Q, Denkinger CM and McMahon SA, 2024. The acceptance of COVID-19 vaccines in Rwanda: a cross-sectional study. BMC Public Health, 24(1): 2875. doi: 10.1186/s12889-024-20417-9

Menegale F, Manica M, Zardini A, Guzzetta G, Marziano V, d'Andrea V, Trentini F, Ajelli M, Poletti P and Merler S, 2023. Evaluation of waning of SARS-CoV-2 vaccine–induced immunity: a systematic review and meta-analysis. JAMA Network Open, 6(5): e2310650–e2310650. doi: 10.1001/jamanetworkopen.2023.10650

Meslé MM, Brown J, Mook P, Hagan J, Pastore R, Bundle N, Spiteri G, Ravasi G, Nicolay N, Andrews N and Dykhanovska T, 2021. Estimated number of deaths directly averted in people 60 years and older as a result of COVID-19 vaccination in the WHO European Region, December 2020 to November 2021. Eurosurveillance, 26(47): 2101021. doi: 10.2807/1560-7917.ES.2021.26.47.2101021

Mohapatra RK, El-Shall NA, Tiwari R, Nainu F, Kandi V, Sarangi AK, Mohammed TA, Desingu PA, Chakraborty C and Dhama K, 2022b. Need of booster vaccine doses to counteract the emergence of SARS-CoV-2 variants in the context of the Omicron variant and increasing COVID-19 cases: An update. Hum. Vaccin. Immunother., 18(5): 2065824. doi: 10.1080/21645515.2022.2065824

Mohapatra RK, Kuppili S, Kumar Suvvari T, Kandi V, Behera A, Verma S, Biswal SK, Al-Noor TH, El-ajaily MM, Sarangi AK and Dhama K, 2022a. SARS-CoV-2 and its variants of concern including Omicron: a never ending pandemic. Chem. Biol. Drug Design, 99(5): 769–788. doi: 10.1111/cbdd.14035.

Mohapatra RK, Mahal A, Mishra S, Rabaan AA and Sah R, 2023a. Possible threat of the Omicron subvariant BF. 7 to FIH Hockey World Cup 2023 in particular and the South-East Asia Region in general. Int.J. Surgery, 109(3):646–647. doi: 10.1097/JS9.0000000000000241

Mohapatra RK, Mishra S, Kandi V, Branda F, Ansari A, Rabaan AA and Kudrat-E-Zahan M, 2023e. Analyzing the emerging patterns of SARS-CoV-2 Omicron subvariants for the development of next-gen vaccine: An observational study. Health Sci. Rep., 6(10): e1596. doi: 10.1002/hsr2.1596

Mohapatra RK, Mishra S, Pintilie L and Tuglo LS, 2023c. Potentially pandemic MERS-CoV constantly circulating in the Middle East threatens the globe: Preparedness and prevention with commentaries on the 'one health'model. Int. J. Surgery Open, 58: 100670. doi: 10.1016/j.ijso.2023.100670

Mohapatra RK, Padhi BK, Kandi V, Mishra S, Rabaan AA, Mohanty A and Sah R, 2023b. Camel virus (MERS) reported from Qatar: a threat to the FIFA-2022 and Middle East. QJM: Int. J. Med., 116(2):150–152. doi: 10.1093/qjmed/hcac271

Mohapatra RK, Verma S, Kandi V, Sarangi AK, Seidel V, Das SN, Behera A, Tuli HS, Sharma AK and Dhama K, 2023d. The SARS-CoV-2 Omicron variant and its multiple sub lineages: transmissibility, vaccine development, antiviral drugs, monoclonal antibodies, and strategies for infection control–a review. Chemistry Select, 8(9): e202201380. doi: 10.1002/slct.202201380

Natalini A, Simonetti S, Sher C, D'Oro U, Hayday AC and Di Rosa F, 2022. Durable CD8 T cell memory against SARS-CoV-2 by Prime/Boost and multi-dose vaccination: Considerations on inter-dose time intervals. Int.l J. Mol. Sci., 23(22): 14367. doi: 10.3390/ijms232214367

Newport MJ, Goetghebuer T, Weiss HA, Whittle H, Siegrist CA and Marchant A, 2004. Genetic regulation of immune responses to vaccines in early life. Genes Immun., 5(2): 122–129. doi: 10.1038/sj.gene.6364051

Nyberg T, Ferguson NM, Nash SG, Webster HH, Flaxman S, Andrews N, Hinsley W, Bernal JL, Kall M, Bhatt S and Blomquist P, 2022. Comparative analysis of the risks of hospitalisation and death associated with SARS-CoV-2 omicron (B. 1.1. 529) and delta (B. 1.617. 2) variants in England: a cohort study. Lancet, 399(10332): 1303–1312. doi: 10.1016/S0140-6736(22)00462-7

Our world in data (2024), Total COVID-19 vaccine doses administered. Available online at: https://ourworldindata.org/covid-vaccinations, Accessed on 12 August 2024.

Panda S, Singh PK, Mishra S, Mitra S, Pattnaik P, Adhikary SD and Mohapatra RK, 2023. Indian biosimilars and vaccines at crossroads–replicating the success of pharmagenerics. Vaccines, 11(1): 110. doi: 10.3390/vaccines11010110

Parker EP, Kampmann B, Kang G and Grassly NC, 2014. Influence of enteric infections on response to oral poliovirus vaccine: a systematic review and meta-analysis. J. Infect. Dis., 210(6): 853–864. doi: 10.1093/infdis/jiu182

Patil N, Ranjan A, Gaurav, Mukherjee D, Panda BK, Diksha, Komal, Narang RK and Singh A, 2024. Navigating Biosimilar Regulatory Pathways in Emerging Markets: Insights from Brics Nations. Appl. Clin. Res. Clin. Trials Regul. Aff. doi: 10.2174/0126673371316219240929170401

Plotkin SA, 2013. Complex correlates of protection after vaccination. Clin. Infect. Dis., 56(10): 1458–1465. doi: 10.1093/cid/cit048.

Pollard AJ and Bijker EM, 2021. A guide to vaccinology: from basic principles to new developments. Nat. Rev. Immunol., 21(2): 83–100. doi: 10.1038/s41577-020-00479-7

Pulendran B, Li S and Nakaya HI, 2010. Systems vaccinology. Immunity, 33(4): 516–529. doi: 10.1016/j.immuni.2010.10.006

Rami F, Searight HR, Morrissey MB, Charvonia A, Indart M and Brown LM, 2023. Health inequities and social determinants of health in refugee and immigrant communities. Am. Psychol., 78(2): 160. doi: 10.1037/amp0001113

Riumallo-Herl C, Chang AY, Clark S, Constenla D, Clark A, Brenzel L and Verguet S, 2018. Poverty reduction and equity benefits of introducing or scaling up measles, rotavirus and pneumococcal vaccines in low-income and middle-income countries: a modelling study. BMJ Glob. Health, 3(2): e000613. doi: 10.1136/bmjgh-2017-000613

Rodrigo C, Fernando D and Rajapakse S, 2014. Pharmacological management of tetanus: an evidence-based review. Critical Care, 18: 1–10. doi:10.1186/cc13797.

Rodrigues CM and Plotkin SA, 2020. Impact of vaccines; health, economic and social perspectives. Front. Microbiol., 11: 1526. doi: 10.3389/fmicb.2020.01526

Roslund MI, Nurminen N, Oikarinen S, Puhakka R, Grönroos M, Puustinen L, Kummola L, Parajuli A, Cinek O, Laitinen OH and Hyöty H, 2024. Skin exposure to soil microbiota elicits changes in cell-mediated immunity to pneumococcal vaccine. Sci. Rep., 14(1): 18573. doi: 10.1038/s41598-024-68235-8.

Sah R, Mohapatra RK, Mishra S, Chinnam S, Rabaan AA, Alshahrani NZ, Mohanty A, Al-Ahdal T, León-Figueroa DA and Padhi BK, 2023. Cocktail of FIFA 2022 Vis-A-Vis camel beauty pageant championship; potential health threat of MERS among players and fans-a possible global spread. Travel Med. Infect. Dis., 52: 102541. doi: 10.1016/j.tmaid.2023.102541

Satapathy BS, Pattnaik G, Sahoo RN, Pattanaik S, Sarangi AK, Kandi V, Mishra S, Rabaan AA, Mohanty A, Sah R and Mohapatra RK, 2023. COVID-19 vaccines and their underbelly: Are we going the right way?. Health Sci. Rep., 6(9): e1540. doi: 10.1002/hsr2.1540

Shahapur PR, Shahapur R, Bagali S, Karigoudar R, Wavare S, Jyothi P, Kandi V, Suvvari TK, Mittal RJ and Jadhav M, 2022. Breakthrough infections: Clinical profile and outcomes of covid-19 vaccinated and unvaccinated people from a tertiary care hospital. Cureus, 14(12). doi: 10.7759/cureus.32089.

Sharun K and Dhama K, 2021. COVID-19 vaccine diplomacy and equitable access to vaccines amid ongoing pandemic. Arch. Med. Res., 52(7): 761–763. doi: 10.1016/j.arcmed.2021.04.006.

Shearley AE, 1999. The societal value of vaccination in developing countries. Vaccine, 17: S109–S112. doi: 10.1016/S0264-410X(99)00303-5

Siegers KE, van Herwaarden AE, de Waard JH, Del Nogal B, Hermans PW, van Tienoven D, Berbers GA, de Jonge MI and Verhagen LM, 2022. The metabolic hormone adiponectin affects the correlation between nutritional status and pneumococcal vaccine response in vulnerable indigenous children. Plos one, 17(7): e0270736. doi: 10.1371/journal.pone.0270736.

Stein C, Nassereldine H, Sorensen RJ, Amlag JO, Bisignano C, Byrne S, Castro E, Coberly K, Collins JK, Dalos J and Daoud F, 2023. Past SARS-CoV-2 infection protection against re-infection: a systematic review and meta-analysis. Lancet, 401(10379): 833–842. doi: 10.1016/S0140-6736(22)02465-5

Sullivan SG and Cowling BJ, 2015. "Crude vaccine effectiveness" is a misleading term in test-negative studies of influenza vaccine effectiveness. Epidemiology, 26(5): e60. doi: 10.1097/EDE.0000000000000343

Troiano G and Nardi A, 2021. Vaccine hesitancy in the era of COVID-19. Pub. health, 194: 245–251. doi:10.1016/j. puhe.2021.02.025.

USFDA (2020), FDA Takes Key Action in Fight Against COVID-19 By Issuing Emergency Use Authorization for First COVID-19 Vaccine. Available online at: https://www.fda.gov/news-events/press-announcements/fda-takes-key-action-fight-against-covid-19-issuing-emergency-use-authorization-first-covid-19, Accessed on 20 September 2024.

USFDA (2021), FDA Approves First COVID-19 Vaccine. Available online at: https://www.fda.gov/news-events/press-announcements/fda-approves-first-covid-19-vaccine, Accessed on 20 September 2024.

Van Damme P and Van Herck K, 2007. A review of the long-term protection after hepatitis A and B vaccination. Travel Med. Infect. Dis., 5(2): 79–84. doi: 10.1016/j.tmaid.2006.04.004

van der Heiden M, Duizendstra A, Berbers GA, Boots AM and Buisman AM, 2017. Tetanus Toxoid carrier protein induced T-helper cell responses upon vaccination of middle-aged adults. Vaccine, 35(42): 5581–5588. doi: 10.1016/j.vaccine.2017.08.056

van Dorst MM, Pyuza JJ, Nkurunungi G, Kullaya VI, Smits HH, Hogendoorn PC, Wammes LJ, Everts B, Elliott AM, Jochems SP and Yazdanbakhsh M, 2024. Immunological factors linked to geographical variation in vaccine responses. Nat. Rev. Immunol., 24(4): 250–263. doi: 10.1038/s41577-023-00941-2.

Verguet S, Murphy S, Anderson B, Johansson KA, Glass R and Rheingans R, 2013. Public finance of rotavirus vaccination in India and Ethiopia: an extended cost-effectiveness analysis. Vaccine, 31(42): 4902–4910. doi: 10.1016/j.vaccine.2013.07.014

Watson OJ, Barnsley G, Toor J, Hogan AB, Winskill P and Ghani AC, 2022. Global impact of the first year of COVID-19 vaccination: a mathematical modelling study. Lancet Infect. Dis., 22(9): 1293–1302. doi: 10.1016/S1473-3099(22)00320-6

Waugh S and Cameron CE, 2024. Syphilis vaccine development: Aligning vaccine design with manufacturing requirements. Hum. Vaccin. Immunother., 20(1): 2399915. doi: 10.1080/21645515.2024.2399915.

WHO (2023), COVID-19 advice for the public: Getting vaccinated. Available online at: https://www.who.int/emergencies/diseases/novel-coronavirus-2019/covid-19-vaccines/advice, Accessed on 17 September 2024.

WHO (2024a), Coronavirus disease (COVID-19) pandemic. Available online at: https://www.who.int/europe/emergencies/situations/covid-19, Accessed on 17 September 2024.

WHO (2024b), Regulation and Prequalification. Available online at: https://www.who.int/teams/regulation-prequalification/eul/covid-19, Accessed on 20 September 2024.

WHO (2024c), Biologicals. Available online at: https://www.who.int/health-topics/biologicals#tab=tab_1, Accessed on 19 October 24.

Willis DE, Moore R, Selig JP, CarlLee S, Gurel-Headley MP, Cornett LE and McElfish PA, 2024. COVID-19 booster uptake: are hesitant adopters less likely to get a booster shot than nonhesitant adopters?. Behav. Med., 50(3): 260–268. doi: 10.1080/08964289.2023.2249168

Wouters OJ, Shadlen KC, Salcher-Konrad M, Pollard AJ, Larson HJ, Teerawattananon Y and Jit M, 2021. Challenges in ensuring global access to COVID-19 vaccines: production, affordability, allocation, and deployment. Lancet., 397(10278): 1023–1034. doi:10.1016/S0140-6736(21)00306-8.E.

Yamin D, Yechezkel M, Arbel R, Beckenstein T, Sergienko R, Duskin-Bitan H, Yaron S, Peretz A, Netzer D and Shmueli E, 2023. Safety of monovalent and bivalent BNT162b2 mRNA COVID-19 vaccine boosters in at-risk populations in Israel: a large-scale, retrospective, self-controlled case series study. Lancet Infect. Dis., 23(10): 1130–1142. doi: 10.1016/S1473-3099(23)00207-4

Yarlagadda H, Patel MA, Gupta V, Bansal T, Upadhyay S, Shaheen N and Jain R, 2022. COVID-19 vaccine challenges in developing and developed countries. Cureus, 14(4). doi: 10.7759/cureus.23951.

Zimmermann P and Curtis N, 2019. Factors that influence the immune response to vaccination. Clin. Microbiol. Rev., 32(2): 1110–1128. doi: 10.1128/cmr.00084-18.

7

Vaccine Development Strategies in India and Its Global Impact

Basundhara Lenka and Snehasish Mishra*

School of Biotechnology, Kalinga Institute of Industrial Technology (KIIT) Deemed to be University, Bhubaneswar-751024, Odisha, India

Abstract

Indian vaccine diplomacy during the pandemic added dimensions to geopolitics afresh while augmenting the domestic vaccine demands. Indian vaccines are a strong connecting link since 1960s for international relations. The public-sector multinational manufacturers have mostly contributed to Indian vaccine diplomacy significantly. Indian vaccine manufacturing companies like Biological E., Panacea Biotech, Bharat Biotech, etc. support the R&D and accelerate vaccine manufacturing and commercialisation worldwide. As a developing nation, India enjoys a good global positioning and exports vaccines for global healthcare, especially its neighbouring countries. India's intensified efforts to develop vaccines against active infections enhanced its global impact and introduced novel vaccine technology to the world. Highly effective vaccines were supplied free-of-cost during the COVID-19 pandemic to hundreds of countries that helped save global citizens. The primary objective was to enhance adaptive immunisation, prevent disease susceptibility and ensure herd immunity among the population. Vaccine administration is dose-dependent for its efficacy, while the cost factor needed to be resolved through optimised resource management. Since 2021, vaccine diplomacy of India has spread at global scale with successful mass vaccination campaign that started in a short duration (about six months) after the pandemic broke out. During the critical period of COVID-19 pandemic, India initiated the 'generous supply' of vaccines, supporting vaccine equity policy. This article details the associated Indian initiatives in this direction and the global impact.

Keywords: COVID-19, Vaccine diplomacy, Covaxin, Ayushman Bharat, Vaccination

1. Introduction

Decentralised vaccine production capabilities in the developing countries have evolved rapidly. While helping in the cost control and minimising undesirable excess production for the targeted socioeconomic needs, it also enhances the sense of health security against the emerging epidemics (Plotkin *et al.*, 2017). Vaccine production efficiency differs globally owing to the factors like resources availability, the available expertise, the production platform available and the production practices, market access, inspection and quality compliance, related regulatory framework for drug approval, and the existing surveillance and review of the long-term effect of the applied dose to the subject. Despite the numerous challenges, developing countries are increasingly investing in vaccine development (Makenga *et al.*, 2019). With this in light, India has been a glaring example that has set high standards.

1.1. Vaccine Development and Commercialisation in India

Indian vaccines have significantly occupied a comfortable global market niche since 1960s under Expanded Programme on Immunisation (EPI) and make vaccines available across the globe irrespective of their socioeconomic status and geographical location, displacing many multinational players that produced generic vaccines (Gupta *et al.*, 2013). Indian public-sector manufacturers have contributed about 53% to the Global Alliance for Vacancies and Immunisation (GAVI) since 2008. This contribution dropped to 29% in 2010 after the manufacturing of numerous vaccines like pneumococcal conjugates and rotavirus by multinational companies. Indian vaccine manufacturers currently compete with multinational companies in complex vaccines development (Chandrasekharan *et al.*, 2019), including through the biologics and biosimilars routes (Panda *et al.*, 2023).

India vaccine development initiatives collaborated flexibly with multiple stakeholders that emphasised on productivity and commercialisation enhancement. India's indigenous research needs to be multidisciplinary and should create multi-stakeholders with complementing opportunities. It called for diverse discussions on manufacturing infrastructure, intellectual property rights, skilled workforce, funding and R&D collaboration, good vaccine production support, development and commercialisation (Gupta *et al.*, 2013).

1.2. Indian vaccine diplomacy

Vaccine diplomacy is all about vaccine expertise, state-of-art manufacturing platforms and good associated infrastructure that helps provide humanitarian aid internationally, generates goodwill and improves foreign policy goals.

Indian vaccine diplomacy fits well into science diplomacy to forge partnerships among nations and strengthens global scientific network. As the largest vaccine manufacturing country, India has secured an enviable position in exporting vaccines widely (including the low and medium-income countries with low or no purchasing capacity) ensuring standard healthcare worldwide. India supplied huge quantity of vaccines to numerous nations free-of-cost during the COVID-19 pandemic and saved the population from the severity and fatality of the malady (Ministry of External Affairs, India, 2023). Indian government initiated a vaccine production series with the Neighbourhood First Policy of the Ministry of External Affairs, India (2021). As its constituent, India donated various vaccines to neighbourhood countries like Bhutan and Nepal that earned goodwill and fortified healthy ties. COVID-19 pandemic reinforced India's vaccine research and production capabilities. To expedite the vaccine research programme, various governmental agencies like the Department of Biotechnology (DBT) and the Indian Council of Medical Research (ICMR) collaborated with private-sector companies through funding and expertise-sharing. This led to successful development of thirty vaccines of which three were at clinical trials stages by November 2020 (Chakraborty and Agoramoorthy, 2020). Indian vaccine research and development strategies have reached wider across the globe, encouraging funding and R&D facilities (Chakraborty and Agoramoorthy, 2020).

2. Purpose and Key Objectives of India's Vaccination Programmes

The foremost plan of all the vaccination programmes is to enhance adaptive immunity, reduce disease susceptibility and increase the overall vaccine efficacy among the targeted population (WHO, 2005). Human subjects are administered with multiple vaccine doses which would be more effective in enhancing disease resistivity for longer duration and reducing the complications in vaccine-preventable diseases.

2.1. Indian Vaccination Strategies

The manner in which Indian vaccination programmes strategised to protect human health reflects its technological innovation, capabilities to collaborate on expertise and the available skilled manpower. However, vaccination strategies needed to be more adaptive. Vaccine preventable diseases (VPD) like rubella, measles, rotavirus, varicella and rabies were not included under risk-groups thereby stifling the healthcare system from convincing the susceptible (risk-group) subjects to administer the vaccine (Gopalakrishnan, 2020). Vaccine administration with higher scope to reduce the disease burden is an age-group based strategy (Bonanni *et al.*, 2014). VPD mostly needed single cohort immunisation, like the diphtheria-tetanus-pertussis (DTP) vaccine, that begins at infant stage and is recommended to receive at a specific infancy age. In addition, adults and youngsters are recommended for vaccination simultaneously as a double cohort strategy to strengthen their immune system (Pollard and Bijker, 2021). Mass vaccination programmes introduce vaccines into a population that also generates herd immunity in a minimum time period to efficiently eradicate a VPD (Heymann and Aylward, 2006). Mass vaccination strategies are developed in response to a continuing epidemic or pandemic, like the polio vaccination in 1950, measles and yellow fever in Latin America, Africa and sub-Saharan Africa (2003), and more recently the COVID-19 (Heymann and Aylward, 2006). Feasibility of immunisation strategies in India involves the demographic composition of the population stating the disease susceptibility. Additionally, the underlying social and biological factors influence the expected transmission and infection rates (Doherty *et al.*, 2016; Scarbrough Lefebvre *et al.*, 2015).

According to WHO report (2005), human disease burden is defined on the provided valuable data regarding a particular disease and the preventive measures based on the prevalence rate, the mortality rate, hospitalisation and disability factors. Various mathematical models were employed to infer the disease burden, transmission rate and infection criticality in instances where the required data were inadequate, to devise vaccination strategies (Keeling *et al.*, 2013). Besides, vaccination feasibility against a specific disease, funding and monitoring its public health impact also strengthen immunisation initiatives.

2.2. VPD Surveillance

Effective surveillance, diagnostics and validation through proper techniques are the basic prerequisites before enlisting an illness under VPD. Sharing of global resources on expertise, instrumentation, biomarker discovery and diagnostic intermediaries shall boost the efforts further. Post-marketing surveillance by public institutions would not be effective in adopting a vaccination programme without capacity-building within the vaccine manufacturers to acquire data that could be used to document vaccine safety and efficacy (Gupta *et al.*, 2013). New vaccines need to be introduced systemically and decision on its administration could be taken after community-based surveillance for a hastened and effective drive. Datasets from the contiguous population (from neighbouring countries too) may be analysed to support the process to introduce new vaccines and reinforce immunisation programmes.

2.3. The Indian Indigenous Vaccines Development Strength

Supported by the Indian government, vaccine industries in India (like Bharat Biotech, Panacea Biotech and Biological E.) have had healthy growth trends recently. Serum Institute of India (SII) is a large private vaccine manufacturing farm in India with a capacity to produce 1.3 billion vaccine doses annually, while exporting its product to more than 140 countries. Indian vaccine technology compliments the technologies of the West (Bharti and Bharti, 2021). SII supplies large amount of DTP and measles vaccines to the United Nation agencies like PAHO (Pan American Health Organisation) and UNICEF. One in every two children is immunised globally by at least one SII-synthesised vaccine which demonstrates the global acceptability and popularity that SII enjoys. SII claims, the measles vaccine developed from MRC-5 cells instead of chick embryo had up to 10–20-folds enhanced efficacy as compared to the GlaxoSmithKline and Merck collaborated constituted vaccine (Douglas and Samant, 2018). Private sector vaccine companies in India have profusely invested on their production facilities. Focussing on vaccinology R&D, SII currently produces pneumococcal conjugate vaccine, rotavirus vaccine, Human Papilloma virus vaccine, polyvalent meningococcal conjugate vaccine, vaccine combinations containing acellular pertussis, and others (Douglas and Samant, 2018).

2.4. Vaccine Production Capacity of Indian Public and Private Sectors

An effective vaccination programme influences the commercial and economic activities of a nation by providing a feeling of health security and wellbeing. Indian private sector provided 75% of the preventive and curative measures for both urban and rural India, with increasing vaccination rates. The costing between the vaccines of the public and private sectors differs. Private sector vaccination programme was expensive; it put extra financial burden on vaccinating the public at private hospitals. The government proactively intervened and set their equitable pricing in vaccine administration billing by private clinicians (Gupta *et al.*, 2013). Indian COVID-19 vaccination strategy was unique in numerous manners through several modifications in the guidelines, since a VPD of unknown dimensions and clinical manifestations was being addressed (Mandal *et al.*, 2021). Yet, the plans seemed inadequate, and vaccination policies still had a scope for further improvement. Primarily it related to India's huge geography and demography which needed identifying the susceptible population and targeted vaccination to control and overcome the adverse effects of the pandemic.

India galloped to develop SARS-CoV-2 vaccines to tackle the pandemic situation. More than 150 Indian educational institutions worked on SARS-CoV-2 vaccine development and produced vaccines like inactivated vaccines (IAcV), replicating viral vectors (RVV), DNA and RNA vaccines, live-attenuated vaccines (LAVs) and protein components. Table 1 lists a few such vaccine R&D efforts of Indian institutions. SARS-CoV-2 reportedly had similar genetic constituents with two deadly corona viruses, MERS and SARS-CoV-1. Thus, combined vaccine production strategy to formulate novel vaccines for SARS-CoV-2 could be adopted to simultaneously combat SARS and MERS viruses (Salvatori *et al.*, 2020).

Table 1: Development and manufacturing status of human vaccines by Indian institutions

Indian institution	Vaccine candidate	Status
ICGEB, New Delhi	Dengue vaccine	Development is underway of efficacious, safe and cost-effective tetravalent dengue vaccines
THSTI, Gurgaon; IAVI	HIV vaccines	Design of vaccines are under research to trigger the production of neutralising antibodies to encounter HIV
ICGEB, New Delhi	Malaria vaccine	Phase I clinical trials of JAIVAC-1 vaccine for *P. falciparum* and PvDBPII vaccine for *P. vivax* is completed in BBIL, Hyderabad
AIIMS, New Delhi; CDC and NIH, USA	Rotavirus vaccine	Phase III clinical trial of rotavirus vaccine 116E underway at three sites: SAS, New Delhi; CMC, Vellore; KEM Hospital, Pune
UDSC; THSTI, New Delhi	Tuberculosis vaccine	Recombinant BCG 85c (Rbcg85c), vaccine showed significant result against tuberculosis
AIIMS, New Delhi	Typhoid vaccine	Vi-conjugate typhoid vaccine technology collaborating with USV Ltd. Mumbai
NIV, Pune	Hepatitis A	Transfer agreement signed with BBIL for further development
IMTECH, Chandigarh; NICED, Kolkata	Cholera vaccine	Live cholera oral vaccine (strain VA1.4) phase II trial completed; Phase III trial will start soon
NII, New Delhi	Japanese encephalitis vaccine	Developed and transferred Vero cell-derived Japanese encephalitis vaccine to Panacea Biotech
IOP and IMM, New Delhi	Leishmania vaccine	Live-attenuated *L. donovani* vaccine against visceral leishmaniasis (lab-tested)

Source: Gupta *et al.* (2013)

Abbreviations used: THSTI: Translational Health Science Technology Institute, ICGEB: International Centre for Genetic Engineering and Biotechnology; NII: National Institute of Immunology; IOP: Institute of Pathology; IMTECH: Institute of Microbial Technology; AIIMS: All India Institute of Medical

Sciences; NICED: National Institute of Cholera and Infectious Diseases; BBIL: Bharat Biotech International Ltd.; IMM: Institute of Molecular Medicine; JEV: Japanese encephalitis virus; CDC: Centres for Disease Control & Prevention; NIV: National Institute of Virology; HIV: Human immunodeficiency virus; NIH: National Institutes of Health; UDSC: Delhi University, South Campus; IAVI: International AIDS Vaccine Initiative

Indian vaccination strategy was designed to gain long-term benefits from COVID-19 vaccine administration in the shortest possible duration for the public to benefit from it and remain protected during COVID-19. Indian Health Ministry reported only around 7% vaccination drive carried out by the private sector since 1 May 2021 during the pandemic, although they were allotted about 25% of the total vaccine supply (Times of India, 2021). This could be attributed to the critical differential pricing. Less allocation of vaccine supply to private sectors or very small proportion of the vaccination of the public by the private sector was more beneficial (Wouters *et al.*, 2021).

India has successfully supplied about 20% of the generic therapeutics and preventives across the globe, and has played a crucial role in a significant transition of global pharmaceutical sector from the conventional generics to biologics, biosimilars and biomimics (Panda *et al.*, 2023). Indian pharmaceutical companies have put significant efforts over the years and have established a positive impact in branding global pharmaceutical industry. The reduced treatment expenses, the achievements in biologic and biosimilar products have progressively improved Indian healthcare system. The potential of biosimilars in effectively treating chronic diseases and regulating the international biosimilars and vaccines market has been phenomenal. Indian biosimilars especially by Biocon, Bengaluru (Indian biopharmaceutical giant) are being increasingly approved by the international regulators thereby facilitating their successful entrance into the US market (Mazumdar-Shaw, 2018). Several Indian companies including Dr. Reddy's, Enzene Biosciences Ltd. and Biocon successfully tested numerous biosimilars and biologics to treat and manage inflammation and respiratory distress due to COVID-19 (Panda *et al.*, 2023).

In addition to these encouraging success stories, the biosimilar manufacturing companies need to religiously comply with the current good manufacturing practices (cGMPs) in producing the desired products adequately, and good clinical practices (GCPs) in diligently administer these. To continue the good show, biopharmaceuticals manufacturers in India should learn from the rejections and need to follow the international guidelines (especially that of the USFDA and the EMA) that are revised from time-to-time. Although the Indian guidelines are also revised frequently, but these still do not comply with the internationally-set standards on various counts including the animal testings (Clinical Trial II). The set Indian guidelines for animal testing do not mandate to provide enough data on the complementing efficacy of the bioactive compound being tested on human subjects. For instance, the monoclonal antibodies (mAbs) testing on rats measures the immunological response potential on animals but it fails to provide the data on how the biosimilars would influence the human subjects in response to dissimilar metabolic processes (Dolinar *et al.*, 2014). As rodents reportedly lack complementing receptors, mAbs do not exhibit any toxic response. However, such safety testing could be measured through 3D cell culture (xenograft model) during the clinical trial, which seems to be having more similarity in the *in vivo* tissue organs with regard to gene expression profiles (Panda *et al.*, 2023).

Indian Immunologicals Limited (IIL), a public-sector biopharmaceuticals company for preventives, is an emerging vaccine manufacture company which has taken encouraging strides in tackling the numerous infectious disease challenges especially encountered in animals like the foot and mouth disease (FMD) in cattle, the rabies in canine animals and other emerging diseases, thereby creating employment opportunities for about 750 people (Behera *et al.*, 2023). IIL has become the leading supplier of FMD vaccines to the Government of India under the National Animal Disease Control programme (NADCP), and has produced an array of FMD vaccines for supply across the globe. An initiative of the National Dairy Development Board (NDDB), IIL's new Biosafety Level 3 (BSL-3) state-of-the-art facility in Hyderabad manufactures fill-finish drug and vaccine substances (Chanda *et al.*, 2024), with an investment of 700 crore. IIL produces more than 150 vaccine products and strongly believes in the 'One Health' approach that emphasises on the interconnectedness of the health and wellbeing of animals, humans and the environment. IIL is aggressively signing Memoranda of Understanding (MoUs) with various R&D institutions and facilities across the length and breadth of India, and is expanding its vaccine manufacturing capabilities to significantly contribute in improving vaccine production capacities within India and ensure global health and wellbeing (Kaur *et al.*, 2021).

2.5. Vaccinating Indian Adults

Indian adult immunisation strategy follows several guidelines which include Geriatric Society of India guidelines, CDC (Centres for Disease Control) guidelines, Association of Physicians of India-Expert panel guidelines and the World Health Organisation (WHO) guidelines (WHO recommendations for Routine Immunisation, 2021; Verma *et al.*, 2015; Dash *et al.*, 2020). Vaccine like influenza is recommended to administer to the population above 50 years, human papilloma virus for 9-26 years age-group, and MMR (measles, mumps and rubella), DPT and Zoster to persons above 60 years (Verma *et al.*, 2015). Physicians emphasise on adult vaccination on priority and recommend certain vaccine administration guidelines. Pneumococcal vaccine for the diabetic in 2–64 years age-group was prescribed by the Research Society in a Study on the Diabetics in India (Chawla *et al.*, 2020). Vaccination could potentially reduce the susceptibility to infectious diseases and the associated high mortality and morbidity (Bajaj, 2018).

3. Economic and Social Impacts of Indian Vaccination Drives

Vaccination helps prevent the manifestation of an infection and reduces the risk of secondary health impacts. Valued in lines with health-centric outcome, Indian vaccination strategy is appreciated far and wide. International bodies like UNICEF (United Nations International Children's Emergency Fund), GAVI, the Vaccine Alliance and the WHO have all supported and appreciated Indian vaccination programme. Global health experts and economists agreed that broad-based vaccination could potentially ensure health, social and economic benefits (Bloom *et al.*, 2017). Vaccines reduce disease susceptibility, promote health benefits by preventing the pathogens from infecting, guarantees health and wellbeing, and provide a sense of health safety. It is evident that an array of non-targeted pathogens could also be controlled through the combined action of multivalent vaccines. For instance, pneumonia vaccination prevented long-term sequelae like lungs deformity in children. Similarly, vaccination reduced secondary health impacts like vision and hearing impairments in meningitis patients (Bloom *et al.*, 2017). Vaccination prevents health-related anxiety and depression, and ensures a healthier and happier (due to health security) life.

3.1. Socioeconomic Impacts of Vaccination

While vaccination has health benefits, it also enhances the economic wellbeing of individuals as well as a nation. Mass education about vaccination and its benefits could be integrated in to the school academic curricula to transform it in to a way of life. A vaccinated child is more likely to attend school and extra-curricular activities regularly with better functional abilities than its unvaccinated counterpart. Similarly, a vaccinated adult is protected from VPDs and is likely to enjoy more productive hours thereby boosting the income (Gupta *et al.*, 2013). The elderly are top-prioritised during a vaccination drive due to old-age related complications, so that they remain healthy, enjoy their retired life, and more importantly participate in suitable economic and social activities (Bloom *et al.*, 2017).

The social, economic and physical health benefits of vaccination are measured through economic assessments and are expressed in terms of social wellbeing. Mental peace and wellbeing benefits in the vaccinated individuals would lead to increase the economic wellbeing at individual households. Vaccination decreases the negative consequences of VPD and reduces the risk of economic slowdown and poverty. Vaccination has intergenerational societal benefits. At the macro-economy level, a vaccination programme and its associated economic benefits increase the governmental tax receipts and reduce healthcare expenses. Cervical cancer prevention through HPV (human papillomavirus) vaccination enhances the survival chances of a mother to care for the children (Bloom *et al.*, 2017).

4. India's Vaccination Programme and Healthcare Services

Vaccination schedule in the developing countries including India requires updating the individual immunisation calendar and regular visits to the clinics (or community healthcare centres). The Health ministry in India has played a crucial role in making strong decisions on updating immunisation schedule, integrating it with the national health policy and planning, and social mobilisation (Patel and Nowalk, 2010). Strengthening the vaccination infrastructure is required to make a strong roadmap for vaccine administration across the various age-groups (Gupta *et al.*, 2013). Cervical cancer (about 85% of the cases caused by HPV) was the most significant fatal disease in female folks in the low- and middle-income countries (LMICs) as per reports (Bosch *et al.*, 2013). Numerous adverse events encountered in HPV vaccine during the clinical trials had led to shutting it down and discontinue by the government (Wigle *et al.*, 2016). The role of local healthcare infrastructure, geopolitics, involvement of international bodies and public trust to support vaccination drives are significant factors.

Vaccination needs to be encouraged to avoid a likely major surgery later. Antimicrobial stewardship (AMS) programmes, annual health check, wellness centres could facilitate and increase the vaccination coverage (Hermsen *et al.*, 2021). Pneumococcal vaccine helps prevent major infections and is strongly recommended to avoid cochlear implants to lessen hospitalisation bills and reduce the duration of hospitalisation (Scelfo *et al.*, 2021). Doorstep healthcare services were conveniently provided by mobile vaccination vans that reduced hospitalisation during the COVID-19 pandemic (Mantel and Cherian, 2020). The household level nursing care facilitates vaccination by visiting the house of the subject, educate on benefits of vaccination during routine consultation, improve public perception and enhance vaccine uptake. A pulmonologist could prescribe the administration of pneumococcal vaccine to asthma patients during COPD (chronic obstructive pulmonary disease). Also, the counsellors play a major role in counselling the relatives of a patient regarding the benefits of vaccines and the need to vaccinate them during acute emergencies (Gurnani *et al.*, 2018). Vaccination is effectively reinforced in public through reminder apps, SMS (short messaging services) notification and time-to-time prescription (Perri-Moore *et al.*, 2016). The Indian government is currently aggressive following the hepatitis B vaccination. It should additionally emphasise on other vaccines too and recommend including as many such vaccines under the *Ayushman Bharat* scheme. Alongside other healthcare services, the Indian *Ayushman Bharat* initiative could focus on all the age groups for vaccination (Lahariya, 2018).

5. Indian Vaccine Innovations

Indian vaccine R&D initiatives have largely been very much reassuring in recent times. Although a few of the initiatives are in infancy now, its vaccine initiatives included the development of DNA vaccines to express specific proteins and stimulate adaptive immunity in the host. India developed and formulated routine cultured, processed and inactivated vaccines against the expressed bacterial and viral antigens (Gupta *et al.*, 2013). The strategy to develop live attenuated vaccine is incapacitating the microbial infectivity while still retaining its ability to trigger robust immune responses. Subunit vaccines include the formulated recombinant proteins or purified toxoids to stimulate the desired immune responses. Appropriate polysaccharides are conjugated with the antigen protein to enhance the immune responses (Chen *et al.*, 2022).

5.1. Institutional Vaccine Innovation and Formulation in India

Multivalent vaccine formulation involves two or more antigens, which minimises the need of multiple shots of individual vaccines. This is an area of research interest currently among the various Indian entities in developing advanced vaccines. The prioritised candidate pathogens in these initiatives include dengue virus, tuberculosis (TB), enterotoxigenic *E. coli* (ETEC), respiratory syncytial virus (RSV), Zika virus, Norovirus, Human Immunodeficiency Virus (HIV), chickenpox, herpes zoster virus, malaria and HPV (Ghosh, 2019). India has spread its wings on the strategies to develop vaccines to minimise the chances of infection during the recent pandemic and future occurrences, and is making efforts to develop vaccines against the diseases that also include the neglected tropical diseases (NTD). Vaccine development against pneumonia (by *S. pneumoniae*) is at the research and development stage at SII (Ghosh, 2019). Two Indian vaccine manufacturing companies, Biological E. Ltd. and

Tergene Biotech have collaborated to develop multivalent pneumococcus vaccine (Jain *et al.*, 2024). Live-attenuated vaccine against tetravalent chimera of dengue virus is being manufactured by Sanofi Pasteur, France which has high public acceptance and a strong market presence (Ghosh, 2019). Indian company Panacea Biotech collaborated with the National Institute of Health (NIH), USA to develop dengue vaccines. The Drug Controller General of India (DCGI) approved the dengue vaccine for early human clinical trials (Mani *et al.*, 2013). Bharat Biotech Ltd., Hyderabad and SII, Pune have collaborated to develop HPV vaccines (Yadav *et al.*, 2020).

India is maintaining its pace and marching with great strides on developing vaccines against malarial parasites *Plasmodium falciparum* and *Plasmodium vivax* HIV vaccine developed in India is being tested for its efficacy at HIV Vaccine Translational Research (HVTR) Lab of the Translational Health Science and Technology Institute (THSTI), NCR Biotech Science Cluster, Faridabad, Haryana. However, vaccine development against TB (except the existing BCG) has yet not been very encouraging. As BCG vaccine reportedly has several limitations, efforts to develop effective TB vaccines are needed (Schrager *et al.*, 2018). India needs to endeavour to develop vaccines against diseases like chikungunya virus, Ebola virus, Zika virus and norovirus too (Schrager *et al.*, 2018). Bharat Biotech has successfully developed two competent vaccines (one recombinant and one inactivated) against Zika virus (Pattnaik *et al.*, 2020) which needs to be validated further. Bharat Biotech has successfully also produced vaccine against chikungunya infection.

6. Vaccination and Indian Foreign Diplomacy

India's vaccine manufacturing strength has not only saved the population from COVID-19 pandemic across the globe, but has also maintained strong international relations with the countries and has improved its status in global geopolitics. India has tied up with its neighbouring countries and has initiated vaccine diplomacy in line with the 'changing the world order' strategy (Bharti and Bharti, 2021). Post the recent pandemic, India plays a significant role in changing the fate especially of the global healthcare. Mr Narendra Modi, the Indian Prime Minister stated that 'after the pandemic, a new world order is about to take shape and India has a big role to play in the emerging new world order' (Bharti and Bharti, 2021). India's vaccine diplomacy has actively been implemented in Central Asia, Africa and Southeast Asia thereby enhancing (or at least stabilised) their economic growth.

India's vaccine diplomacy to support the world during the COVID-19 pandemic was based on five points. These are, 1. agreements on reality, 2.

conditions of good life, 3. healthy relations between parties, 4. minimum conditionality, and 5. ordered coexistence (Srivastava and Sharma, 2014). The popularity and high standards of Indian pharmaceutical industry was obvious in making qualitative and affordable therapeutics and preventives and fulfilling about 60% of the global vaccine demand even before the COVID-19 pandemic (Sharun and Dhama, 2021). India is recognised as the world's emerging vaccine manufacturing country that was capable to produce the most cost-effective vaccines.

6.1. Maitri Programme

As a part of its vaccine diplomacy, India launched the 'Vaccine Maitri Programme' to supply vaccines to its neighbours. In addition, India supported worldwide immunisation programmes in numerous deprived countries (about 100 in number) under the COVID-19 Vaccines Global Access Facility. India supplied about 666.6 lakh COVID-19 vaccine doses to 95 countries (Bharti and Bharti, 2021). India's COVAX partnership contributed around 19.8 million COVID-19 vaccine doses to more than 43 countries, as per the reports (Kumraj et al., 2021). India supplied vaccine doses to Nepal (1.1 million), Maldives (200 thousand on 21 March 2021), Afghanistan (500 thousand on 7 February 2021), Bhutan (550 thousand on 28 March 2021) and Myanmar (1.7 million on 11 February 2021) under the 'Maitri Programme' vaccine diplomacy. Khadga Prasad Sharma Oli, the Nepali Prime Minister appreciated and thanked India for supplying the vaccines at a 'critical time'. India also arranged several trainings on vaccine administration in Bhutan, Nepal, Maldives, Morrocco, Brazil and Bangladesh. India's vaccine diplomacy is encouraging and is praised across the globe by nations, and numerous international leaders.

Global endorsement of India's vaccine diplomacy has raised its global profile and stature. As a result of the vaccines supplied to Asian, European, African and Caribbean countries around the world, the WHO DG commended India's efforts for 'supporting vaccine equity'. More than 60 countries started vaccinating the frontline workers and other priority groups under the COVAX partnership commitment, as Indian vaccination strategies gained popularity (Koller *et al.*, 2021). India's neighbourhood vaccine supply strategy through 'Maitri Programme' has improved bilateral ties that were somehow strained earlier. As China offered its vaccines to its neighbours too as a competing neighbour, India's vaccine diplomacy faced difficulties against China's expansive efforts to influence relationship with the neighbouring countries (Gauttam *et al.*, 2020).

The western countries stood steadfast with India during the pandemic which strengthened the relation of India. As events unfolded, Adar Poonawala, Chief executive, SII, revealed that the US did not supply the required raw materials in time to develop vaccines as a result of which the manufacturing slowed down in the last two months then (Bown and Bollyky, 2022). The USA joined India along with other QUAD members (Australia and Japan) on 12 March 2021 QUAD summit. A main objective of the action plan drafted there was to support India, and provide resources and infrastructures to develop best quality vaccines.

6.2. Impact of COVID-19 on India's Neighbourhood Policy

The double-mutant coronavirus variant the Delta variant (WHO-coded B.1.61) emerged in April 2021 in the second wave of COVID-19 that played havoc and the world witnessed a very critical situation. About 300,000 fresh confirmed cases and almost 5000 deaths in a short span were reported during the period. India provided vaccines to the neighbouring countries and supported them as the wave emerged, but multiple waves that continued later for more than a year was catastrophic and created a more devastating situation. Experts criticised India and its preparedness during the second wave, hinting at the lack of consistency of the vaccine and the oxygen supplies to the hospitalised patients.

India dominated in vaccine diplomacy since the second COVID-19 wave. French President Macron supported Indian vaccine diplomacy at the India-EU virtual summit and stated that 'India does not need lectures on vaccine supplies' (Bharti and Bharti, 2021). India's vaccination programme for the adult and the elderly was expedited in May 2021. Sadly, more than 400 thousand fresh confirmed cases daily and 3000 deaths, primarily due to lack of beds and oxygen in hospitals, were reported in India then (Filip *et al.*, 2022). India finally was triumphant through its vaccination drives and instilled vaccine nationalism in the citizens. India's vaccine drive started in January 2021, and mass vaccination followed after six months. The three major vaccines manufactured and/or approved immediately by India were, Covishield, Covaxin and Sputnik V. There was 90% vaccine coverage (either single-shot or with the booster-dose) in next six months. India manufactured 570 million vaccine doses at that time and targeted to complete the mass vaccination campaign among Indian residents by 2021 end (Bharti and Bharti, 2021).

6.3. India's Vaccine Diplomacy and International Affairs

With no solutions at hand during the pandemic, Covaxin that was freely supplied by India was probably a Good Samaritan option for especially the economically backward countries to protect their citizens. Canadian Prime Minister Justin Trudeau, former US president Donald Trump and the president of France Emmanuel Macron appreciated Indian vaccine diplomacy. The WHO Director General, Tedros Adhanom Ghebreyesus praised India's COVID-19 vaccine efforts. He intended to work with India to encourage vaccine production for most of the vulnerable diseases in the world to protect global citizens (Ariyawardana, 2022). Jerome Kim, the Director General of International Vaccine Institute opined that 'about 70% of the vaccines used around the world for extended immunisation programmes were made in India'. As stated by Antonio Guterres, former Secretary General of the UN, India's vaccine manufacturing potential is regarded as the 'best asset' (Altindis, 2022).

The two Indian vaccine manufacturing companies that were majorly active and successful during the COVID-19 were Bharat Biotech and Serum Institute of India to cater to global demand, alongside a few other manufacturers. Vaccines are mass produced in India against pertussis, tuberculosis, tetanus, measles and diphtheria. AstraZeneca partnered with SII to produce sizable portion of COVID-19 vaccines (Bown and Bollyky, 2022). While Bharat Biotech introduced Covaxin, Johnson and Johnson started vaccine production in India about the same time. The big advantage of Indian vaccines in terms of the logistics was these could be stored at a conventional refrigerated condition (at 2–8°C) without losing its viability/efficacy. In contrast, vaccines by others like that of Pfizer and Moderna (mRNA vaccines) required a sub-zero temperature, a major logistics challenge especially for the tropical countries and other Low- and Medium-Income Countries (LMICs). Table 2 lists some of the major COVID-19 vaccines produced in India.

Table 2: Lists of potential COVID-19 vaccines in India (Kumar *et al.*, 2021)

Name	Company	Storage temp.	Vaccine design strategy
Covishield	Serum Institute of India, Pune	2–8°C	Non-replicating chimpanzee adenovirus vaccine vector (ChAdOx1)
Covaxin	Bharat Biotech Ltd, Hyderabad	2–8°C	Inactivated virus vaccine
Sputnik V	Dr. Reddy's Laboratories, Hyderabad	-18°C	Inactivated human adenovirus Ad5 and Ad26 with spike protein inserts
ZyCoV-D	Zydus Cadila, Cadila Healthcare, Ahmedabad	2–8°C	Plasmid DNA vaccine
HDT-301	Gennova Biopharmaceuticals Ltd, Pune	2–8°C	mRNA vaccine

7. Vaccination strategies of India during the COVID-19

Surveys have reported that people in the low- and medium-income countries (LMICs) neither had the purchasing capacity nor did they opt for vaccination as they doubted the safety and efficacy of the vaccines (Lane *et al.*, 2018; Mohapatra *et al.*, 2023), and were not in favour of the vaccination programme (Agrawal *et al.*, 2020). Such public perceptions slowed down the expected vaccination rates initially in the developing world thereby affecting the overall vaccination coverage (Bogart *et al.*, 2021). The reported fear and distrust coupled with the deliberate misinformation through media were the critical hurdles in vaccination campaigns as slated by the governments (Yoda and Katsuyama, 2021).

India initiated its COVID-19 vaccination programme on 16 January 2021, after the Indian government and WHO approved the vaccines for 'emergency use'. The government of India appealed to the Supreme court that the drive was neither mandatory nor related to social service purpose for the general public, but it was voluntary (Reley and Jahnavi, 2022). Indian government established a National Expert Group on Vaccine Administration (NEGVAC) to regulate the COVID-19 vaccine administration (Ministry of Health and Family Welfare, 2021). An advisory committee that involved experts from specialised branches set the clinical criteria for COVID-19 immunisation prioritising the comorbid patients. For instance, the vaccine administration was prioritised for congenital cardiovascular diseases or associated ailments. Besides, it was agreed that the vaccines should be first administered to the frontline workers, healthcare personnel and people over 50 years of age. People in 50-60 years age-groups were priorities due to the high risk of mortality and morbidity among them (the deadline set for the calculation of age was 1 January 2021). Someone missing from the vaccination list by any chance could be easily identified through the 'COWIN' app launched by the Indian government and could register for self-vaccination (Kumar *et al.*, 2021). In no case, the journey was at all easy. Large population, limited healthcare infrastructure and geographic constraints were the added challenges faced in India during the mass vaccination drive (Patel and Nowalk, 2010). India had nevertheless successfully administered vaccines to about 461.5 million people of 18 years or above age group by 31 July 2021.

7.1. Indian Vaccination Drives and Public Reviews: A Case Study

Case studies of vaccination programme in Gujarat revealed several factors that influenced COVID-19 vaccine acceptance (Fig. 1; Tolia *et al.*, 2022). Public opinions during the survey revealed significant illusive perceptions on the mass vaccination drive in India. Many participants on the survey opined that

'I already had corona once. Now, I am safe at least for the last three to four months. I have antibodies in the body, so need not be revaccinated'. Another opinion was that 'I have heard all this kind of news of vaccine inefficacy. I do have hesitancy and fear. You will not believe it; forget about the vaccine, I have not even taken a test to check whether I have contracted corona or not till today!'. Religious and cultural aspects also influenced the public on deciding whether to administer the COVID-19 vaccines. As Indians are religiously sentimental, these factors had glaring effect on the vaccine uptake preferences. Religious leaders influenced the public in their day-to-day life irrespective of their educational background or lifestyles. Some survey respondents stated 'religious leaders will educate local people or the community explaining them about vaccination if they are educated about the underlying process'.

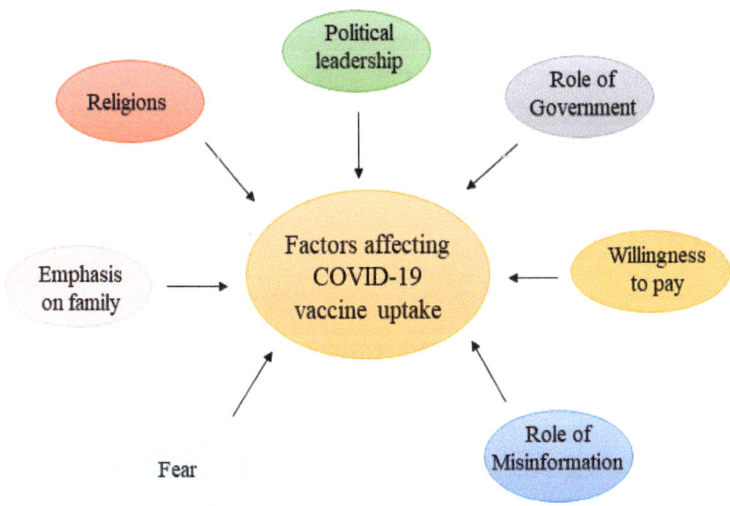

Fig. 1: The major factors that affected the vaccination drive in India during the pandemic

7.1.1. Impact of Cultural Differences on Vaccination Drive

Vaccine ingredients might hurt religious sentiments. For instance, Islam raised the 'halal' (permissible) aspect with regard to the vaccine uptake. Islamic followers continued with the opposite opinion and refused to vaccinate as it did not follow Islamic laws. 'The main reason why I am apprehensive about the vaccine is that I do not know exactly what was there in it. I will accept only if the ingredients are halal (and not haram)'. However, many others slowly-but-steadily were strongly determined and preferred to vaccinate themselves as the campaign progressed. 'On vaccine ingredients, it will not matter to me what was inside. We are given medicine like cough syrup when ill. It contains alcohol which is haram, but we overlook this aspect then. We take such medicines regularly, so we cannot claim that we have not taken alcohol. I will accept vaccine as vaccine only and avoid over-thinking on such aspects'.

Indian families were hesitant to vaccinate their children on numerous pretexts, like 1. vaccines are not yet tested in children, 2. vaccines might have side-effects, 3. children are mostly at home so there was no need to vaccinate them, 4. doctor consultation was needed first. Some others opined that 'when it comes to children, one has to be very careful as they have a long life ahead. It will be a big problem if some major side-effect occurred. After doctor consultation, it should be ensured that they are mentally and physically capable of being vaccinated, only then the vaccine may be administered'. Others opined that they would prioritise the elderly family members for vaccination. As the elderly had lower immunity, they had a higher risk to be infected and should follow precautions to avoid potential side-effects. The opinion was like 'elders should be vaccinated as their immune system was weak. Also, there might be comorbidities. However, doctor's advice before being vaccinated was vital', and 'I feel like the elderly should vaccinate, but they need to ascertain if they had other major clinical conditions like high blood pressure, diabetes or cancer, and they should be advised on the same by the family doctor first'.

7.1.2. Political and Social Media Dimensions

Politics plays a major role in influencing the public to participate in any mass drive in India including vaccination, reviewers opined. As a goodwill gesture and to instil faith in the public, the Prime Minister of India was the first to administer the vaccine. He connected to the public through 'Mann ki Baat' broadcasted by the All India Radio (AIR), Doordarshan National and Doordarshan News. 'Honourable Prime Minister of India and the Chief Minister of Delhi took the vaccines, so that the public could follow suit'. People felt reassured and vaccinated themselves being aware about the benefits. Administering vaccine personally and suggesting others to follow the same would significantly boost public perceptions. Celebrities too are strongly influential like the popular politicians. The government utilised available resources effectively and wisely to carry forward the vaccination programme. The timely delivery of safe and hygienic vaccines was appreciated by one and all. The government undertook various initiatives to guide people, create awareness about the vaccines using Hindi and other vernacular (like Gujarati and Marathi) in layman language. A caller tune of 30 seconds was also put to spread the awareness, informing about the slots when available. Although irritating at times, it had positive influence and was helpful in delivering the necessary information as the situation infolded and became grimmer. To reduce the vaccine hesitancy and enhance vaccination coverage, the following ideas were suggested in the conducted surveys:

a) Providing adequate information to the general public especially among the rural areas and weaker sections
b) Preventing the offline as well as online misleading information through check and balance
c) Supplying vaccines seamlessly to private hospitals for easy availability for the public who could afford
d) Collecting and providing data in desired segments (like state-wise) on measures taken in the country
e) Collaborating with the NGOs to enhance the service to the public
f) Supplying vaccine to the private corporate employees on a priority
g) Ensuring the transparency concerning vaccine administration

Nearly all the participants agreed for a paid vaccination as they trusted the private health institutes more than the government counterparts. They believed on the a) vaccine affordability, b) hygiene and safety, c) not to amplify government's burden, d) helping the needy instead who could not afford purchasing it, and e) reservations about the vaccination centres being run by the government. 'I paid for my parents' vaccination; the reason was not safety, hygiene or anything of that sort. The reason was that I did not feel to burden the government with additional 500 rupees', a respondent said. 'If supposed to be vaccinated, I would pay for it as I could afford it'. Another statement was 'The most important and genuine reason behind not to choose government health centre was someone needy could avail the vaccination free-of-cost there and I can get the same on payment from a private hospital'.

The participants in the surveys also conveyed that they had misconceptions about vaccines from the social media. 'There are stories related to vaccine floating around stating that the genetic makeup changed if the vaccine was administered. We are surrounded by lots of misinformation about vaccine as we do not have all information related to the vaccine'. The fear of vaccine efficacy and side-effects seemed to be genuine as the vaccine trial process was incomplete. It was approved for 'Emergency Use' only due to the prevailing hard times then. 'My grandmother and mother both have high blood pressure and diabetics. As I insisted on vaccination, they were concerned about vaccination side-effects. So, they remained hesitant'. A teenager stated 'I am afraid as we are young. I do not think corona easily enters the body if necessary COVID-appropriate measures could be followed. We have already improved our health due to the lockdown. So, I do not feel the need to vaccinate as it might instead cause damage'. Many had doubts on the vaccine, and instead tilted to

Ayurveda for three reasons, 1. Ayurveda contains natural ingredients only, 2. It is relatively easily accessible, 3. They have least side-effect, if any. One response was 'I choose Ayurveda when I have a health issue as my brother's wife, brother-in-law and father-in-law are all Ayurvedic physicians. Ayurvedic medicines only could treat illnesses completely, and I am apprehensive about other drugs'.

8. Indian Vaccine Expertise and Outlook

India's vaccine manufacturing industry enjoys larger internal market. Vaccine manufacturing strategy supports the government's Universal immunisation programme (UIP). Besides UIP strategy, few other governmental initiatives were undertaken to strengthen the productivity and infrastructure (Ghosh, 2019). Vaccine manufacturing, marketing and its supply in Indian market increased rapidly in recent times as reflected in the pharma sales volume. Vaccine trade in India created awareness and spread its benefits among the middle-class educated family reassuring them to buy vaccines from open market at an affordable price. 27 million people were immunised through the government's UIP programme (Ghosh, 2019). While common man was vaccinated at a lower price under UIP programme, the industry benefited from vaccines export. A vaccine needs WHO approval before it was released. Indian vaccine suppliers are in a good position to export adequate amount of the production annually. Some vaccines are developed to act against numerous pathogens simultaneously (multivalent vaccines). Certain infectious diseases spread rapidly in a region, thus effective vaccines need to be developed against active ongoing infections (Mohapatra *et al.*, 2024). Indian efforts have also ignited international collaborations alongside promising local institutions that needed increased fund allocation and enhanced global effect. India has set vaccine technology standards for the world to emulate.

9. Conclusion

Indian vaccine manufacturing, distribution and diplomacy strategies had a great sight with strong vision ingrained with a focus on the affordable supply of vaccines, therapeutics and drugs around the globe. India supplies vaccine to the UNICEF covering its major vaccines requirements under the EPI programme. Some wholesale distributors are committed to provide these at a cheaper price. National Regulatory Authority supports new techniques and creates opportunities for Indian manufacturers in the international market. They could also provide high-quality vaccines at affordable rates within the country easily then. All global studies and reports could be made public among the vaccine manufacturers, participating institutions, and the general public for awareness building, and a focussed and targeted global innovative action plan. These are key strategies to determine future goals for public health management at the global scale. The widely applicable Indian vaccine diplomacy offers tips to emulate and strategise at the global level too.

References

Agrawal A, Kolhapure S, Di Pasquale A, Rai J and Mathur A, 2020. Vaccine hesitancy as a challenge or vaccine confidence as an opportunity for childhood immunisation in India. Infect. Dis. Ther., 9: 421–432. doi: 10.1007/s40121-020-00302-9

Altindis E, 2022. Inequitable COVID-19 vaccine distribution and the intellectual property rights prolong the pandemic. Expert Rev. Vaccines, 21(4): 427–430. doi: 10.1080/14760584.2022.2014819

Ariyawardana SN, 2022. India's vaccine diplomacy and changing geopolitics in the global south. J. Soc. Sci. Humanit. Rev., 7(3): 142–161. doi: 10.4038/jsshr.v7i3.107

Bajaj S, 2018. RSSDI clinical practice recommendations for the management of type 2 diabetes mellitus 2017. Int. J Diabetes Dev. Ctries., 38: 1–115. doi: 10.1007/s13410-018-0604-7

Behera JK, Mishra P, Jena AK, Behera B and Bhattacharya M, 2023. Human health implications of emerging diseases and the current situation in India's vaccine industry. Sci. One Health, 2: 100046. doi: 10.1016/j.soh.2023.100046

Bharti SS and Bharti SS, 2021. India's Vaccine Diplomacy: Role in New Order and Challenges. Tor. Int. Stud., 1(14): 93–104. doi: 10.12775/TIS.2021.007

Bloom DE, Brenzel L, Cadarette D and Sullivan J, 2017. Moving beyond traditional valuation of vaccination: needs and opportunities. Vaccine, 35: A29–A35. doi: 10.1016/j.vaccine.2016.12.001

Bogart LM, Ojikutu BO, Tyagi K, Klein DJ, Mutchler MG, Dong L, Lawrence SJ, Thomas DR and Kellman S, 2021. COVID-19 related medical mistrust, health impacts, and potential vaccine hesitancy among Black Americans living with HIV. JAIDS J. Acquir. Immune Defic. Syndr., 86(2): 200–207. doi: 10.1097/QAI.0000000000002570

Bonanni PAOLO, Sacco CRISTIANA, Donato ROSA and Capei RAFFAELLA, 2014. Lifelong vaccination as a key disease-prevention strategy. Clin. Microbiol. Infect., 20: 32–36. doi: 10.1111/1469-0691.12537

Bosch FX, Broker TR, Forman D, Moscicki AB, Gillison ML, Doorbar J, Stern PL, Stanley M, Arbyn M, Poljak M and Cuzick J, 2013. Comprehensive control of human papillomavirus infections and related diseases. Vaccine, 31: H1–H31. doi: 10.1016/j.vaccine.2013.10.003

Bown CP and Bollyky TJ, 2022. How COVID-19 vaccine supply chains emerged in the midst of a pandemic. World Econ, 45(2): 468–522. doi: 10.1111/twec.13183

Chakraborty C and Agoramoorthy G, 2020. India's cost-effective COVID-19 vaccine development initiatives. Vaccine, 38(50): 7883–7884. doi: 10.1016/j.vaccine.2020.10.056

Chanda MM, Purse BV, Sedda L, Benz D, Prasad M, Reddy YN, Yarabolu KR, Byregowda SM, Carpenter S, Prasad G and Rogers DJ, 2024. Bluetongue risk map for vaccination and surveillance strategies in India. Pathogens, 13(7): 590. doi: 10.3390/pathogens13070590

Chandrasekharan S, Amin T, Kim J, Furrer E, Matterson AC, Schwalbe N and Nguyen A, 2015. Intellectual property rights and challenges for development of affordable human papillomavirus, rotavirus and pneumococcal vaccines: Patent landscaping and perspectives of developing country vaccine manufacturers. Vaccine, 33(46): 6366–6370. doi: 10.1016/j.vaccine.2015.08.063

Chawla R, Madhu SV, Makkar BM, Ghosh S, Saboo B, Kalra S and RSSDI-ESI Consensus Group, 2020. RSSDI-ESI Clinical Practice Recommendations for the Management of Type 2 Diabetes Mellitus 2020Table. No title available. Indian J. Endocrinol. Metab., 24(1): 1–122. doi: 10.4103/ijem.IJEM_225_20

Chen S, Yang L, Ou X, Li JY, Zi CT, Wang H, Hu JM and Liu Y, 2022. A new polysaccharide platform constructs self-adjuvant nanovaccines to enhance immune responses. J. Nanobiotechnol., 20(1): 320. doi: 10.1186/s12951-022-01533-3

Dash R, Agrawal A, Nagvekar V, Lele J, Di Pasquale A, Kolhapure S and Parikh R, 2020. Towards adult vaccination in India: a narrative literature review. Hum. Vaccin. Immunother., 16(4): 991–1001. doi: 10.1080/21645515.2019.1682842

Doherty M, Schmidt-Ott R, Santos JI, Stanberry LR, Hofstetter AM, Rosenthal SL, Cunningham AL, 2016. Vaccination of special populations: Protecting the vulnerable. Vaccine, 34(52): 6681–6690. doi: 10.1016/j.vaccine.2016.11.015.

Dolinar RO, Edelman S, Heinemann L, Home P, Goyal S, Polonsky WH and Schellekens H, 2014. Impact of biosimilar insulins on clinical practice: meeting report. J Diabetes Sci. Technol., 8(1): 179–185. doi: 10.1177/1932296813518267

Douglas RG, Samant VB, 2018. The vaccine industry. Plotkin's Vaccines, 41–50. doi: 10.1016/B978-0-323-35761-6.00004-3

Filip R, Gheorghita Puscaselu R, Anchidin-Norocel L, Dimian M and Savage WK, 2022. Global challenges to public health care systems during the COVID-19 pandemic: a review of pandemic measures and problems. J Pers. Med., 12(8): 1295. doi: 10.3390/jpm12081295

Gauttam P, Singh B and Kaur J, 2020. COVID-19 and Chinese global health diplomacy: geopolitical opportunity for China's hegemony?. Millennial Asia, 11(3): 318–340. doi: 10.1177/0976399620959771

Ghosh PK, 2019. Human vaccines in India: Present and future perspectives. MGM J. Med. Sci., 6(3): 137–147. Doi: 10.4103/mgmj.mgmj_11_20

Gopalakrishnan S, 2020. Vaccination programme in India-the present status: a review. Int J Community Med Public Health, 7(9): 3746. doi: 10.18203/2394-6040.ijcmph20203953

Gupta SS, Nair GB, Arora NK, Ganguly NK, 2013. Vaccine development and deployment: opportunities and challenges in India. Vaccine, 31: B43–B53. doi: 10.1016/j.vaccine.2012.11.079

Gurnani V, Haldar P, Aggarwal MK, Das MK, Chauhan A, Murray J, Arora NK, Jhalani M, Sudan P, 2018. Improving vaccination coverage in India: lessons from Intensified Mission Indradhanush, a cross-sectoral systems strengthening strategy. bmj, 363: k4782. doi: 10.1136/bmj.k4782

Hermsen ED, Jenkins R, Vlaev I, Iley S, Rajgopal T, Sackier JM, Loubser P, Pronk N, Wilkinson E, Chow Y, Gunther C, 2021. The role of the private sector in advancing antimicrobial stewardship: recommendations from the Global Chief Medical Officers' Network. Popul. Health Manag., 24(2): 231–240. doi: 10.1089/pop.2020.0027

Heymann DL, Aylward RB 2006. Mass Vaccination: When and Why. In: SA Plotkin (Eds) Mass Vaccination: Global Aspects — Progress and Obstacles. Current Topics in Microbiology and Immunology, Springer, Berlin, Heidelberg: 1–16. doi: 10.1007/3-540-36583-4_1

Jain SS, Singh VK, Kante RK, Jana SK and Patil RH, 2024. Current trends in development and manufacturing of higher-valent pneumococcal polysaccharide conjugate vaccine and its challenges. Biologicals, 87: 101784. doi: 10.1016/j.biologicals.2024.101784

Kaur H, Kaur M, Bhattacharyya A, Prajapat M, Thota P, Sarma P, Kumar S, Kaur G, Sharma S, Prakash A and Saifuddin PK, 2021. Indian contribution toward biomedical research and development in COVID-19: A systematic review. Indian J. Pharmacol., 53(1): 63–72. doi: 10.4103/ijp.ijp_168_21

Keeling M, Tildesley M, House T and Danon L, 2013. The mathematics of vaccination. Math. Today, 49: 40–43.

Koller CN, Schwerzmann CJ, Lang ASA, Alexiou E and Krishnakumar J, 2021. Addressing different needs: The challenges faced by India as the largest vaccine manufacturer while conducting the world's biggest COVID-19 vaccination campaign. Epidemiologia, 2(3): 454–470. doi: 10.3390/epidemiologia2030032

Kumar VM, Pandi-Perumal SR, Trakht I, Thyagarajan SP, 2021. Strategy for COVID-19 vaccination in India: the country with the second highest population and number of cases. npj Vaccines, 6(1): 60. doi: 10.1038/s41541-021-00327-2.

Kumraj G, Pathak S, Shah S, Majumder P, Jain J, Bhati D, Hanif S, Mukherjee S and Ahmed S, 2022. Capacity building for vaccine manufacturing across developing countries: the way forward. Hum. Vaccin. Immunother., 18(1): 2020529. doi: 10.1080/21645515.2021.2020529

Lahariya C, 2018. 'Ayushman Bharat'program and universal health coverage in India. Indian pediatr., 55(6): 495–506. doi: 10.1007/s13312-018-1341-1

Lane S, MacDonald NE, Marti M, Dumolard L, 2018. Vaccine hesitancy around the globe: Analysis of three years of WHO/UNICEF Joint Reporting Form data-2015–2017. Vaccine, 36(26): 3861–3867. doi: 10.1016/j.vaccine.2018.03.063

Makenga G, Bonoli S, Montomoli E, Carrier T, Auerbach J, 2019. Vaccine production in Africa: a feasible business model for capacity building and sustainable new vaccine introduction. Front. Public Health, 7: 56. doi: 10.3389/fpubh.2019.00056

Mandal S, Arinaminpathy N, Bhargava B, Panda S, 2021. Responsive and agile vaccination strategies against COVID 19 in India. The Lancet Global Health, 9(9): e1197–e1200. doi: 10.1016/S2214-109X(21)00284-9

Mani S, Tripathi L, Raut R, Tyagi P, Arora U, Barman T, Sood R, Galav A, Wahala W, de Silva A, Swaminathan S, 2013. Pichia pastoris-expressed dengue 2 envelope forms virus-like particles without pre-membrane protein and induces high titer neutralizing antibodies. PLoS one, 8(5): e64595. doi: 10.1371/journal.pone.0064595

Mantel C and Cherian T, 2020. New immunization strategies: adapting to global challenges. Bundesgesundheitsbl, 63: 25–31. doi: 10.1007/s00103-019-03066-x

Mazumdar-Shaw K, 2018. Leveraging affordable innovation to tackle India's healthcare challenge. IIMB Manag. Rev., 30(1): 37–50. doi: 10.1016/j.iimb.2017.11.003

Ministry of External Affairs,2021(May 28). Government of India. Vaccine Supply. https:// www.mea.gov.in/vaccine-supply.htm

Ministry of External Affairs,2023(June 15). Government of India. Vaccine Supply.

Ministry of Health and Family Welfare, 2021. COVID-19 Vaccine Operational Guidelines. Available online:https://main.mohfw.gov.in/sites/default/files/COVID19VaccineOG111Chapter16.pdf (accessed on 12 November 2021).

Mohapatra RK, Kandi V, Gaidhane AM, Zahiruddin QS, Rustagi S, Satapathy P, Mishra S and Tuglo LS, 2024. Global domination of the recently VoI-classified'JN. 1′ outcompeting other variants–Comparing the vaccines' efficacy. Clinical Infection in Practice, 22:100358. https://doi.org/10.1016/j.clinpr.2024.100358

Mohapatra RK, Verma S, Kandi V, Sarangi AK, Seidel V, Das SN, Behera A, Tuli HS, Sharma AK and Dhama K, 2023. The SARS-CoV-2 Omicron variant and its multiple sub-lineages: transmissibility, vaccine development, antiviral drugs, monoclonal antibodies, and strategies for infection control–a review. ChemistrySelect., 8(9):e202201380. https://doi.org/10.1002/slct.202201380

Panda S, Singh PK, Mishra S, Mitra S, Pattnaik P, Adhikary SD and Mohapatra RK, 2023. Indian biosimilars and vaccines at crossroads–replicating the success of pharmageneries. Vaccines, 11(1): 110. doi: 10.3390/vaccines11010110

Patel AR and Nowalk MP, 2010. Expanding immunization coverage in rural India: a review of evidence for the role of community health workers. Vaccine, 28(3): 604–613. doi: 10.1016/j.vaccine.2009.10.108

Pattnaik A, Sahoo BR and Pattnaik AK, 2020. Current status of Zika virus vaccines: successes and challenges. Vaccines, 8(2): 266. doi: 10.3390/vaccines8020266

Perri-Moore S, Kapsandoy S, Doyon K, Hill B, Archer M, Shane-McWhorter L, Bray BE, Zeng-Treitler Q, 2016. Automated alerts and reminders targeting patients: a review of the literature. Patient Educ. Couns., 99(6): 953–959. doi: 10.1016/j.pec.2015.12.010

Plotkin S, Robinson JM, Cunningham G, Iqbal R, Larsen S, 2017. The complexity and cost of vaccine manufacturing–an overview. Vaccine, 35(33): 4064–4071. doi: 10.1016/j.vaccine.2017.06.003

Pollard AJ and Bijker EM, 2021. A guide to vaccinology: from basic principles to new developments. Nat. Rev. Immunol., 21(2): 83–100. doi: 10.1038/s41577-020-00479-7

Reley P and Jahnavi P, 2022. No Vaccine, No Salary: Is Mandatory Vaccination for COVID-19 Constitutional under Indian Law?. Indian JL. Pub. Pol'y, 8: 61.

Salvatori G, Luberto L, Maffei M, Aurisicchio L, Roscilli G, Palombo F and Marra E, 2020. SARS-CoV-2 SPIKE PROTEIN: an optimal immunological target for vaccines. J. Transl. Med., 18(1): 222. doi: 10.1186/s12967-020-02392-y

Scarbrough Lefebvre CD, Terlinden A and Standaert B, 2015. Dissecting the indirect effects caused by vaccines into the basic elements. Hum Vaccin Immunother., 11(9): 2142–2157. doi: 10.1080/21645515.2015.1052196

Scelfo C, Menzella F, Fontana M, Ghidoni G, Galeone C and Facciolongo NC, 2021. Pneumonia and invasive pneumococcal diseases: the role of pneumococcal conjugate vaccine in the era of multi-drug resistance. Vaccines, 9(5): 420. doi: 10.3390/vaccines9050420

Schrager LK, Harris RC, Vekemans J, 2018. Research and development of new tuberculosis vaccines: a review. F1000Research, 7: 1732. doi: 10.12688/f1000research.16521.2

Sharun K and Dhama K, 2021. India's role in COVID-19 vaccine diplomacy. J. Travel Med., 28(7): taab064. doi: 10.1093/jtm/taab064

Srivastava J and Sharma A, 2014. International relations theory and world order: Binaries, silences and alternatives. South Asian Survey, 21(1–2): 20–34. doi: 10.1177/0971523115592471

Times of India, 2021. Covid Vaccination India: Since May 1, Private Sector Gave 7% of Jabs Despite 25% Quota. 2021. Accessed July 31, 2021. https://timesofindia.indiatimes.com/india/covid-19-since-may-1-private-sector-gave-7-of-jabs-despite-25 quota/articleshow/84778026.cms

Tolia V, Renin Singh R, Deshpande S, Dave A, Rathod RM, 2022. Understanding factors to COVID-19 vaccine adoption in Gujarat, India. Int. J. Environ. Res. Public Health, 19(5): 2707. doi: 10.3390/ijerph19052707

Verma R, Khanna P and Chawla S, 2015. Adult immunization in India: Importance and recommendations. Hum. Vaccin. Immunother., 11(9): 2180–2182. doi: 10.4161/hv.29342

WHO Recommendations for Routine Immunization, 2021. Accessed June 29, 2021.

Wigle J, Fontenot HB and Zimet GD, 2016. Global delivery of human papillomavirus vaccines. Pediatric Clinics, 63(1): 81–95.

World Health Organization, 2005. Vaccine introduction guidelines. Adding a vaccine to a national immunization programme: decision and implementation. WHO/ IVB/05.18. Geneva, Switzerland; 2005.

Wouters OJ, Shadlen KC, Salcher-Konrad M, Pollard AJ, Larson HJ, Teerawattananon Y and Jit M, 2021. Challenges in ensuring global access to COVID-19 vaccines: production, affordability, allocation, and deployment. The Lancet, 397(10278): 1023–1034. doi: 10.1016/S0140-6736(21)00306-8

Yadav A, Kapoor N, Malviya S and Malhotra SK, 2020. COVID-19 pandemic and the global vaccine strategy. The Scientific Temper: 11(1&2). doi: 10.58414/SCIENTIFICTEMPER.2020.11.1.06

Yoda T and Katsuyama H, 2021. Willingness to receive COVID-19 vaccination in Japan. Vaccines, 9(1): 48. doi: 10.3390/vaccines9010048

8

One Health Approach for Universal Wellbeing and Comprehensive Role of Vaccines

***Manas Ranjan Behera*[1], *Aurobinda Rout*[2], *Ranjan Kumar Mohapatra*[3], and *Snehasish Mishra*[4,*]**

[1]*School of Public Health, KIIT Deemed University, Bhubaneswar-751 024 Odisha, India*
[2]*School of Applied Sciences, KIIT Deemed University, Bhubaneswar Odisha-751 024, India*
[3]*Department of Chemistry, Government College of Engineering Keonjhar-758 002, Odisha, India*
[4]*School of Biotechnology, KIIT Deemed University, Bhubaneswar-751 024 Odisha, India*

Abstract

The world turned into a grossly inhabitable during the infamous COVID-19 pandemic, with community health issues everywhere. Each one felt unsafe if other earthly inhabitants were, be it humans or other living beings. Onset of SARS-CoV-2 set a 'new normal' world order. The ever-evolving and mutating SARS-CoV-2 variants extended the pandemic wave after wave thereby complicating the situation, pushing the global healthcare system to its limits and exposing its underbelly. The continually evolving variants were more aggressively transmissive and infective. As the world still reels under tremendous healthcare pressure, other infectious diseases are emerging as are identified by the World Health Organisation (WHO), creating international health emergency situations. The situation becomes alarming with the increasing zoonotic (spillover) and reverse zoonotic (spillback) factors being more proactive in the disease spread. There is a greater need to vaccinate not only humans but also animals, especially the domesticated ones and known reservoirs/carriers. Vaccines must be developed on priority and equitably distributed as the first step to counter a pandemic or potential pandemic. Vaccination is self-limiting due to increasing reported breakthrough infection cases. A strong link of the environmental health to the overall global health needs to be acknowledged, and due diligent measures taken. Hence, there is a strong need of the One Health approach as a 360° solution, and follow it up at global-scale both in letter and spirit. This chapter discusses spillover and spillback of diseases like SARS-CoV-2 and Mpox as case examples, the mitigation strategies and the need for workable One Health models, and challenges and measures to counter future outbreaks. It stresses on foolproof vaccination strategies across to catalyse individual and herd immunities for universal wellbeing.

Keywords: One health, Zoonosis, Disease prevention, Animal vaccination, Infectious disease

1. Introduction

The world waits anxiously for the COVID-19 pandemic inflicted by SARS-CoV-2 to end that had played havoc for more than two years during the early '20s. Since the first reported case in the Wuhan province of the Chinese mainland, the virus spread around the globe, hitting the social, cultural and economic human lives hard (Mohapatra *et al.*, 2021). Inadequate knowledge on the biology and pathogenesis of SARS-CoV-2 in the initial days caused severe mortalities owing to the pandemic (Mohapatra *et al.*, 2024). Also, no specific therapeutics or preventives were available to tackle COVID-19. Several countries experienced multiple waves that limited public movements and badly affected the global economy (Mohapatra *et al.*, 2022[a]). As SARS-CoV-2 clinical, pathological and immunology aspects were gradually understood through case observations as also laboratory and clinical trials, patient management improved and the associated mortality declined. Multiple variants emerged as the virus mutated, and the World Health Organisation (WHO) labelled them as 'variant of concern', 'variant of interest' and 'variant under monitoring' considering the aetiological significance and factors like their transmissibility and pathogenicity (Mohapatra *et al.*, 2023a). The Delta variant (B.1.617.2) was reportedly the most virulent and highly transmissible among the reported variants. First reported in South Africa, the Omicron variant had the most global spread (Viana *et al.*, 2022, Mohapatra *et al.*, 2022[b]). The BF.7 (BA 5.2.1.7) variant was actively lethal in countries like China, Korea, Japan and a few American and European countries (Mohapatra *et al.*, 2022[c]). Multiple Omicron and recombinant SARS-CoV-2 lineage emerged variants put global healthcare under tremendous pressure (Mohapatra *et al.*, 2022[d]).

Most countries rigorously vaccinated their citizen with a handful of WHO-approved vaccines, meant for 'emergency use' (Satapathy *et al.*, 2023). It was opined that non-uniform vaccination among the developed and the developing nations due to the unequal distribution of vaccines could have led to rapid viral mutations and the global spread of the variants. Also, the vaccine hesitancy among the public adversely impacted the vaccination drive, primarily attributed to the misleading social media propaganda (Mohapatra *et al.*, 2022[b]). The genuine fear and hesitation were mostly attributed to the novel technology adopted in vaccine development manufacturing, and most of the vaccines were passed for 'emergency use' only while their clinical trial phases were still ongoing. Thus, reliable datasets and reports on the long-term efficacy and safety were missing which was a genuine technical concern among even the intellectual lots. Thus, the world was far from being certain over the severity of infections by the viral variants and the protection guarantee of the vaccines. Omicron variant was capable of breaking the immunity barrier easily that resulted in breakthrough infections and the pandemic recurred wherein SARS-CoV-2 reinfected even the fully vaccinated individual (Mohapatra *et al.*, 2022[d]). Studies report that most outbreaks were either asymptomatic or had mild symptoms. Many approved vaccines provided immunological protection for up to six months after the second/booster dose (Yu *et al.*, 2022).

The world has 60% of its population (over 4.3 billion) living in the region where SARS-CoV and SARS-CoV-2 first appeared. Also, they make up 22% of the world's land area and the major cities and towns here are densely populated. Human population growing and invading into the wild might encourage ever more wild-to-human transmission of novel viral diseases. Long-term effect of global climate change and biodiversity loss could intensify interspecies infectious disease outbreaks in future, making the situation more alarming. A decrease in biodiversity could be a cause of the rise in the frequency of virus transmission from an infected host. It is imperative that zoonotic disease surveillance is revamped through coordinated efforts of health authorities to curtail new outbreaks (Zumla *et al.*, 2022). This article discusses zoonotic diseases such as SARS-CoV-2 and human monkeypox (hmpox), zoonosis and reverse zoonosis, their mitigation strategies and the need of one health approach along with the challenges to counter such outbreaks and any future outbreaks.

Indigenous communities worldwide have identified, acknowledged and applied holistic, nature- and society-based approaches to sustainably balance the live players in the ecosystem, the humans, animals and the plants (Hillier *et al.*, 2021; Jack *et al.*, 2020). From the indigenous people, such practices are progressively being popular among other local and cohesive communities across the world that includes peasants, forestry and agrarian groups (Mumford *et al.*, 2023). The importance of such integrated approaches in addressing health, social, financial and ecological issues were noted worldwide by both the mainstream scientific communities (Schultz, 2008) and the policymakers (WHO, 2022[a]).

Environmental factors like the wildlife and ecological systems are often overlooked although these play a crucial role in the complex health issues that affect humans and animals, as identified by the Wildlife Conservation Society. The idea of addressing health issues at the interface of humans, animals and environment was widely promoted during late 1990s and early 2000s by international health agencies, as also the government and academic stakeholders across the world (Coghlan and Hall, 2013; Salk, 2019). Some proactive global players include World Health Organisation (WHO), World Organisation for Animal Health (WOAH), Food and Agriculture Organisation (FAO), United Nations Environment Programme (UNEP), Convention on Biological Diversity (CBD) and United Nations System Influenza Coordination (UNSIC). The idea has gradually snowballed into the 'One Health' concept and is currently widely recognised as a useful approach to address complex health issues (Mackenzie *et al.*, 2014).

2. History of the 'One Health' Approach

One Health approach is an integrative framework that addresses infectious diseases by recognising close connections between humans, animals, plants and the environment. The concept originated in the mid-20th century when Calvin Schwabe, a veterinary surgeon in the US, proposed the idea of 'One Medicine'. Schwabe advocated for a unified, interdisciplinary perspective where veterinary medicine could significantly contribute to general medicine (Zinsstag *et al.*, 2023). He emphasised the necessity of including social sciences and improving communication strategies to enable effective engagement of communities in controlling and preventing infectious diseases (Zinsstag *et al.*, 2023).

The One Health concept was further redefined and broadened in the 21st century to include the ecosystem, encompassing plant health, wildlife and geographical regions. The global SARS-CoV-1 epidemic in 2002-2004 highlighted the dangers posed by zoonotic diseases, accelerating the popularity of 'One Health' (Mackenzie and Jeggo, 2019). It recognises the close interlink among human health, animal health, behavioural patterns and ecological settings (Evans and Leighton, 2014). In the context of One Health, it means that human health depends on a healthy ecosystem. This healthy ecosystem is conceived as a continuum that ranges from the microbiota in the human gut to the larger living environment, lifestyle factors and the global ecological landscape (Zinsstag *et al.*, 2011). Although the term 'One Health' gained widespread use only in 2004, its principles have long been present in historical treatises on traditional medicines in the West and Asia (Mackenzie and Jeggo, 2019; Zinsstag *et al.*, 2011).

One Health approach incorporates all the relevant stakeholders (that include the experts in public health, animal health, agriculture, environment and wildlife sectors), scientific bodies, and the communities at various levels of the society. The fundamental component of this strategy encourages these groups to work together for the common good, which is universal wellbeing (Pepin *et al.*, 2024). An effective implementation of One Health as a policy depends on the coordinated efforts of the policymakers in close consultation with the public service sectors and experts from a wide range of disciplines, while also engaging the general public to incorporate their perspectives (Fig. 1).

One Health is being increasingly recognised as a crucial framework to address complex health and wellbeing challenges at local, national, regional and global levels (de Castañeda *et al.*, 2023). Although the One Health concept is still in its infancy in principle, many researchers, institutions and organisations seem to have vowed to adopt it in its true letter and spirit. One Health model gained greater momentum to enhance the access to best practices and expertise, leading to a stable strategy to address especially the global human health issues. It primarily focuses on addressing the issues related to the emergence, reemergence and spread of zoonotic diseases and their antimicrobial resistance (AMR). The biodiversity loss that the WCS originally highlighted has also been addressed by the ideas of EcoHealth and Planetary Health (Zinsstag *et al.*, 2011; Lerner and Berg, 2017). The core concept of One Health refers to interdisciplinary multi-sectoral approach that aims at strengthening the trust, collaboration, communication and coordination surrounding a specific complex health issue. It applies equally to activities conducted under both EcoHealth and Planetary Health frameworks, despite the perceived differences in scopes among these three concepts.

Accessible resources and guidelines facilitate One Health initiatives across the world (Pelican *et al.*, 2019), and many nations have established national One Health frameworks that oversee the health policy, strategy and implementation (Tangwangvivat *et al.*, 2019). A comprehensive One Health Operational Framework with integrated tools was recently developed by the Food and Agriculture Organisation (FAO) of the United Nations (UN) and the Centers for Disease Control and Prevention of the US (Ghai *et al.*, 2022). One Health is becoming increasingly influenced by both ecological and biodiversity perspective as well as traditional knowledge systems of indigenous people (Ruscio *et al.*, 2015; Garnier *et al.*, 2020). A significant demand for genuine inclusion in One Health is being made by indigenous voices (Hillier *et al.*, 2021; Jack *et al.*, 2020).

The World Bank has provided One Health framework to operationalise One Health in both the donor country and the target country (Stephen and Stemshorn, 2016; Machalaba *et al.*, 2018). This framework comprises five domains considered as the foundation of 'One Health' building blocks, i) One Health stakeholders, roles and responsibilities; ii) financial and personal resources; iii) communication and information; iv) technical infrastructure; and v) governance. This is comparable to the World Health Organisation's health system building blocks (Ferrinho and Fronteira, 2023). This framework could be adopted and replicated in various contexts to ensure improved outcomes at the human-animal-environment interface (Ferrinho and Fronteira, 2023).

Historically driven by domain researchers, 'One Health' mainly focused on the infectious diseases, particularly the zoonotic diseases, as mentioned earlier (Adisasmito *et al.*, 2022). Thus, multiple countries across the globe implemented One Health approach to detect and control zoonotic diseases (Acharya *et al.*, 2021; Rai *et al.*, 2024). The relevance of the approach has become more significant in current times due to the manifold increase in the surge of numerous outbreaks attributed to the emerging and reemerging infectious agents (Rabinowitz *et al.*, 2018). Avian influenza, anthrax, rabies and brucellosis are priority zoonosis in many countries (Yasobant *et al.*, 2019; Wang *et al.*, 2019) and they offer suitable case examples to highlight the relevance of One Health approach (Bengis and Frean, 2014). Scrub typhus, another reemerging vector-borne zoonotic disease originating in the Asian continent (Tilak and Kunte, 2019; Gaba *et al.*, 2021) also is closely linked to environmental factors (Liu *et al.*, 2023; Zangpo *et al.*, 2023). These evidences and the alarming trend of the upsurge of various emerging infectious outbreaks will undoubtedly further validate the utility of 'One Health' in future.

Presently, the scope of One Health has been extended far beyond as reflected in the United Nations Sustainable Development Goals (SDGs), and it is hoped that One Health approach shall assist in meeting the SDGs (Dye, 2018). Six of the SDGs have direct association with the One Health approach. These are, good health & wellbeing (SDG3), clean water and sanitation (SDG6), sustainable cities and communities (SDG11), climate action (SDG13), life below water (SDG14) and life on land (SDG15) (Laaser *et al.*, 2022). Most of these SDGs are interlinked and requires multi-sector approach and collaboration, thereby providing a unique opportunity for One Health initiative (Queenan *et al.*, 2017).

Four global organisations, *viz.*, WHO, WOAH, FAO and UNEP formed the One Health Quadripartite in March 2022 recognising the need for inter-sectoral and international collaboration, which offers a formal and legal framework to address the challenges at the human-animal and ecosystem interface (Rai *et al.*, 2024). This quadripartite has mainstreamed 'One Health', defined by the WHO as *'an approach to designing and implementing programs, policies, legislation and research in which multiple sectors communicate and work together to achieve better public health outcomes'* and focuses the need for One Health approach in six critical areas. These are: a) control and prevention of zoonotic diseases; b) laboratory diagnostics and services; c) management of neglected tropical diseases; d) combatting antimicrobial resistance; e) promoting environmental health; and f) ensuring food safety, that support countries to mitigate, prevent, monitor, detect and control of zoonotic outbreaks while contributing to the SDGs (Pitt and Gunn, 2024). The relevance of the One Health approach is further emphasised by its connection to the six SDGs and thirty-six SDGs target. It was evident by 2023 that significant progress was lacking in several SDG targets closely aligned with the One Health principles, such as, safe drinking water, ecosystem conservation, greenhouse gas emission reduction, vaccine coverage, sustainable fishing, food security and species extinction prevention (Pepin *et al.*, 2024). Thus, applying a One Health approach enables a deeper understanding of both the positive and negative consequences of policy decisions. For instance, a public health intervention might provide immediate benefits for human health, but could also exacerbate environmental degradation, leading to long-term negative health consequences through both direct and indirect manners. This comprehensive perspective helps identify complementary strategies to mitigate adverse effects, and supports a more accurate evaluation of the costs and benefits aspects that are associated with the policy decisions.

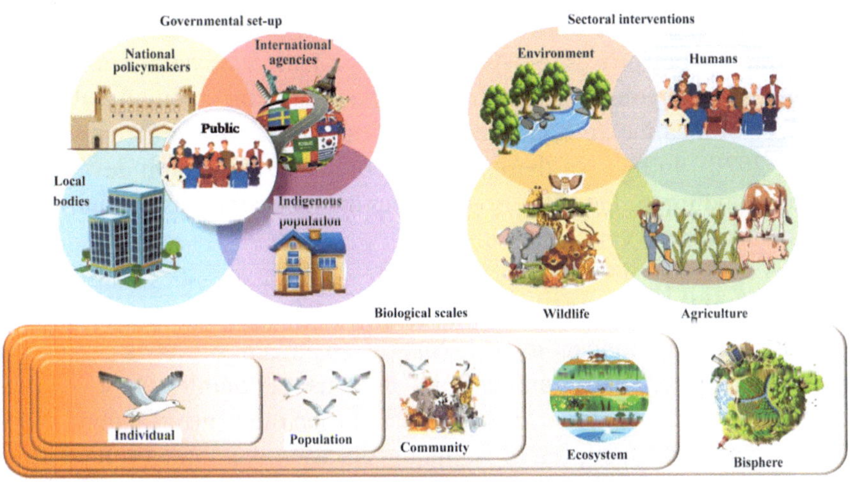

Fig. 1: Depiction of sectoral integration and scales to operationalise 'One Health'

3. The Evolving Global Context

Numerous global crises that the mankind could face in coming times include emerging and reemerging infectious diseases, increased frequency and severity of pandemics, extreme climate conditions, irreversible environmental damage, food insecurity, growing imbalances in health and wellbeing as well as social and economic divide. These are fast approaching their threshold, thus creating immediate impact on individuals, communities and countries. Simultaneously, the awareness on the necessity of collaborative action to achieve a future that is ecologically and environmentally sustainable is growing. Addressing the enormous challenges to ensure justice and equity while ensuring health and wellbeing, understanding and appreciating the fact that colonialism and discrimination with constrained worldviews and systems have widened the disparities is crucial. Such historical human misdemeanors have caused larger environmental degradation, propelled ecosystem collapse and have harmed the communities. These constraints also have posed serious threats to the global capabilities to frame coordinated, long-term action plans to tackle complex situations. Numerous viewpoints describing this scenario have been presented since decades in the form of books (Mumford *et al.*, 2023) and scholarly articles (Garnier *et al.*, 2020; Steffen *et al.*, 2015; Rushton *et al.*, 2021). Further, the policymakers and scientific organisations have outlined potential course of action (Falk *et al.*, 2021; Healy *et al.*, 2022).

The world currently is transforming from economic and commercial standpoints. The world is becoming more and more 'volatile, uncertain, complex and ambiguous' (VUCA), and prone to abrupt shifts (Bennett and Lemoine 2014). As suggested by the VUCA concept, the health and ecosystem processes could benefit from more flexible and responsive approaches to business and social processes. According to Klaus Schwab's theory of the fourth industrial revolution, new technologies will fundamentally alter how people receive healthcare both individually and collectively (Trenovski and Merdzan, 2020). In light of these, an array of social and health development activities including the One Health initiatives must be continuously and rapidly reevaluated.

4. Emerging and Reemerging Zoonotic Diseases

The WHO defines zoonosis as a disease or an infection that is transmitted naturally from vertebrate animals to humans. Zoonotic pathogens are categorised as viral, bacterial, fungal, parasitic or other novel agents (Table 1). Some common examples of zoonotic diseases are viral (yellow fever, rabies and influenza), bacterial (leptospirosis, brucellosis, salmonellosis and plague), fungal (histoplasmosis and cryptococcus), parasitic (schistosomiasis, leishmaniasis, hydatid disease and toxoplasmosis), etc. Livestock has played a key role in the development of civilization since centuries in many forms, like food, cloth, shelter, transport and business. Spillover of zoonoses occurs due to such close interactions between the animals and humans for food, cloth, shelter, transport and business (Rahman *et al.*, 2020; Yadana *et al.*, 2023; Braam *et al.*, 2021).

Historically, the world has witnessed major zoonotic pandemics like the Plague of Justinian (541–543 AD), the Black Death pandemic due to the bubonic plague (1346–1353 AD), the Spanish flu pandemic (1918) and numerous others (Kelly, 2020). More recently zoonotic Nipah virus (NiV) emerged in Malaysia in 1999 transmitted through saps of raw palm through bats, causing severe encephalitis in children (Soman Pillai *et al.*, 2020). Very recently, the world encountered one of the worst forms of pandemic in documented history in the form of COVID-19 in 2019-2020 caused by coronavirus (SARS-CoV-2), as yet another example of how the zoonotic virus emerged from a live market in Wuhan city, China that spread across the globe. It resulted in unforeseen human agony that wreaked havoc worldwide, exposing the underbelly of global healthcare infrastructure.

Table 1: A list of common zoonoses, the etiological agents and the involved non-human host

Bacterial		**Viral**		**Fungal**		**Parasitic**	
Pathogen	**Host**	**Pathogen**	**Host**	**Pathogen**	**Host**	**Pathogen**	**Host**
Brucella	Racoon, hare	Rabies	Dog, bat	*Cryptococcus*	Bat	*Leishmania* sp.	Sandfly
Leptospira	Rat, cattle, buffalo	Influenza	Bat, camel	*Histoplasma capsulatum*	Bat	*Echinococcus granulosis* (hydatid)	Dog
Salmonella	Poultry, egg	Dengue and Chikunguniya	*Aedes* mosquito	–	–	*Schistosoma*	Snail
Yersinia pestis (bubonic plague)	Rat	Japenese encephalitis virus	Pond heron, cattle egrets	–	–	*Toxoplasma*	Cat
–	–	Hanta virus	Bandicoot, rat, shrews	–	–	–	–
–	–	Crimean congo haemorrhagic virus	Shrews, bat	–	–	–	–
–	–	Kyasanur forest disease virus	Sick/dying monkey, bird, ticks	–	–	–	–

The South-East Asia including India is socio-economically, politically and culturally diverse, that experiences major economic, social and environmental changes (Chongsuvivatwong *et al.*, 2011). This has triggered the emergence and reemergence of many zoonotic viral diseases in last couple of decades (Table 2).

Table 2: The sequence of emerging and reemerging zoonotic viral diseases in humans in the Southeast Asian region in last two decades of the 21st Century (January 2000–October 2022)

First report	Virus	Country	Source
2001	Nipah virus	India	WHO, 2021[a]
2003	SARS-CoV	Vietnam	Reynolds *et al.*, 2006
		Singapore	
		Thailand	
		The Philippines	
		Indonesia	
		Malaysia	
2003	Influenza A (H5N1)	Vietnam	WHO, 2021[b]
2004	Influenza A (H5N1)	Thailand	WHO, 2021[b]
2005	Influenza A (H5N1)	Indonesia	WHO, 2021[b]
		Cambodia	
2007	Dengue virus	Cambodia	Yek *et al.*, 2023
2007	Influenza A (H5N1)	Lao PDR	WHO, 2021[b]
		Myanmar	
2008	Chikungunya virus	Malaysia	Khor *et al.*, 2023
2009	Chikungunya virus	Thailand	Tun *et al.*, 2022
2009	Ebola	The Philippines	Hussein, 2023
2009	Influenza A (H1N1)	All South East Asia countries	Malik, 2023
2009	Chikungunya virus	Myanmar	Saba Villarroel *et al.*, 2023
		Indonesia	
2013	Dengue virus	Thailand	Polwiang, 2015
		Lao PDR	WHO, 2022[b]
2013	Chikungunya virus	Singapore	Calvez *et al.*, 2022
		Lao PDR	
2014	Dengue virus	Brunei	Saba Villarroel *et al.*, 2023
2014	MERS-CoV	Malaysia	WHO, 2022[b]
2015	MERS-CoV	Thailand	WHO, 2022[b]
		The Philippines	
2015	Dengue virus	Indonesia	Kaligis *et al.*, 2023
2016	Zika virus	Singapore	Prem *et al.*, 2019
		Thailand	Ruchusatsawat *et al*, 2019
		Vietnam	Nguyen *et al.*, 2020
		India	WHO, 2017

First report	Virus	Country	Source
2017	Chikungunya and Dengue virus	The Philippines	Wimalasiri-Yapa *et al.*, 2019
2019		Malaysia	Mashudi *et al.*, 2022
		The Philippines	Ong *et al.*, 2022
2019	Monkeypox	Singapore	Luo and Han, 2022
2019	Avian Influenza A (H9N2)	India	Potdar *et al.*, 2019
2020	SARS-CoV-2	All South East Asia countries	WHO, 2022[b]
2020	SARS-CoV-2	India	Dey and Dey, 2020
2020	Chikungunya virus	Cambodia	Kril *et al.*, 2021
2020	Dengue virus	Singapore	Merakou *et al.*, 2023
2021	Influenza A (H5N1)	India	WHO, 2021[b]
2022	Monkeypox	Vietnam	Velavan and Mayer, 2022 George *et al.*, 2023
		Thailand	
		The Philippines	
		Indonesia	
		India	
2022	Dengue virus	Vietnam	Huynh *et al.*, 2022
		Timor-Leste	

South-East Asian region is emerging as a dynamic hotspot for numerous zoonotic diseases among humans attributed to disrupted natural ecosystem and climate change due to numerous anthropogenic reasons like dense population, travel and migration, industrialisation, rapid and expanded agriculture, deforestation, disturbed wildlife dynamics, and meat consumption and trade (Gortazar *et al.*, 2014; Fig. 2). It is heartening that the region is increasingly embracing 'One Health' to provide significant insights to understanding the cycle and chain of zoonosis. However, barriers across countries still exist which hinder its successful implementation.

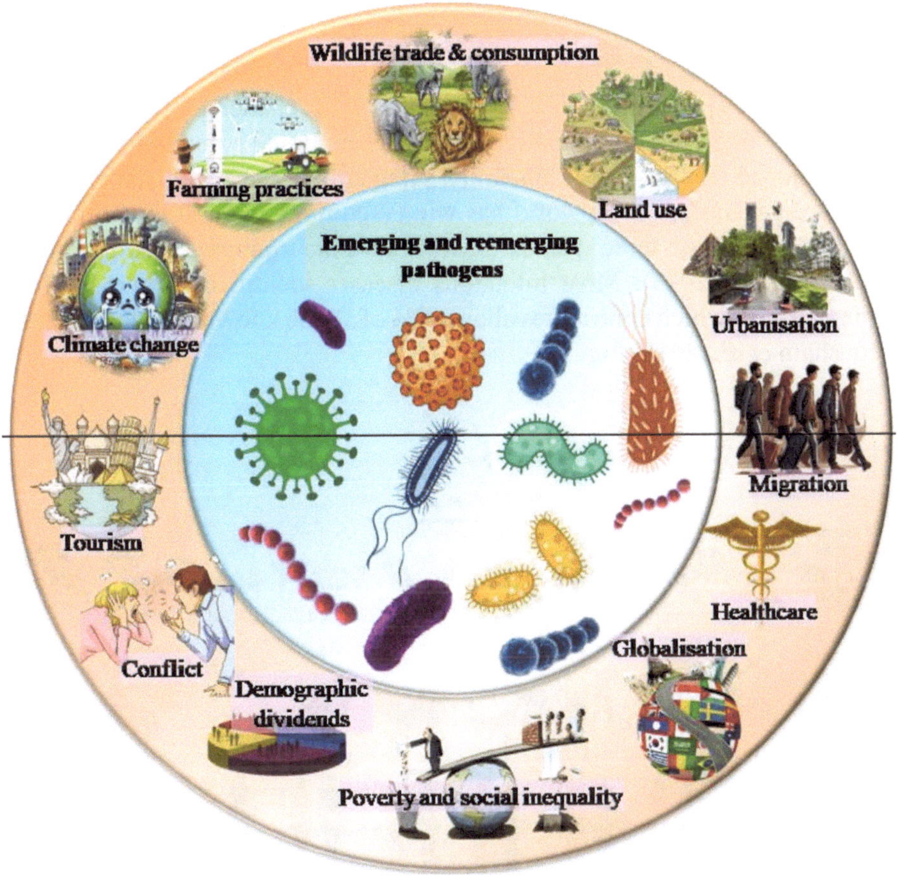

Fig. 2: Anthropogenic factors as drivers of the emerging and reemerging infectious diseases

Thus, emerging infectious diseases pose a serious threat to the society in the 21st century that necessitates global health security (Duff *et al.*, 2021). Recent outbreaks of viral diseases such as Zika, Ebola and COVID-19 emphasise the need for worldwide preparedness and cooperation due to their rapid spill-over potential resulting in overwhelming disasters, if not nipped at bud. Emerging infectious diseases are those that were either newly discovered (emerging) or present in the past but are now spreading worldwide (reemerging). Infectious diseases that were under control in the past but have reemerged as notable public health concern are stated as reemerging infectious diseases (Mostafavi *et al.*, 2022). Nearly 75% of such freshly encountered diseases originate from animals (Petersen *et al.*, 2018; Woolhouse, 2022)

Many of these neither have a preventive nor a curative, and thus public healthcare providers are often the victims. Both the emerging and reemerging forms constantly trigger the urgency of tangible interventions (Johnson and Mueller, 2002). The world has witnessed numerous cohesive interventions to address large outbreaks like SARS, HIN1 (swine flu), H5N1 (avian influenza) and COVID-19 pandemic. As we come across these challenges time and again, it becomes increasingly imperative that evidence-based community strategies are developed for the sake of humanity, safeguarding the health and wellbeing of future generations. The world has witnessed more than 30 new infectious diseases in the last three decades, with the Asian countries leading the list (Behera *et al.*, 2023). Most infectious diseases identified in humans have animal origins which contributes about 60% of all the known human infections (Rousham *et al.*, 2018; Fig. 3).

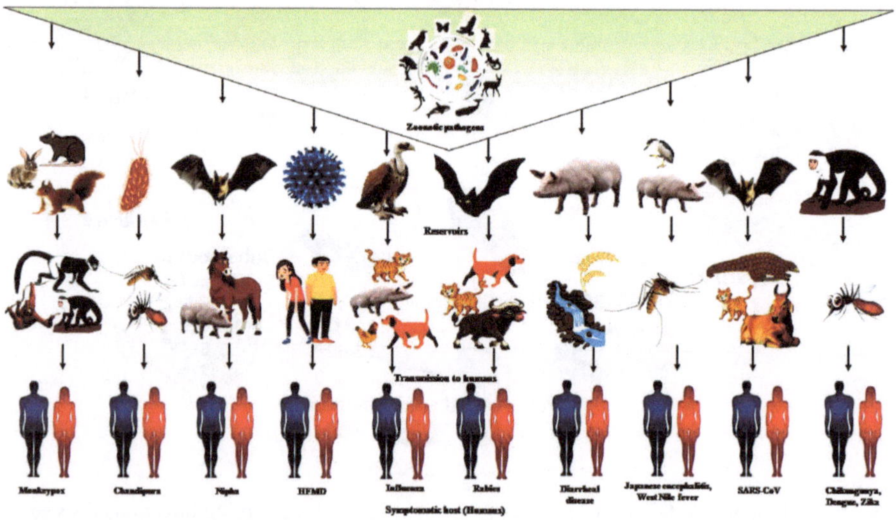

Fig. 3: Spillover events of zoonotic diseases from natural reservoirs to humans through transmuted pathogens

Novel diseases keep on emerging primarily attributed to climate change, altered environment and genetic mutation in microbes. With AMR emerging as a critical public healthcare concern in the South-East Asian nations including India, both preventives and curatives are disrupted. Thus, a functional and focused community healthcare system in place is very much necessary in order to prevent the spread of infectious diseases. Vaccines have made momentous progress to tackle such global health crises.

5. Understanding and Addressing the Zoonoses (Spillover)

Agriculture and food-supply sectors are critical links in preventing critical zoonotic infection. Food safety alongside its security is of greater concern in larger part of the world. Aboriginal population around the woods often consume animal carcasses like that of rodents and marsupials. This increases the risk of animal-to-human disease transmission. Wildlife hunting for food need to be consciously minimised, and in light of this the animal husbandry practices could be improved in vulnerable regions. Bush meat consumption in the urban world is a liking rather than an urgent need, which could be duly and responsibly addressed. Mass campaigns to educate people of the harmful effect of handling and consuming food of animal origin (including bush meat), and the possible deadly consequences of coming in contact with animals that may be carrying the virus could help curb the infectious diseases.

More than half of the infectious diseases that affect humans originate in animals wherein a significant population of these harmful microbes demonstrate animal-human transmissions. Pandemics like the COVID-19 originated in animals (allegedly from a live-food market in Wuhan city, mainland China). Infectious diseases like Ebola originated from the wild animals, attributable to increased deforestation and human intrusion into thick greens in the jungle (Song and Zheng, 2022). Increased use of products of animal origin especially in traditional medicine could aggravate the spread of especially viral diseases in urban set-up which needs efforts to minimise their use (Yinka-Ogunleye *et al.*, 2018). Acknowledging that the previous known pandemics emerged from animals, policy drafting for increased disease surveillance among pets, domestic and wild animals by government agencies is imminent and urgent. Nations need to coordinate to develop integrated fool-proof surveillance systems to detect and counter dreaded infectious diseases (Yong *et al.*, 2020).

As global temperature steadily and gradually rises in recent times, it hints at significant global warming and climate change. The melting of ice in glaciers due to global warming has resulted in an increase in the mean sea level. Unplanned rapid industrialisation with high CO_2 emission, pollution at the local-level and warming and climate change at global scale have adversely affected environmental health and its virginity. All these have negatively impacted the humans, animals and the environment in particular and ecology in general (Sironi *et al.*, 2022). Compounded with it, encountered issues like microbial resistance, vector-borne infections, livestock diseases and the denuding environmental health necessitate negotiating the One Health approach.

Several disturbing severe infections have either emerged or reappeared in current times, posing serious public health threat. As SARS-CoV-2 started spreading and COVID-19 became globally pandemic, the surveillance system and countermeasures to manage outbreak effectively were inadequate thereby exposing the underbelly of the global healthcare preparedness. Although chronic diseases are usually in routine surveillance target, constant rise in fresh outbreaks by the emerging or reemerging infectious diseases has necessitated rapid identification of such pathogens, possibly even before the infections reach humans (Sooksawasdi and Kuiken, 2021). The primary step in accomplishing this is to set up a dynamic surveillance system for both animals and humans, and revamping existing healthcare. Such dynamic surveillance system would monitor the 'hot spots' to detect the epicentre and contain the virus well in advance before the situation become alarming. A globally coordinated surveillance network to alert authorities quickly toward emerging health threats seems a promising strategy to effectively deal with the threat dynamics. NGOs, governmental agencies and philanthropic foundations may need to work together with greater vertical and horizontal reach to accomplish it (Afrooghe *et al.*, 2022).

6. Understanding and Addressing the Reverse Zoonoses (spillback)

Understanding the factors behind the spillback (reverse zoonosis) of viruses from humans to animals through elaborative studies and analyses is warranted. Research is being carried from time to time to decipher and elaborate reverse zoonoses at the human-animal interface. Transmission of the H1N1 virus from humans to the swine, the transmission cycle of *Plasmodium simium* in humans and monkeys, or the circulatory pattern of *Mycobacterium tuberculosis* from humans to elephants are some classical examples in this regard. Researchers have found the reverse zoonotic transmission potentials of SARS-CoV-2 from human to various wild animals like lion, tiger and deer as also the domesticated animals like dog and cats (Sah *et al.*, 2022[b]; Seang *et al.*, 2022; Fig. 4). Investigating the SARS-CoV-2 transmission in the humans and zoo-animal interface is essential to understand the transmission potentials across species. Although statistical model to understand the nature of human-human transmission of Mpox virus has been developed, however its reverse zoonosis remains to be investigated and established. The reemergence nature of diseases like Mpox since its first outbreak in 1970 clearly indicates that such diseases have grossly been neglected which become progressively threatening. With this in view, the confirmation of all the animal candidates behind the reverse zoonosis of each infectious disease is necessitated.

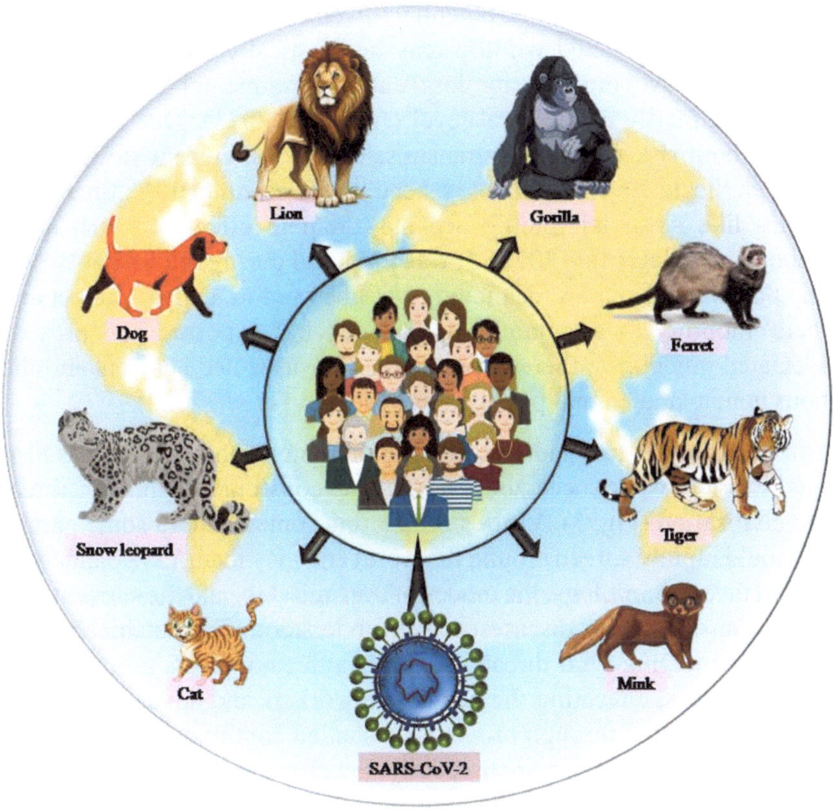

Fig. 4: Reported wild and domesticated animals in SARS-CoV-2 reverse zoonoses, a case instance

To implement a seamless One Health approach strategically, consorted efforts by the front-line environmental researchers, human doctors, animal doctors (veterinarians) and healthcare workers (paramedics) are required. Effective management tools and techniques against reverse zoonosis need to be explored. Easy and rapid risk mitigation tools need to be formulated and proper strategies could be developed to prevent the animals-humans (spillover) and humans-animals (spillback) transmission mechanisms as was prominently encountered in case of SARS-CoV-2 and Mpox viral transmissions. Successful promotion and collaboration among researchers and public healthcare agencies are essential to devise measures against reverse zoonoses. For a far-reaching and deeper sustainable impact, awareness campaigns among the livestock farmers, zoo workers, pet owners and the veterinary professionals may need to be carried out as they frequently come in contact with the vulnerable animals some of which could be silent carriers.

In the event of an evident or a potential reverse zoonosis, population of the vulnerable and suspected wildlife may be drastically reduced or culled, although it may have biodiversity loss and environmental destabilisation consequences primarily at the local level (Jia *et al.*, 2021). Due to species-specificity in both risk factors and transmission modes, current strategies to detect and eradicate reverse zoonoses need to be revamped. Cutting-edge technologies like Artificial Intelligence may help in effectively managing reverse zoonoses (McCarthy, 2022). It was proposed during the SARS-CoV-2 pandemic that state-of-the-art technology shall be used to analyse the pet and pet-owners' mobility to ascertain their chance viral exposure and provide with associated guidelines, thereby protecting the suspected subjects and the contiguous human and animal populations (Shepherd *et al.*, 2022).

In light of the COVID-19 pandemic and the ongoing Mpox outbreak as also numerous historical experiences, zoonotic illnesses constitute a significant threat to human civilisation (Fig. 5). Viruses originating somewhere in some part of the world could rapidly spread around the world and may manifest a pandemic. It is vital that the epidemiology, the modes of transmission, and the surrounding factors about an infectious disease be well understood. To sustainably deal with new or reemerging viral threats, public health campaigns, promotion of preventive measures, educating the healthcare workers and advancing public healthcare preparedness through proactive sustained continuous surveillance, rapid risk assessments, quick response, early detection and contact tracing are critical (Bunge *et al.*, 2022). COVID-19 pandemic served as a reminder of the significance of integrated national healthcare systems connected to the global grid, and enacting global legislation, regulations and frameworks for quick responses. As the pandemic potential of Mpox looms large, The World Health Organisation (WHO) and other global agencies have provided information online on Mpox, discovery of the knowledge gaps, and formulation of research strategies, with regular update. While this is a wise application of the digital world to consider while dealing with outbreaks, at the same time the public may be urged to follow the guidelines that are being updated from time to time (Kumar *et al.*, 2023; Costello *et al.*, 2022).

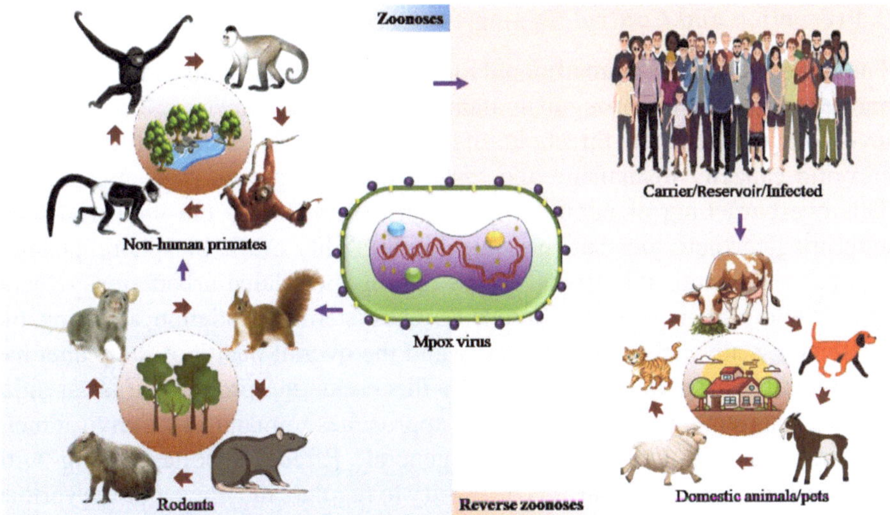

Fig. 5: Reported Mpox reverse zoonoses by wild and domestic animals, another case instance

Devising appropriate clinical management measures to protect frontline healthcare workers including clinicians and prevent the spread to control outbreaks involving highly infectious and transmissible pathogenic diseases is especially important. This shall ensure prevention of the occurrence of secondary cases and thereby curb the diseases from becoming pandemic. Although the exact mode of transmission of the numerous prevailing microbial infectious diseases and outbreaks are under investigation, the general precautionary strategies promulgated during the recent COVID-19 pandemic by SARS-CoV-2 could largely aid in limiting the transmission and severity of such dreaded diseases. An up-to-date, comprehensive, reliable and long-term investigation plan is urgently felt for the reasons of addressing the research gaps and unravelling the unanswered questions regarding the emergence, ecology and the epidemiology of the diseases, improving the surveillance capabilities, and designing appropriate preventive measures, preparedness, and immediate response mechanism. Priorities on understanding the underlying genetic evolution, evolving epidemiology, ecologic niche modelling and pinpointing the animal reservoir(s) for potential global health threats, implementing the One Health concept widely and more proactively, formulating evidence-based rapid responsiveness and best management/control practices to tackle viral outbreaks efficiently needs to be devised, which could ultimately lead to the reduction of the infection risks its humans.

7. Prevention and Control Strategies - MPox as Case Instance

The rapid increase in human population that has accelerated industrialisation and urbanisation has brought humanity to a critical juncture. The pollution levels have reached a threshold that has seemingly exceeded the Earth's carrying capacity to manage and restore the ecology and the environment. This overburdening of natural systems primarily due to the industrial-scale anthropogenic activities has threatened the stability of the biosphere, pushing it beyond its sustainable limits. As the densely populated urban areas expand further and human activities intensify, ecosystem degradation affecting the biodiversity, air quality, water quality and the overall health of the planet has become a growing concern. To address this escalating problem, it is essential to adopt more integrated and strategic approaches to manage the environment in particular and the biosphere in general. Effective policymaking with proactive integrated measures is necessary to regulate the impact of the various sectors associated with the environment. Such efforts should aim at balancing the anthropogenic activities with the planet's ecological limits, ensuring a sustainable ecosystem, the biosphere, and the health of all the species including humans. This holistic approach is crucial in navigating through the challenges of a growing population within a finite ecosystem.

The One Health approach emphasises the interconnectedness of environmental, animal and human health, and aligns well with the traditional medicines practices of the indigenous and tribal communities particularly. These communities exemplify a holistic health model by maintaining a symbiotic relationship with the environment, relying on Mother Nature for both their nutritional and medicinal needs. Traditional healers (like the bhagats and vaidu) use herbal remedies sourced locally from the ecosystem to manage health conditions and treat diseases, reflecting an in-depth understanding about the nature (Mutatkar, 2021). This approach not only focused on treating a disease but also on preventing a disease through spiritual and environmental measures. The 'One Earth, One Family' philosophy further emphasises this perspective and the interconnectedness in managing especially the communicable diseases. Primitive societies of the indigenous population, living in close contact with nature, seemingly had lower incidences of communicable diseases as compared to the modern society. Regular exposure to diverse ecosystems helped strengthen the immune systems of these people while the medicinal plants with antimicrobial properties were utilised to treat the various infections (Sandifer *et al.*, 2015).

Further, these communities also practised physical isolation from distant tribes, which means that they had a deep understanding of the environmental cycles, which must have also helped in limiting the transmission of the diseases. The use of natural remedies, improvement of the environmental hygiene and maintaining a well-balanced ecosystem can complement the medical interventions (Sandifer *et al.*, 2015) under the One Health model. Incorporating these age-old indigenous practices into the contemporary One Health strategies could benefit the efforts to tackle disease prevention efforts in the modern era. By reducing the focus on dense urbanisation and promoting sustainable interactions with nature, the risk of outbreaks of infectious diseases may be reduced to a large extent. Realigning our health practices with those of the indigenous communities offers a holistic and sustainable way to mitigate the spread of communicable diseases, reinforcing the One Health framework's call for integrated human, animal and environmental health and wellbeing.

To prevent and control potentially pandemic infectious diseases in future like the Mpox and SARS-CoV-2 outbreaks, it is essential to understand their zoonotic reservoirs. Diseases like Mpox are receiving enhanced global attention in recent times after multination outbreaks (Saxena *et al.*, 2023). The state-of-art sequencing techniques like the nextgen sequencing and reliable molecular diagnosis of Mpox was needed to prevent its further zoonotic transmission (Petersen *et al.*, 2019, Chakraborty *et al.*, 2022[a]). In light of this, suspected or confirmed Mpox cases could be immediately isolated and healthcare workers may abide by standard precautions on the use of personal protective equipment, hygiene and sanitation, scientific handling of contaminated medical disposables, etc. Mpox severely suppresses the immune system for which the WHO-approved antiviral tecovirimat is prescribed for critical patients as its availability is low at the global scale. Repurposed drug brincidofovir has been effective in treating Mpox that was originally approved for smallpox (Chakraborty *et al.*, 2022[b], Ortiz-Saavedra *et al.*, 2022). However, patients treated with tecovirimat testified no adverse effect while they developed elevated liver enzymes with brincidofovir treatment (Adler *et al.*, 2022). Jynneos and Acam2000 are two approved smallpox vaccines that have testified effective against Mpox (Sah *et al.*, 2022[a]). Nevertheless, patients with Mpox symptoms on supportive therapy need to be isolated and have their prodromal (like chills, lymphadenopathy, malaise, myalgias, headache, etc.) and rash stages assessed. Healthcare workers dealing with Mpox patients should adopt regular contact and droplet precautions to prevent its spread. Current Mpox outbreak necessitates healthcare providers, especially those working in sexual health and dermatological clinics, to be trained on it. Exploratory pharmaceutical countermeasures may also be invoked (Kumar *et al.*, 2023).

Manifestation of Mpox symptoms may vary in humans compared to animals. The data on the clinical presentation of Mpox in animals is scarce as most of the international guidelines and recommendations focus on human symptoms and pet owners (Afrooghe *et al.*, 2022). As an emerging zoonotic pathogen and reports of human-to-dog (spillback) transmission (reverse zoonosis) in Mpox (Seang *et al.*, 2022), enhanced screening of animals including pets and obtaining more evidence of human-to-animals transmission of Mpox virus was felt necessary (Beig *et al.*, 2022; Mohapatra *et al.*, 2022[e]; Sykes *et al.*, 2022). Numerous Mpox cases in pets may remain undiagnosed if the owners and veterinarians would solely rely on the clinical manifestations in decision-making on the health status of the exposed animals. Asymptomatic carriage of Mpox virus in humans is also being increasingly documented (Farahat *et al.*, 2022). Subclinical carriage of Mpox virus in non-human species and zoonotic transmission from asymptomatic animals as possible contributor to the global illness burden in humans is yet to be unravelled. More studies to determine the clinical profile of Mpox in animals and whether or not sub-clinical infection/transmission occurs in species other than humans shall be required (Shepherd *et al.*, 2022). To comprehend the potential risk of further zoonotic ingress among the human population and to appraise on the development of control measures to reduce the spread (in humans and animals both), it is important to understand the likelihood of reverse zoonotic transmission via pets associated with the ongoing Mpox outbreak (Seang *et al.*, 2022; Sykes *et al.*, 2022). Monitoring of pets living in the same household as the confirmed human Mpox cases is an important step in comprehending the danger posed by the Mpox virus (Shepherd *et al.*, 2022; Yuan *et al.*, 2023).

8. Strategising Animal Vaccination

Vaccination plays a pivotal role in protecting human as well as animal health. It helps prevent the transmission of zoonotic diseases, as also mitigate reverse zoonosis. Zoonosis refers to the transfer of diseases from animals to humans (spillover) while reverse zoonosis occurs when a pathogen is transmitted from humans to animals (spillback). These highlight the intricate interconnection between human, animal and the environmental health, emphasising the need for a comprehensive approach like the One Health framework (Goraichuk *et al.*, 2021). With pressures of global population growth and the associated environmental degradation, animal vaccination has become ever more important to maintain ecological balance and minimise the outbreaks of zoonotic infectious diseases. Vaccinating the domestic animals, livestock and the wildlife is crucial to prevent the spread of infectious diseases that could infect across species. For instance, rabies as a well-known viral zoonotic disease is controlled through vaccination programmes in both the domesticated and wild canine animals like dogs, protecting not just the animals but also the humans (Pattnaik *et al.*, 2023). Similarly, diseases like the foot-and-mouth disease (FMD), brucellosis and bovine tuberculosis in the cattle population could manifest severe ecological as well as economic consequences if left unattended (Morand, 2020).

Animal vaccination helps reduce the risk of the zoonotic spillover events, minimise disease transmission across species, and also plays an important role in agriculture and food security, ensuring that the ecosystem remains healthy. Livestock diseases could trigger mass mortality among animal population, causing food shortage, economic crisis and added environmental stress, as more land shall be required to compensate for the lost resources. This is especially true in rapidly developing nations like India where agriculture and livestock are the major players in socioeconomy. India's National Animal Disease Control Programme (NADCP) that aims at eliminating the diseases like FMD and brucellosis is one such initiatives to prevent livestock disease outbreaks (Sekiguchi *et al.*, 2022).

Zoonotic infectious diseases like avian influenza, Ebola and COVID-19 have drawn attentions towards the serious threat posed by animal-to-human disease transmission. These diseases could spread through direct contact with infected animals, consuming the contaminated animal products, or the inadvertent exposure to the pathogens in the environment (Abebe, 2020). Anthropogenic activities like deforestation, habitat destruction and large-scale (industrial) intensive farming increase the likelihood of zoonotic spillovers by disrupting the ecosystem and frequently exposing the humans to wildlife. The COVID-19 pandemic, suspected to have zoonotic origins, has reinforced the global need for stronger animal health measures, including animal vaccinations. Reverse zoonosis is also a growing concern as human populations that continue to expand and occur more frequently. Infections like Methicillin-resistant *Staphylococcus aureus* (MRSA), influenza and tuberculosis have the ability to transmit from humans to the domesticated, farmed and wildlife animals (González-Barrio, 2022). This two-way exchange of pathogens endangers not only the human health but also the livestock and the biodiversity. Vaccination, coupled with hygiene of the dwelling places and biosecurity practices, is essential in mitigating the transmission of pathogens in both directions, *i.e.*, spillover and spillback.

Animal vaccination has been highly effective in controlling deadly diseases at the global scale. For instance, while vaccination campaigns have nearly eradicated rinderpest worldwide mass rabies vaccination efforts in countries like the US have significantly reduced human fatalities due to rabies (Rupprecht *et al.*, 2024). Strict vaccination protocols among the livestock in Europe have helped curb the spread of diseases like bovine tuberculosis (Milián-Suazo *et al.*, 2022). The need for efficient animal vaccination programmes in India is even more urgent given the country's large livestock population and its dependence on agriculture. India ranks among the top global producers of foods of animal origin like beef, milk and poultry, making its economy highly vulnerable owing to the likely livestock disease outbreaks (Kumar *et al.*, 2021). Owing to the vast spread of the country, challenges persist especially in vaccinating animals in the rural and remote regions too due to logistics reasons. Wildlife vaccination also needs critical enforcement in India due to habitat encroachment and rising human-wildlife conflicts due to encroachment and deforestation. For instance, vaccinating the animals in the wild like monkeys and stray dogs against diseases like the Mpox and rabies could help prevent the transmission in thickly green and densely populated regions (Monath, 2013).

Wildlife vaccination is becoming ever more important in today's socio-economic context. The interactions between the wild animals and humans are constantly on a rise as human population grows that encroaches on the natural habitats, increasing the risk of zoonotic spillovers. Vaccinating the wildlife could act as a barrier, preventing zoonotic pathogens from spreading to humans. For example, vaccinating wild primates in Africa against Ebola protects the animals and reduces the risk of disease transmission to humans due to habit of bushmeat consumption (Devaux *et al.*, 2019). Similarly, wildlife vaccination helps safeguard the biodiversity, and is critical in maintaining the ecosystem balance. Hence, vaccination programmes for both the domesticated and wild animals are indispensable to prevent the spread of zoonotic diseases, ensuring food security and maintaining ecological stability. As human activities disrupt the natural ecosystems and population growth increases, the role of animal vaccination in assuring global health becomes even more imminent. However, the mode of vaccination for the wild animals in the wild remains a challenging task. There have been suggestions to either vaccinate by feeding them with the formulated edible vaccine mixed feed, or capturing the individual suspected carrier or an infected animal and vaccinating it, or randomly vaccinate the animals that are zoonosis agents and leave them in the wild to further facilitate herd immunity. In any case, the drive needs to be followed up numerous times suitably throughout the year. Table 3 provides a list of the numerous vaccine that have been developed across the globe to vaccinate both the domesticated and wild animals.

Table 3: A list of the various vaccines for animal health and wellbeing developed globally

Vaccine	**Target animal**	**Concerned disease**	**Specific usage region**
Rabies vaccine	Dog, cat, wild bat and fox	Rabies	Global
FMD vaccine	Cattle, sheep, goat, pig	Foot and mouth disease (FMD)	Especially Asia and Africa
Brucellosis vaccine (RB51)	Cattle, goat, sheep	Brucellosis	Especially USA, Europe and India
Bovine tuberculosis vaccine	Cattle	Tuberculosis	Europe, India and Africa
Rinderpest vaccine	Cattle and buffalo	Rinderpest[#]	Africa and Asia
Canine distemper vaccine	Dog, wild carnivore	Canine distemper	Global
Leptospirosis vaccine	Dog, pig, cattle	Leptospirosis	Global
Newcastle disease vaccine	Poultry	Newcastle disease	Global
Avian influenza vaccine	Poultry, wild bird	Avian influenza (bird-flu)	Asia and Europe
Anthrax vaccine	Cattle, sheep, goat, horse	Anthrax	Africa and Asia
Clostridial vaccine	Cattle, sheep, goat	Clostridial diseases (blackleg, tetanus)	Global
Porcine reproductive and respiratory syndrome (PRRS) vaccine	Pig	PRRS	Global
Infectious bursal disease vaccine	Poultry	Infectious bursal disease	Global
Bovine viral diarrhoea (BVD) vaccine	Cattle	Bovine viral diarrhoea	Global
Bluetongue vaccine	Sheep, cattle	Bluetongue	Europe and Asia
Salmonella vaccine	Poultry, pig, cattle	Salmonellosis	Global
Equine influenza vaccine	Horse	Equine influenza	Global
Rabies oral vaccine (wildlife)	Fox, raccoon, wolf	Rabies (oral vaccine for wildlife)	Europe and North America
Ebola vaccine (wildlife)	Primates in the wild	Ebola	Africa
Classical swine fever (CSF) vaccine	Pig	Classical swine fever	Asia and Europe
African horse sickness vaccine	Horse	African horse sickness	Africa
Actinobacillus pleuropneumonia vaccine	Pig	Pleuropneumonia	Global
Parvovirus vaccine	Dog	Canine parvovirus	Global
Lyme disease vaccine	Dog	Lyme disease	North America and Europe

[#]eradicated in 2011

It is essential to assess the zoonotic microbial flora of animals coexisting with humans to restrict any microbial spillover (zoonosis) from animals to humans and vice versa, *i.e.*, spillback (reverse zoonosis). Effective measures like vaccination particularly of a susceptible host (or a carrier/reservoir) would be increasingly beneficial to control the transmission, and possibly also reduce the risk of mutation (Forni *et al.*, 2022). Similar to the numerous variants of the COVID-19 virus (SARS-CoV-2), the Mpox virus also has been noticed to be prevailing in different variants that include A, A.1, A.2 and B.1. However, the prevailing Mpox variant that is in circulation during the current outbreak had been identified as the B.1 variant (Chakraborty *et al.*, 2022[c]). The 2022 Mpox outbreak was primarily associated with the infections among the homosexuals/gay males (who had sex with other men). It points to the fact that Mpox may be more prevalent in the geographical regions that have relatively high population of such sexually promiscuous individuals. Given the increased prevalence of HIV among the homosexuals, few of the cases could be suffering from immunodeficiency thereby predisposing them to serious Mpox infections and critical complications. Further, the immunocompromised status of the infected individuals favours the proliferation of the virus, and further facilitates mutations. Despite the evidences of Mpox being transmitted from humans to dogs (reverse zoonosis), it is still unclear as to if the virus could transmit from the infected dogs and other animals. In view of this, it was suggested to isolate the pet animals and refrain them from coming in close contact with an Mpox infected member in the family. Moreover, insightful studies to understand the mechanism of viral transmissions to humans through pets are required.

Unlike the SARS-CoV-2 which was associated with both the spillover and spillback infections in animals during the current pandemic, Mpox infection in a wide range of animals appears to be uncommon due to less available reports. Hence, animal surveillance for Mpox seems imminent. Earlier studies have identified that wild animals including rodents, squirrels, dormice and non-human primates (like chimpanzees, African gorillas, marmosets and monkeys) may act as the Mpox carriers (Falendysz *et al.*, 2017; Beer *et al.*, 2019). The CDC, Atlanta in the US suggested that animals (especially the mammals) like squirrels, prairie dogs, marmots, groundhogs, giant-pouched rats, chinchillas, hedgehogs, shrews, monkeys, apes and dogs may be predisposed to Mpox infection. Although Gerbils, Guinea pigs, hamsters, raccoons, mice, rats, domestic rabbits, cats, cattle, camels, skunks, voles, badgers, coyotes and foxes may suffer from infections with other orthopox viruses, it is not clear yet as to whether they could be Mpox infected (Chapman *et al.*, 2010). As a few animals like goats, sheep, pigs, reptiles, amphibians and birds are not yet reported to suffer from Orthopoxvirus infections, their Mpox susceptibility is an area for investigation.

Despite the availability of animal vaccines against SARS-CoV-2 and its variants, there is no such vaccine counterpart available for pets and wild animals against Mpox (Parnian *et al.*, 2024). The currently approved Mpox vaccines that are available over-the-counter are only for human use. Moreover, these human vaccines are still not available in the low and middle-income countries (LMIC). It is extremely important therefore to produce an animal vaccine against Mpox virus to restrict the animal-animal and animal-human transmissions. This step could potentially prevent a future emergence of any Mpox variants too. It was suggested that high-risk animals are screened for Mpox viral infection. A considerable number of people were noted to acquire Mpox infection from pet prairie dogs pointing to a possible pet animal-to-human transmission (Chauhan *et al.*, 2023). According to American Veterinary Medical Association (AVMA), domestic cats could also suffer from Mpox viral infection (Rodriguez, 2024). Given the understanding of the possibility of multipronged transmission of the Mpox virus, human, pet animal and wild animal vaccination were suggested to stop viral transmission and the emergence of variants (Mohapatra *et al.*, 2023b). In North America, Raccoons were vaccinated against rabies by dropping edible baits from helicopters (Mohapatra *et al.*, 2023b).

Different vaccination strategies were previously suggested. One among them is vaccinating a susceptible species with a longer life span that confers long-term immunity (Saied, 2022). The other strategy suggested was to vaccinate a susceptible animal with a shorter life span. Vaccines that could provide immunity and that could be transmitted horizontally (in a single generation) and vertically (through generations) were also suggested. A vaccine that may provide herd immunity among wild animals was also recommended as a potential approach. However, the live-attenuated vaccine used for developing herd immunity is associated with the risk of revitalising especially the viruses and resulting in reemergence of the aetiological agent and reinfection.

Animal health programmes face diverse financial and logistics challenges worldwide. The role of biosimilars in animal vaccines development with their enhanced affordability and reach is becoming increasingly significant (Panda *et al.*, 2023). Biosimilars-based animal vaccine development allows for more accessible vaccination options, especially in resource-limited regions like the low- and middle-income countries (LMIC) and rural India, thereby enhancing their availability and affordability. Broader immunisation coverage in case of domesticated animals, the livestock and the wildlife could be achieved through the use of biosimilars in strategic vaccination drives, thus helping to prevent zoonotic and reverse zoonotic transmission and ultimately strengthening the One Health framework.

9. The One Health Approach

The abiotic components and the biotic community of the environment (within the ambit of ecology) are closely related with larger vertebrates (humans and animals) that significantly impact each other. These impacts could extend to intra- and inter-species disease transmission. The mobility of humans and animals has increased in dimensions as the modes of transportation have advanced, and it could facilitate infectious diseases becoming more active in global spread. The environmental factors contributing to the vulnerability of humans to contracting a disease include, among others, polluted air, water and soil, biotic and abiotic interactions, and deforestation. The 'One Health' approach demands an interlinked network connecting the physicians, veterinarians, researchers and environmentalists to forge a 360° solution for environmental, animal and human health. One Health system proposes functional collaborations between various disciplines directly or indirectly working toward human, animal and environmental health. Such coordinated efforts at local, national and international levels help establish more effective infectious disease surveillance, establishing the microbial behavioural pattern and disease prevention. Cutting-edge molecular tools of advanced life sciences involving nutrigenomics (that relates to the interaction and evolution of genetic set-up with the changing/altered food habits) and metagenomics (that account for the genome pool of a particular ecological niche) could facilitate a fool-proof One Health in place.

Given that the microbes including viruses reemerge in various forms of variants, it appears that the humans need to learn to live with these in the 'new normal'. However, the scenario is extremely complex as the microbes could further mutate into more lethal forms and transmit through animals (zoonosis) and elsewhere in the environment and establish themselves to infect the humans later. Such microbial behaviour could potentially lead to evolution of novel microbial species that could prove to be disastrous to the ecology in general and the ecosystem in particular (Tiwari *et al.*, 2020). Thus, it is important for the local and national governments to envision more comprehensive 'One Health' approach to tackle the pandemic situations now, and in future too. Fig. 6 provides a comprehensive systems biology approach towards a disease-alert society in line with 'One Health' that could prove to be extremely beneficial for all the living beings in the long run.

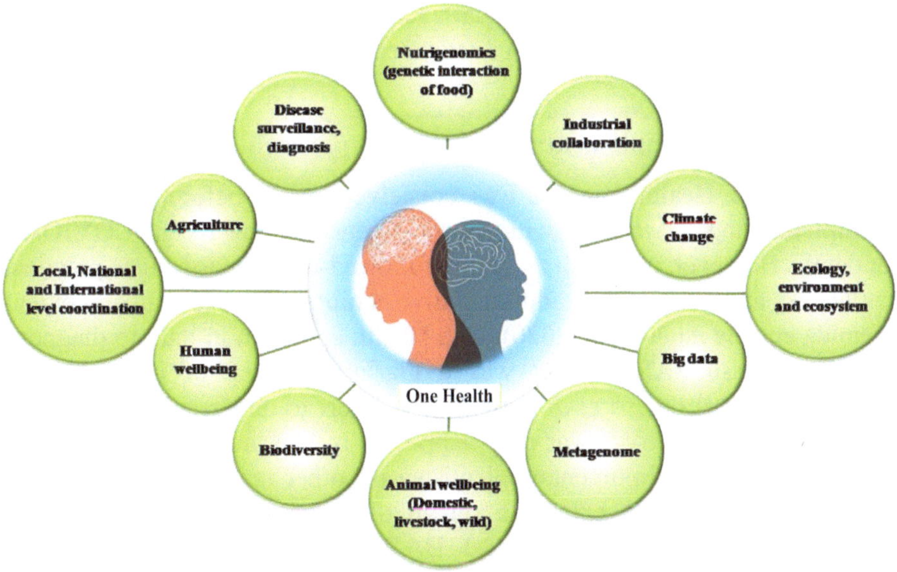

Fig. 6: Systems biology approach towards a disease-alert society in line with 'One Health'

For instance, the animal origin of COVID-19 is being studied by two independent researcher groups; one considers bat as the primary source while the other considers pangolin. There is every possibility that the virus might have been transmitted from the bats and pangolins to humans, or possibly through other intermediate animal hosts like the domesticated wild yak. Any precise conclusion on the genesis of the SARS-CoV-2 virus seems to be impossible without extensive *in vitro* and *in vivo* investigations with long-term monitoring of the zoonosis (Amao *et al.*, 2022; Rudan *et al.*, 2022). In any case, the animals are certainly and progressively becoming more integrated in human health and wellbeing.

Due to their growing proximity, humans are increasingly at risk of contracting zoonotic infections (Jorwal *et al.*, 2020). The spread of Mpox infection during the ongoing COVID-19 pandemic as a coinfection and similar numerous occurrences in history make it imminent and urgent that recent travel and immunisation history of the suspected and vulnerable population be provided to healthcare professionals, particularly during outdoor vacationing or upon returning from an endemic region (Bhattacharya *et al.*, 2022). Chemical sanitisation (such as alcohol-based) along with the use of soap and water for disinfection could be encouraged (Okyay *et al.*, 2022). In case of Mpox, it is recommended that visitors of the endemic countries isolate themselves from sick or dead animals (like rodents and marsupials), and avoid eating/

handling wildlife meat (like bush meat). The suspected samples from humans or animals could be handled only in dedicated specialised laboratories (Bunge *et al.*, 2022).

10. Right Time to Implement 'One Health' Approach

Although One Health concept was conceived much before, the urgency of implementing it was felt with the emergence of the recent COVID-19 pandemic. However, it was not diligently followed-up earlier owing to practical bottlenecks and political and administrative complacencies to a greater extent (Hemida and Ba Abduallah, 2020). One Health approach in Italy to diagnose and characterise SARS-CoV-2 was a glaring instance of its successful implementation (Lorusso *et al.*, 2020). The effort to understand the ecology of the virus SARS-CoV-2 was duly supported by the proactive involvement of veterinarians, environmental scientists and other stakeholders. With the view to understand the extensive spread of Omicron and its sublineages including the BA.1, BA.1.1, BA.1.2.1, BA.2, BA.3, BA.4 and BA.5 variants and BF.7 that was active later, it was important to control the transmission by enforcing effective surveillance strategies by following the One Health approach in true letter and spirit (Montagutelli *et al.*, 2022). The One Health approach was recommended to control the spread of SARS-CoV-2 and all its variants considering the cases of coronaviruses originating from animals in earlier instances (Korath *et al.*, 2022). It was also stressed that the adaptability and survival of the novel virus in various animal reservoirs like cats, dogs, cattle, birds and pigs may potentially be the most critical factor responsible for epidemics and pandemics in future. Studies noted that the Omicron variant could have emerged from the spilling (spillover as well as spillback) of the genetically-modified viruses across animals (like rats) and humans. The One Health approach is suggested to improve the understanding of such virus spillovers, its transformation into novel variants and its entry into the human body (Montagutelli *et al.*, 2022).

It is critical that policymakers focus more on the threats that arise due to the emerging and reemerging zoonotic diseases (Okyay *et al.*, 2022). Preparedness to tackle especially the zoonotic viral diseases in future, and preventing the appearance and reappearance of zoonoses necessitated an understanding of their genesis like their natural reservoir, primary host or range of hosts, intermediate hosts and the spillover events (like spillover time and frequency of infection, reservoir to human, etc.). Zoonosis, medication and vaccine development need to be prioritised and bolstered (Nguyen *et al.*, 2021; Haider *et al.*, 2022). Multidisciplinary collaborative research to curb the global spread of infections has been time and again advocated. Alongside, deciphering the deadly genes from the whole genome sequence, genome evolution and phylogenetics, altered and evolving epidemiological patterns and genomic diagnostics of the aetiological agents are also required.

The recent COVID-19 pandemic should serve as a wake-up call for the healthcare fraternity to take time-oriented action to stop the spread of the numerous potential infectious agents as independent cases. For instance, comparing the transmission of Mpox virus via the aerosol droplets to that of COVID-19 could be a critical mistake (Jia *et al.*, 2021; Raheel *et al.*, 2022). Effective techniques to rapidly isolate and quarantine patients exhibiting the symptoms of the infectious diseases are the immediate pressing needs. Understanding the epidemiology is crucial especially for the very aggressive spillover infections and aggressively mutated forms that are likely to spread fast (Sah *et al.*, 2022[b]). One approach is to create a worldwide, freely accessible database, similar to Global health repository on the GitHub. Countries with advanced healthcare systems may extend their expertise in the outbreak-hit regions to effectively contain and manage the health-wise fragile situation at source. Until more specific and rapid screening tests were available, widespread screening programmes in line with the US that focussed on all the members of the Orthopoxvirus family may be implemented to effectively track and control (Seang *et al.*, 2022). Many infectious diseases put everyone at risk due to their varying transmission mechanisms. During differential diagnosis, such infectious dreaded diseases could be assessed especially in the highly vulnerable patients (Afrooghe *et al.*, 2022; Yuan *et al.*, 2022).

Any human, animal or environmental factor could disturb the delicate interrelationship between them and destabilise the ecosystem thereby making it more vulnerable to diseases. For instance, a disarray in the resident human microbiome (microflora or commensals that are resident in or on the body) disturbs the body defense system and predisposes a person to diseases by opportunistic extraneous pathogens. Such instances also include the diseases being transmitted through the animal reservoirs, like SARS-CoV by palm civet cats, MERS-CoV by dromedary camels and Ebola by monkeys among others. All these case transmissions have confirmed a disturbed ecosystem interrelationship leading to the manifestation of the diseases. However, the originating and the potential reservoir animal in case of the SARS-CoV-2 and human Mpox has been a matter of debate necessitating further investigations in recent times as these are not yet absolutely confirmed. One Health approach may potentially facilitate the process to identify the originating pathogens and facilitate zeroing on the potential reservoirs that enable the aetiological agents to survive in the environment. Thus, the understandings on the animal-human (POHA) and animal-human-environment (ROHA) interactions in line with the One Health strategy is necessary to be improved (Aggarwal and Ramachandran, 2020).

11. Challenges in Implementing 'One Health'

Most of the countries across the globe could face challenges in the practical implementation of the One Health approach due to its inherent complexities. Thus, a detailed knowledge and diligent leadership to adhere to the principles and practices of One Health in its true letter and spirit are essential (El Zowalaty and Järhult, 2020). The recent COVID-19 pandemic witnessed a revamped industry-academia interaction platform especially between the Government-sponsored research agencies and the vaccine companies to fight against infectious diseases as definite positive fallout which was explored well. The research and development initiatives provided critical information on countering the COVID-19 more effectively, promoted mechanisms for fair and equitable global distribution of the preventives (vaccines) and therapeutics (medicines) in a more effective manner, as also highlighted the bottlenecks in the prevailing licensing conditions (Light, 2005).

Facilitating One Health response in a seamless manner within an institutional framework calls for the consideration of adequate and effective global response measures against the emerging and reemerging infectious diseases (such as the COVID-19 pandemic). It also necessitates strict quality control measures in live animal markets which were presumed to be the source of numerous outbreaks as also experienced during the COVID-19 pandemic. This could especially be challenging in the low- and middle-income countries (LMIC) as such (live animal) markets are crucial link in food distribution systems, and business and sustenance life lines. To add to owe, the resources to detect and monitor infectious diseases such as the COVID-19 were scarce in these regions. The dynamic and ever-evolving socioeconomy further makes the situation ever more critical. Rapid environmental surveillance of such markets within the local, regional and international regulatory frameworks is essential. To reduce the transmission risk of such diseases in the future, examining and evaluating the extent of the existing enforcement of the set guidelines and regulations, and probing the dynamics in the culturally and socially acceptable food distribution and consumption practices are essential too (Loh *et al.*, 2020; Ghai *et al.*, 2022).

One Health approach could prove to be the panacea to ensure good health and wellbeing of all even in the resource-poor nations, especially against the relatively-neglected ailments like leprosy and filariasis (and many other neglected tropical diseases) that are more prevalent in the poorer section of the society. Through concerted efforts across the various healthcare stakeholders, One Health approach could facilitate in the reduction of environmental factors that play an active and critical role in disease transmission (Ghai *et al.*, 2022). For instance, the first-ever mpox case in humans was recorded in 1970 although the virus was first reported in 1958 in laboratory monkeys. Human transmission of mpox initially being limited to the African subcontinent, it reemerged and has since then been reported elsewhere including numerous non-endemic nations including India recently. However, the identification of the animal reservoir, the secondary host(s), the underlying risk factors and the ecological conditions that favoured its emergence and reemergence is yet to be ascertained even after more than six decades of its existence. Although monkey is undoubtedly its primary host, however reports on chimpanzee, rodents, black-tailed prairie dog, etc. as its numerous other zoonotic hosts also exist. Serological evidence suggested that rodents could be the critical carrier of Mpox and human transmitter. In similar views, the duration and prevention potential of post-vaccination immunity of the smallpox vaccine in containing the Mpox epidemic is not yet well-deciphered.

All in all, although the concept is enduring One Health approach is an uneasy road to tread as it requires concerted equally sincere and active participation of all the stakeholders, cutting across the cultural, social, economic and geographical barriers. One Health could be purportedly of two types, Prudential One Health Approach (POHA) and Radical One Health Approach (ROHA) with due ethical concerns considerations. While POHA approach is primarily human-centric, the ROHA approach in contrast is a 360° approach involving the humans, animals and the environment (Sironi *et al.*, 2022). POHA that majorly addresses the humans, animals and human-animal interactions issues is considered as a classical approach, while its extended One Health approach in form of ROHA involves the interactions between humans, animals and the environment (Schmiege *et al.*, 2020). Thus, in essence, POHA considers the only the biotic community while ROHA considers the ecosystem in all its completeness (the biotic community as well as the active abiotic constituents within the ecological settings).

12. Conclusion

Global healthcare system is under tremendous pressure and is being challenged even among the haves, leave alone the have-nots. The recent COVID-19 pandemic had been a strong wake-up call for the humanity to find innovative, concerted and coordinated efforts to address global healthcare issues and further strengthen the infrastructure. Novel viruses and their lethal variants are emerging and reemerging with more deadly forms of their mutants on one hand, while there is the occurrence of chain of events of zoonosis and reverse zoonosis that link the domesticated or the wild animal in the human-centric health chain on the other hand. Although vaccines are available or are being developed for the many infectious diseases, yet their reach to the desired location (of vulnerable or potentially infected regions of animal and human habitats) is at stake. Further, their efficacy also becomes doubtful particularly while dealing with the ever-mutating and ever-evolving viral strains. Also, a skewed (non-equitable) distribution of the available vaccines is a logistics challenge to address. Instead of looking for therapeutics and preventives for the growing incidents of epidemic and pandemic cases especially in the face of documented breakthrough infection, it is prudent to advocate for the One Health approach to nip the issue at the bud. Strict surveillance and control measures under the 'OH' strategy could potentially provide with a 360° solution to the perpetual human agony.

It seems that the world presently is off-track in achieving majority of the UN's set SDGs targets, even by 2050. Ongoing global health crises, the associated multitude issues and sustainability challenges are complex by nature, that require coordinated efforts across different sectors under the One Health umbrella. One Health approach could be formulated as a valuable framework to understand the aetiology, epidemiology and effective control measures against infectious diseases. The benefits of multidisciplinary collaborations in resolving a complex clinical condition involving the biomedical and clinical science domains in diagnostic laboratories, therapeutics and preventives are quite well known. Such collaborative approaches are equally essential within the One Health paradigm.

Addressing the multifactorial challenges posed by infectious diseases requires contributions from an array of diverse professionals, including the healthcare providers, veterinarians, social scientists and the ecologists. The broader objectives of the One Health Quadripartite include fostering the intersectoral cooperation and developing simple yet effective policy guidelines for governments, healthcare planners and the relevant international organisations as important milestones. Achieving these objectives shall necessitate sufficient funding to support in designing multidisciplinary research programmes and their successful implementation, along with rigorous evaluation of their outcomes. Given the prevalence of infectious diseases worldwide that is escalating, research initiatives could be targeted towards a specific geographical region (as the epicenter of an infectious disease) or a particular infectious disease to generate robust evidence, while maintaining a global perspective.

The underlying approach of the One Health approach to effectively address these pressing health challenges is to promote the 'think global and act local' philosophy.

References

Abebe GM, 2020. Emerging and re-emerging viral diseases: the case of coronavirus disease-19 (COVID-19). Int. J. Virol. AIDS, 7(067). doi: 10.23937/2469-567x/1510067

Acharya KP, Subedi D and Wilson RT, 2021. Rabies control in South Asia requires a One Health approach. One health, 12: 100215. doi: 10.1016/j. onehlt.2021.100215

Adisasmito WB, Almuhairi S, Behravesh CB, Bilivogui P, Bukachi SA, Casas N, Becerra NC, Charron DF, Chaudhary A, Zanella JRC and Cunningham AA, 2022. One Health: A new definition for a sustainable and healthy future. PLoS pathogens, 18(6): e1010537. doi: 10.1371/journal.ppat.1010537

Adler H, Gould S, Hine P, Snell LB, Wong W, Houlihan CF, Osborne JC, Rampling T, Beadsworth MB, Duncan CJ and Dunning J, 2022. Clinical features and management of human monkeypox: a retrospective observational study in the UK. Lancet Infect. Dis., 22(8): 1153–1162. doi: 10.1016/ S1473-3099(22)00228-6

Afrooghe A, Damavandi AR and Ahmadi E, 2022. Reverse zoonosis and monkeypox: Time for a more advanced global surveillance system for emerging pathogens. New Microbes New Infect., 48: 101013. doi: 10.1016/j.nmni.2022.101013

Aggarwal D and Ramachandran A, 2020. One health approach to address zoonotic diseases. Indian J Community Med., 45(Suppl 1): S6–S8. doi: 10.4103/ijcm.IJCM_398_19

Amao LK, Olatunji DI, Igbodo G, Okoli SC, Amaechi I, Goni MI, Ehiakhamen O, Aderinola O, Ogunleye A, Ogunbode O and Adeleye A, 2022. Trend and enhanced surveillance of Monkeypox during COVID-19 pandemic in Nigeria. J. Public Health Africa, 13(1): 2184. doi: 10.4081/jphia.2022.2184

Beer EM and Rao VB, 2019. A systematic review of the epidemiology of human monkeypox outbreaks and implications for outbreak strategy. PLoS Negl. Trop. Dis., 13(10): e0007791. doi: 10.1371/journal.pntd.0007791

Behera JK, Mishra P, Jena AK, Behera B and Bhattacharya M, 2023. Human health implications of emerging diseases and the current situation in India's vaccine industry. Sci. One Health, 2: 100046. doi: 10.1016/j.soh.2023.100046

Beig M, Mohammadi M, Monfared FN and Nasereslami S, 2022. Monkeypox: An emerging zoonotic pathogen. World J. Virol., 11(6): 426. doi: 10.5501/wjv.v11.i6.426

Bengis RG and Frean J, 2014. Anthrax as an example of the One Health concept. Rev Sci Tech, 33(2): 593–604.

Bennett N and Lemoine GJ, 2014. What a difference a word makes: Understanding threats to performance in a VUCA world. Bus. horiz., 57(3): 311–317. doi: 10.1016/j. bushor.2014.01.001

Bhattacharya M, Dhama K and Chakraborty C, 2022. Recently spreading human monkeypox virus infection and its transmission during COVID-19 pandemic period: A travelers' prospective. Travel Med. Infect. Dis., 49: 102398. doi: 10.1016/j.tmaid.2022.102398

Braam DH, Jephcott FL and Wood JLN, 2021. Identifying the research gap of zoonotic disease in displacement: a systematic review. Glob Health Res. Policy, 6: 1–12. doi: 10.1186/ s41256-021-00205-3

Bunge EM, Hoet B, Chen L, Lienert F, Weidenthaler H, Baer LR and Steffen R, 2022. The changing epidemiology of human monkeypox—A potential threat? A systematic review. PLoS Negl. Trop. Dis., 16(2): e0010141. doi: 10.1371/journal.pntd.0010141

Calvez E, Miot EF, Keosenhom S, Vungkyly V, Viengphouthong S, Bounmany P, Brey PT, Marcombe S and Grandadam M, 2022. Low Transmission of Chikungunya Virus by Aedes aegypti from Vientiane Capital, Lao PDR. Pathogens, 12(1): 31. doi: 10.3390/pathogens12010031

Chakraborty C, Bhattacharya M, Nandi SS, Mohapatra RK, Dhama K and Agoramoorthy G, 2022[a]. Appearance and re-appearance of zoonotic disease during the pandemic period: long-term monitoring and analysis of zoonosis is crucial to confirm the animal origin of SARS-CoV-2 and monkeypox virus. Vet. Quart., 42(1): 119–124. doi: 10.1080/01652176.2022.2086718

Chakraborty C, Bhattacharya M, Sharma AR and Dhama K, 2022[c]. Evolution, epidemiology, geographical distribution, and mutational landscape of newly emerging monkeypox virus. GeroScience, 44(6): 2895–2911. doi: 10.1007/s11357-022-00659-4

Chakraborty S, Chandran D, Mohapatra RK, Alagawany M, Nahed A, Sharma AK, Chakraborty C and Dhama K, 2022[b]. Clinical management, antiviral drugs and immunotherapeutics for treating monkeypox. An update on current knowledge and futuristic prospects. Int. J. Surg., 105: 106847. 10.1016/j.ijsu.2022.106847

Chapman JL, Nichols DK, Martinez MJ and Raymond JW, 2010. Animal models of orthopoxvirus infection. Vet. Pathol., 47(5): 852–870. doi: 10.1177/0300985810378649

Chauhan RP, Fogel R and Limson J, 2023. Overview of diagnostic methods, disease prevalence and transmission of MPOX (formerly monkeypox) in humans and animal reservoirs. Microorganisms, 11(5): 1186. doi: 10.3390/microorganisms11051186

Chongsuvivatwong V, Phua KH, Yap MT, Pocock NS, Hashim JH, Chhem R, Wilopo SA and Lopez AD, 2011. Health and health-care systems in southeast Asia: diversity and transitions. The Lancet, 377(9763): 429–437. doi: 10.1016/S0140-6736(10)61507-3

Costello V, Sowash M, Gaur A, Cardis M, Pasieka H, Wortmann G and Ramdeen S, 2022. Imported monkeypox from international traveler, Maryland, USA, 2021. Emerg. Infect. Dis., 28(5): 1002–1005. doi: 10.3201/eid2805.220292

Coghlan B, Hall D 2012. The Development of One Health Approaches in the Western Pacific. In: J Mackenzie, M Jeggo, P Daszak, J Richt (eds) One Health: The Human-Animal-Environment Interfaces in Emerging Infectious Diseases. Current Topics in Microbiology and Immunology, Springer, Berlin, Heidelberg: 366: 93–111. doi: 10.1007/82_2012_270

de Castañeda RR, Villers J, Guzmán CAF, Eslanloo T, de Paula N, Machalaba C, Zinsstag J, Utzinger J, Flahault A and Bolon I, 2023. One Health and planetary health research: leveraging differences to grow together. Lancet Planet. Health, 7(2): e109–e111. doi: 10.1016/S2542-5196(23)00002-5

Devaux CA, Mediannikov O, Medkour H and Raoult D, 2019. Infectious disease risk across the growing human-non human primate interface: a review of the evidence. Front. Public Health, 7: 305. doi: 10.3389/fpubh.2019.00305

Dey JK and Dey SK, 2020. SARS-CoV-2 pandemic, COVID-19 case fatality rates and deaths per million population in India. J. Bioinfo., Comput. Syst. Biol., 2(1): 5000110.

Duff JH, Liu A, Saavedra J, Batycki JN, Morancy K, Stocking B, Gostin LO, Galea S, Bertozzi S, Zuniga JM and Alberto-Banatin C, 2021. A global public health convention for the 21st century. Lancet Public Health, 6(6): e428–e433. doi: 10.1016/S2468-2667(21)00070-0

Dye C, 2018. Expanded health systems for sustainable development. Science, 359(6382): 1337–1339. doi: 10.1126/science.aaq1081.

El Zowalaty ME and Järhult JD, 2020. From SARS to COVID-19: A previously unknown SARS-related coronavirus (SARS-CoV-2) of pandemic potential infecting humans–Call for a One Health approach. One health, 9: 100124. doi: 10.1016/j.onehlt.2020.100124

Evans BR and Leighton FA, 2014. A history of One Health. Rev Sci Tech, 33(2): 413–420. doi:10.20506/rst.33.2.2298

Falendysz EA, Lopera JG, Doty JB, Nakazawa Y, Crill C, Lorenzsonn F, Kalemba LSN, Ronderos MD, Mejia A, Malekani JM and Karem K, 2017. Characterization of Monkeypox virus infection in African rope squirrels (Funisciurus sp.). PLoS Negl. Trop. Dis., 11(8): p.e0005809. doi: 10.1371/journal.pntd.0005809

Falk J, Colwell R, El-Beltagy A, Gleick P, Kennel C, Lee YT, Luers A, Murray C, Serageldin I, Takeuchi K and Watanabe C, 2021. Beyond 2020: converging crises demand integrated responses: statement by the RACC International Advisory Committee following the RACC-12 International Forum. Sustain. Sci., 16: 691–693. doi: 10.1007/s11625-020-00876-w

Farahat RA, Khan SH, Dergaa I, Rabaan AA, Dhama K and Memish ZA, 2022. Asymptomatic transmission of monkeypox: Implications for mass gatherings?. New Microbes New Infect., 49: 101056. doi: 10.1016/j.nmni.2022.101056

Ferrinho P and Fronteira I, 2023. Developing one health systems: a central role for the one health workforce. Int. J. Environ. Res. Public Health, 20(6): 4704. doi: 10.3390/ijerph20064704.

Forni D, Cagliani R, Clerici M and Sironi M, 2022. Disease-causing human viruses: novelty and legacy. Trends Microbiol., 30(12): 1232–1242. doi: 10.1016/j.tim.2022.07.002

Gaba S, Gupta M, Gaba R and Lehl SS, 2021. Scrub typhus: An update. Curr Trop Med Rep, 8: 133–140. doi: 10.1007/s40475-021-00234-5.

Garnier J, Savic S, Boriani E, Bagnol B, Häsler B and Kock R, 2020. Helping to heal nature and ourselves through human-rights-based and gender-responsive One Health. One Health Outlook, 2: 1–18. doi: 10.1186/s42522-020-00029-0

George AE, Heera AB, Harikrishnan H, Reghukumar A, Varghese SA, Chandran R, Ashok P, Nair SS and Maheswariamma A, 2023. The dermatological evolution of the first case of monkeypox reported in India. Indian J. Dermatol. Venereol. Leprol., 89(4): 578–581. doi: 10.25259/IJDVL_753_2022

Ghai RR, Wallace RM, Kile JC, Shoemaker TR, Vieira AR, Negron ME, Shadomy SV, Sinclair JR, Goryoka GW, Salyer SJ and Barton Behravesh C, 2022. A generalizable one health framework for the control of zoonotic diseases. Scientific reports, 12(1): 8588. doi: 10.1038/s41598-022-12619-1

González-Barrio D, 2022. Zoonoses and wildlife: one health approach. Animals, 12(4): 480. doi: 10.3390/ani12040480

Goraichuk IV, Arefiev V, Stegniy BT and Gerilovych AP, 2021. Zoonotic and reverse zoonotic transmissibility of SARS-CoV-2. Virus Res., 302: 198473. doi: 10.1016/j.virusres.2021.198473

Gortazar C, Reperant LA, Kuiken T, de la Fuente J, Boadella M, Martínez-Lopez B, Ruiz-Fons F, Estrada-Peña A, Drosten C, Medley G and Ostfeld R, 2014. Crossing the interspecies barrier: opening the door to zoonotic pathogens. PLoS pathogens, 10(6): e1004129. doi: 10.1371/journal.ppat.1004129

Haider N, Guitian J, Simons D, Asogun D, Ansumana R, Honeyborne I, Velavan TP, Ntoumi F, Valdoleiros SR, Petersen E and Kock R, 2022. Increased outbreaks of monkeypox highlight gaps in actual disease burden in Sub Saharan Africa and in animal reservoirs. Int. J. Infect. Dis., 122: 107–111. doi: 10.1016/j.ijid.2022.05.058

Healy JP, Jensen A, Power MB, McKibben B, Cohen G and Basu G, 2022. COVID-19 and climate change: crises of structural racism. J. Clim. Chang. Health, 5: 100092. doi: 10.1016/j.joclim.2021.100092

Hemida MG, Ba Abduallah MM, 2020. The SARS-CoV-2 outbreak from a one health perspective. One Health, 10:100127. doi: 10.1016/j.onehlt.2020.100127

Hillier SA, Taleb A, Chaccour E and Aenishaenslin C, 2021. Examining the concept of One Health for indigenous communities: A systematic review. One Health, 12: 100248. doi: 10.1016/j.onehlt.2021.100248

Hussein HA, 2023. Brief review on ebola virus disease and one health approach. Heliyon, 9 (8): e19036, doi: 10.1016/j.heliyon.2023.e19036

Huynh LN, Tran LB, Nguyen HS, Ho VH, Parola P and Nguyen XQ, 2022. Mosquitoes and Mosquito-Borne Diseases in Vietnam. Insects, 13(12): 1076. doi: 10.3390/insects13121076

Jack JC, Gonet J, Mease A and Nowak K, 2020. Traditional knowledge underlies one health. Science, 369(6511): 1576–1576. doi: 10.1126/science.abe2401

Jia P, Dai S, Wu T and Yang S, 2021. New approaches to anticipate the risk of reverse zoonosis. Trends Ecol. Evol, 36(7): 580–590. doi: 10.1016/j.tree.2021.03.012

Johnson NP and Mueller J, 2002. Updating the accounts: global mortality of the 1918-1920" Spanish" influenza pandemic. Bull. Hist. Med., 76(1): 105–115. Doi: 10.1353/bhm.2002.0022

Jorwal P, Bharadwaj S and Jorwal P, 2020. One health approach and COVID-19: A perspective. J Family Med. Prim. Care, 9(12): 5888–5891. doi: 10.4103/jfmpc.jfmpc_1058_20

Kaligis EC, Ratag BT and Langi FF, 2023. Analysis of Dengue Hemorrhagic Fever Surveillance Data (2012-2021) in Indonesia. Indones. J. Public Health Prev. Med., 2(1). doi: 10.35790/ijphpm.v2i1.51398

Kelly BD, 2020. Plagues, pandemics and epidemics in Irish history prior to COVID-19 (coronavirus): what can we learn?. Ir. J. Psychol. Med., 37(4): 269–274. doi: 10.1017/ipm.2020.25

Khor CS, Teoh BT, Sam SS, Khoo HY, Azizan NS, CheMatSeri A, Chin KL, Hamim ZR, Mohamed-Romai-Noor NA, Yaacob CN and Abd-Jamil J, 2023. Epidemiological serosurvey of chikungunya fever post outbreak at Tanjung Sepat, Malaysia. J. Infect. Dev. Ctries., 17(01): 118–124. doi: 10.3855/jidc.16613

Korath AD, Janda J, Untersmayr E, Sokolowska M, Feleszko W, Agache I, Adel Seida A, Hartmann K, Jensen-Jarolim E and Pali-Schöll I, 2022. One Health: EAACI Position Paper on coronaviruses at the human-animal interface, with a specific focus on comparative and zoonotic aspects of SARS-CoV-2. Allergy, 77(1): 55–71. doi: 10.1111/all.14991

Kril V, Aïqui-Reboul-Paviet O, Briant L and Amara A, 2021. New insights into chikungunya virus infection and pathogenesis. Ann. Rev. Virol., 8(1): 327–347. doi: 10.1146/annurev-virology-091919-102021

Kumar K, Garg L, Singh RK and Chander M, 2021. Challenges in the Indian livestock sector and suggested interventions: An overview. J Entomol. Zool. Stud., 9(1): 422–428.

Kumar S, Subramaniam G and Karuppanan K, 2023. Human monkeypox outbreak in 2022. J Med. Virol, 95(1).

Laaser U, Bjegovic-Mikanovic V, Seifman R, Senkubuge F and Stamenkovic Z, 2022. One health, environmental health, global health, and inclusive governance: What can we do?. Front. Public Health, 10: 932922. doi: 10.3389/fpubh.2022.932922

Lerner H and Berg C, 2017. A comparison of three holistic approaches to health: one health, ecohealth, and planetary health. Front. Vet. Sci., 4: 163. doi: 10.3389/fvets.2017.00163

Light DW, 2005. Making practical markets for vaccines: Why I decided that the Center for Global Development Report, Making Markets for Vaccines, offers poor advice to government and foundation leaders. PLoS Medicine, 2(10): e271. doi: 10.1371/journal.pmed.0020271

Liu L, Xiao Y, Wei X, Li X, Duan C, Jia X, Jia R, Guo J, Chen Y, Zhang X and Zhang W, 2023. Spatiotemporal epidemiology and risk factors of scrub typhus in Hainan Province, China, 2011–2020. One Health, 17: 100645. doi: 10.1016/j.onehlt.2023.100645.

Loh HC, Seah YK and Looi I, 2021. The COVID-19 pandemic and diet change. Progress Microbes Mol. Biol., 4(1). doi: 10.36877/pmmb.a0000203

Lorusso A, Calistri P, Mercante MT, Monaco F, Portanti O, Marcacci M, Cammà C, Rinaldi A, Mangone I, Di Pasquale A and Iommarini M, 2020. A "One-Health" approach for diagnosis and molecular characterization of SARS-CoV-2 in Italy. One Health, 10: 100135. doi: 10.1016/j.onehlt.2020.100135

Luo Q and Han J, 2022. Preparedness for a monkeypox outbreak. Infect. Med., 1(2): 124–134. doi: 10.1016/j.imj.2022.07.001

Machalaba CC, Salerno RH, Barton Behravesh C, Benigno S, Berthe FC, Chungong S, Duale S, Echalar R, Karesh WB, Ormel HJ and Pelican K, 2018. Institutionalizing One Health: from assessment to action. Health security, 16(S1): S37–S43. doi: 10.1089/hs.2018.0064

Mackenzie JS, McKinnon M, Jeggo M 2014. One Health: From Concept to Practice. In: A Yamada, L Kahn, B Kaplan, T Monath, J Woodall, L Conti (Eds) Confronting Emerging Zoonoses, Springer, Tokyo: 163-189 doi: 10.1007/978-4-431-55120-1_8

Mackenzie JS and Jeggo M, 2019. The one health approach—why is it so important?. Tropical Med. Infect. Dis, 4(2): 88. doi: 10.3390/tropicalmed4020088

Malik YA, 2023. Impact of influenza in south-east Asia. Int. J. Infect. Dis., 130: S40–S41. doi: 10.1016/j.ijid.2023.04.095

Mashudi DN, Ahmad N and Mohd Said S, 2022. Level of dengue preventive practices and associated factors in a Malaysian residential area during the COVID-19 pandemic: a cross-sectional study. Plos one, 17(4): e0267899. doi: 10.1371/journal.pone.0267899

McCarthy MW, 2022. Recent advances in the diagnosis monkeypox: implications for public health. Expert Rev. Mol. Diagn., 22(7): 739–744. doi: 10.1080/14737159.2022.2116979

Merakou C, Fortuna C, Amendola A, Marsili G, Argentini C, Fiorentini C, Benedetti E, Riccardo F, Del Manso M, Bella A and Caporali MG, 2023. Diagnosis of dengue virus infections in Italy from November 2015 to November 2021: a national reference laboratory surveillance report. Int. J. Infect. Dis., 130: S117. doi: 10.1016/j.ijid.2023.04.289

Milián-Suazo F, González-Ruiz S, Contreras-Magallanes YG, Sosa-Gallegos SL, Bárcenas-Reyes I, Cantó-Alarcón GJ and Rodríguez-Hernández E, 2022. Vaccination strategies in a potential use of the vaccine against Bovine tuberculosis in infected herds. Animals, 12(23): 3377. doi: 10.3390/ani12233377

Mohapatra RK, Kandi V, Gaidhane AM, Zahiruddin QS, Rustagi S, Satapathy P, Mishra S and Tuglo LS, 2024. Global domination of the recently VoI-classified'JN. 1' outcompeting other variants–Comparing the vaccines' efficacy. Clinical Infection in Practice, 22:100358. https://doi.org/10.1016/j.clinpr.2024.100358

Mohapatra RK, Kandi V, Tuli HS, Chakraborty C, Dhama K, 2022d. The recombinant variants of SARS-CoV-2: Concerns continues amid COVID-19 pandemic. J Med Virol., 94(8): 3506. doi: 10.1002/jmv.27780

Mohapatra RK, Kandi V, Verma S and Dhama K, 2022c. Challenges of the omicron (B. 1.1. 529) variant and its lineages: a global perspective. Chembiochem, 23(9): e202200059. doi: 10.1002/cbic.202200059

Mohapatra RK, Kuppili S, Kumar Suvvari T, Kandi V, Behera A, Verma S, Biswal SK, Al-Noor TH, El-ajaily MM, Sarangi AK and Dhama K, 2022a. SARS-CoV-2 and its variants of concern including Omicron: a never ending pandemic. Chem Biol Drug Des., 99(5): 769–788. doi: 10.1111/cbdd.14035

Mohapatra RK, Mishra S, Azam M and Dhama K, 2021. COVID-19, WHO guidelines, pedagogy, and respite. Open Med., 16(1): 491–493. doi: 10.1515/med-2021-0266

Mohapatra RK, Mishra S, Kandi V, Sarangi AK, Ansari A, Chakraborty C, Biswal SK and Dhama K, 2022e. Monkeypox plays a similar role like SARS-CoV-2; intensive animal screening is crucial after the first human-to-dog transmission report–Correspondence. Int. J. Surg., 106: 106925. doi: 10.1016/j.ijsu.2022.106925

Mohapatra RK, Mishra S, Tuglo LS, Kutikuppala LVS, Mohapatra PK, Kandi V, Panda SK, Desai DN, 2023b. Need of Monkeypox animal vaccine and its global distribution: right time to address? Int. J. Surg., 110(12):8164-6. doi: 10.1097/JS9.0000000000000100

Mohapatra RK, Tiwari R, Sarangi AK, Islam MR, Chakraborty C and Dhama K, 2022b. Omicron (B. 1.1. 529) variant of SARS-CoV-2: concerns, challenges, and recent updates. J Med. Virol., 94(6): 2336. doi: 10.1002/jmv.27633

Mohapatra RK, Verma S, Kandi V, Sarangi AK, Seidel V, Das SN, Behera A, Tuli HS, Sharma AK and Dhama K, 2023a. The SARS-CoV-2 Omicron variant and its multiple sub-lineages: transmissibility, vaccine development, antiviral drugs, monoclonal antibodies, and strategies for infection control–a review. ChemistrySelect., 8(9):e202201380. https://doi.org/10.1002/slct.202201380

Monath TP, 2013. Vaccines against diseases transmitted from animals to humans: a one health paradigm. Vaccine, 31(46): 5321–5338. doi: 10.1016/j.vaccine.2013.09.029

Montagutelli X, van der Werf S, Rey FA, Simon-Loriere E, 2022. SARS-CoV-2 Omicron emergence urges for reinforced One-Health surveillance. EMBO Mol Med.,14(3):e15558. 10.15252/emmm.202115558

Morand S, 2020. Emerging diseases, livestock expansion and biodiversity loss are positively related at global scale. Biological Conservation, 248: 108707. doi: 10.1016/j.biocon.2020.108707

Mostafavi E, Ghasemian A, Abdinasir A, Mahani SAN, Rawaf S, Vaziri MS, Gouya MM, Nguyen TMN, Al Awaidy S, Al Ariqi L and Islam MM, 2022. Emerging and re-emerging infectious diseases in the WHO Eastern Mediterranean region, 2001-2018. Int. J. Health Policy Manag., 11(8): 1286–1300. doi: 10.34172/ijhpm.2021.13

Mumford EL, Martinez DJ, Tyance-Hassell K, Cook A, Hansen GR, Labonté R, Mazet JA, Mumford EC, Rizzo DM, Togami E and Vreedzaam A, 2023. Evolution and expansion of the One Health approach to promote sustainable and resilient health and well-being: A call to action. Front. Public Health, 10: 1056459. doi: 10.3389/fpubh.2022.1056459

Mutatkar RK, 2021. Tribal health & culture: Symbiotic model of One Health. Indian J Med. Res., 153(3): 327–332. doi: 10.4103/ijmr.IJMR_593_21

Nguyen CT, Moi ML, Le TQM, Nguyen TTT, Vu TBH, Nguyen HT, Pham TTH, Le THT, Nguyen LMH, Phu Ly MH and Ng CFS, 2020. Prevalence of Zika virus neutralizing antibodies in healthy adults in Vietnam during and after the Zika virus epidemic season: a longitudinal population-based survey. BMC Infect. Dis., 20: 1–10. doi: 10.1186/s12879-020-05042-2

Nguyen PY, Ajisegiri WS, Costantino V, Chughtai AA and MacIntyre CR, 2021. Reemergence of human monkeypox and declining population immunity in the context of urbanization, Nigeria, 2017–2020. Emerg. Infect. Dis., 27(4): 1007–1014. doi: 10.3201/eid2704.203569

Okyay RA, Bayrak E, Kaya E, Şahin AR, Koçyiğit BF, Taşdoğan AM, Avcı A and Sümbül HE, 2022. Another epidemic in the shadow of Covid 19 pandemic: a review of monkeypox. proteins, 6(2): 95–99. doi: 10.14744/ejmo.2022.2022

Ong J, Soh S, Ho SH, Seah A, Dickens BS, Tan KW, Koo JR, Cook AR, Richards DR, Gaw LYF and Ng LC, 2022. Fine-scale estimation of effective reproduction numbers for dengue surveillance. PLoS Comput. Biol., 18(1): e1009791. doi: 10.1371/journal.pcbi.1009791

Ortiz-Saavedra B, León-Figueroa DA, Montes-Madariaga ES, Ricardo-Martínez A, Alva N, Cabanillas-Ramirez C, Barboza JJ, Siddiq A, Coaguila Cusicanqui LA, Bonilla-Aldana DK and Rodriguez-Morales AJ, 2022. Antiviral treatment against monkeypox: a scoping review. Trop. Med. Infect. Dis., 7(11): 369. doi: 10.3390/tropicalmed7110369

Panda S, Singh PK, Mishra S, Mitra S, Pattnaik P, Adhikary SD and Mohapatra RK, 2023. Indian biosimilars and vaccines at crossroads–replicating the success of pharmagenerics. Vaccines, 11(1): 110. doi: 10.3390/vaccines11010110

Parnian R, Heydarifard F, Mousavi FS, Heydarifard Z and Zandi M, 2024. Innate Immune Response to Monkeypox Virus Infection: Mechanisms and Immune Escape. J. Innate Immun., 16(1): 413–424. doi: 10.1159/000540815

Pattnaik P, Mahal A, Mishra S, Alkhouri A, Mohapatra RK and Kandi V, 2023. Alarming Rise in Global Rabies Cases Calls for Urgent Attention: Current Vaccination Status and Suggested Key Countermeasures. Cureus, 15(12). doi: 10.7759/cureus.50424

Pelican K, Salyer SJ, Behravesh CB, Belot G, Carron M, Caya F, De La Rocque S, Errecaborde KM, Lamielle G, Latronico F and Macy KW, 2019. Synergising tools for capacity assessment and One Health operationalisation. Rev Sci Tech, 38(1): 71. doi: 10.20506/rst.38.1.2942

Pepin KM, Carlisle K, Anderson D, Baker MG, Chipman RB, Benschop J, French NP, Greenhalgh S, McDougall S, Muellner P and Murphy E, 2024. Steps towards operationalizing One Health approaches. One Health, 18: 100740. doi: 10.1016/j.onehlt.2024.100740

Petersen E, Abubakar I, Ihekweazu C, Heymann D, Ntoumi F, Blumberg L, Asogun D, Mukonka V, Lule SA, Bates M and Honeyborne I, 2019. Monkeypox—Enhancing public health preparedness for an emerging lethal human zoonotic epidemic threat in the wake of the smallpox post-eradication era. Int. J Infect. Dis., 78: 78–84.

Petersen E, Petrosillo N, Koopmans M, Beeching N, Di Caro A, Gkrania-Klotsas E, Kantele A, Kohlmann R, Lim PL, Markotic A and López-Vélez R, 2018. Emerging infections—an increasingly important topic: review by the emerging infections task force. Clin Microbiol. Infect., 24(4), 369–375. doi: 10.1016/j.cmi.2017.10.035

Pitt SJ and Gunn A, 2024. The one health concept. Br. J. Biomed. Sci., 81: 12366. doi: 10.3389/bjbs.2024.12366

Polwiang S, 2015. The estimation of imported dengue virus from Thailand. J. Travel Med., 22(3): 194–199. doi: 10.1111/jtm.12193

Potdar V, Hinge D, Satav A, Simões EA, Yadav PD and Chadha MS, 2019. Laboratory-confirmed avian influenza A (H9N2) virus infection, India, 2019. Emerging Infect. Dis., 25(12): 2328–2330. doi: 10.3201/eid2512.190636

Prem K, Lau MS, Tam CC, Ho MZ, Ng LC and Cook AR, 2019. Inferring who-infected-whom-where in the 2016 Zika outbreak in Singapore—a spatio-temporal model. J. Royal Soc. Interf., 16(155): 20180604. doi: 10.1098/rsif.2018.0604

Queenan K, Garnier J, Nielsen LR, Buttigieg S, Meneghi DD, Holmberg M, Zinsstag J, Rüegg S, Häsler B and Kock R, 2017. Roadmap to a One Health agenda 2030. CABI Reviews, 2017: 1–17. doi: 10.1079/ pavsnnr201712014.

Rabinowitz PM, Pappaioanou M, Bardosh KL and Conti L, 2018. A planetary vision for one health. BMJ global health, 3(5): e001137. doi: 10.1136/ bmjgh 2018 001137

Raheel H, Raheel M, Ali Fahim MA and Naeem U, 2022. Monkeypox and spillover effects: Stigmas, solutions and strategies. Ann. Med. Surg., 81:104346. doi: 10.1016/j.amsu.2022.104346.

Rahman MT, Sobur MA, Islam MS, Ievy S, Hossain MJ, El Zowalaty ME, Rahman AT and Ashour HM, 2020. Zoonotic diseases: etiology, impact, and control. Microorganisms, 8(9): 1405. doi: 10.3390/microorganisms8091405

Rai BD, Tessema GA, Fritschi L and Pereira G, 2024. The application of the One Health approach in the management of five major zoonotic diseases using the World Bank domains: A scoping review. One Health, 18: 100695. doi: 10.1016/j.onehlt.2024.100695

Reynolds MG, Anh BH, Thu VH, Montgomery JM, Bausch DG, Shah JJ, Maloney S, Leitmeyer KC, Huy VQ, Horby P and Plant AJ, 2006. Factors associated with nosocomial SARS-CoV transmission among healthcare workers in Hanoi, Vietnam, 2003. BMC Public Health, 6: 1–9. doi: 10.1186/1471-2458-6-207

Rodriguez J, 2024. One Health Ethics and the Ethics of Zoonoses: A Silent Call for Global Action. Vet. Sci., 11(9): 394. doi: 10.3390/vetsci11090394

Rousham EK, Unicomb L and Islam MA, 2018. Human, animal and environmental contributors to antibiotic resistance in low-resource settings: integrating behavioural, epidemiological and One Health approaches. Proc. Royal Soc. B: Biological Sciences, 285(1876): 20180332. doi: 10.1098/rspb.2018.0332

Ruchusatsawat K, Wongjaroen P, Posanacharoen A, Rodriguez-Barraquer I, Sangkitporn S, Cummings DA and Salje H, 2019. Long-term circulation of Zika virus in Thailand: an observational study. Lancet Infect. Dis., 19(4): 439–446. doi: 10.1016/S1473-3099(18)30718-7

Rudan I, 2022. The COVID-19 pandemic: SARS-CoV-2, childhood hepatitis and monkeypox raise five new questions for the global health research community. J. Global Health, 22: 01002. doi: 10.7189/jogh.12.01002

Rupprecht CE, Buchanan T, Cliquet F, King R, Müller T, Yakobson B and Yang DK, 2024. A Global Perspective on Oral Vaccination of Wildlife against Rabies. J. Wildlife Dis., 60(2): 241–284. doi: 10.7589/JWD-D-23-00078

Ruscio BA, Brubaker M, Glasser J, Hueston W and Hennessy TW, 2015. One Health–a strategy for resilience in a changing arctic. Inter. J. Circumpolar Health, 74(1): 27913. doi: 10.3402/ijch.v74.27913

Rushton J, McMahon BJ, Wilson ME, Mazet JA and Shankar B, 2021. A food system paradigm shift: from cheap food at any cost to food within a one health framework. NAM perspectives, 2021. doi: 10.31478/202111b

Saba Villarroel PM, Gumpangseth N, Songhong T, Yainoy S, Monteil A, Leaungwutiwong P, Missé D and Wichit S, 2023. Emerging and re-emerging zoonotic viral diseases in Southeast Asia: One Health challenge. Front. Public Health, 11: 1141483. doi: 10.3389/fpubh.2023.1141483

Sah R, Hada V, Mohanty A, Alshahrani NZ, Chakraborty S, Bhattacharya M, Chakraborty C and Dhama K, 2022[a]. Recent first report of human-to-dog transmission of Monkeypox virus emphasizes an urgent need of enhancing surveillance and strengthen further explorative research to reveal its real magnitude of reverse zoonosis from other animals including pets as like that happened with SARS-CoV-2/COVID-19 pandemic–Correspondence. Int. J. Surg., 106: 106949. doi: 10.1016/j.ijsu.2022.106949

Sah R, Humayun M, Baig E, Farooq M, Hussain HG, Shahid MU, Cheema HA, Chandran D, Yatoo MI, Sharma AK and Dhama K, 2022[b]. FDA's authorized "JYNNEOS" vaccine for counteracting monkeypox global public health emergency; an update–Correspondence. Int. J Surg., 107: 106971. doi: 10.1016/j.ijsu.2022.106971

Saied AA, 2022. Besides human booster doses: Could vaccinating highly susceptible animals to SARS-CoV-2 be the needed urgent strategic step?. Int. J. Surg., 104: 106761. doi: 10.1016/j.ijsu.2022.106761

Salk JD, 2019. Planetary health: A new reality. Challenges, 10(1): 7. doi: 10.3390/challe10010007

Sandifer PA, Sutton-Grier AE and Ward BP, 2015. Exploring connections among nature, biodiversity, ecosystem services, and human health and well-being: Opportunities to enhance health and biodiversity conservation. Ecosyst. Serv., 12: 1–15. doi: 10.1016/j.ecoser.2014.12.007

Satapathy BS, Pattnaik G, Sahoo RN, Pattanaik S, Sarangi AK, Kandi V, Mishra S, Rabaan AA, Mohanty A, Sah R and Mohapatra RK, 2023. COVID-19 vaccines and their underbelly: Are we going the right way?. Health Sci. Rep., 6(9):e1540. doi: 10.1002/hsr2.1540

Saxena SK, Ansari S, Maurya VK, Kumar S, Jain A, Paweska JT, Tripathi AK and Abdel-Moneim AS, 2023. Re-emerging human monkeypox: a major public-health debacle. J. Med. Virol., 95(1): e27902. doi: 10.1002/jmv.27902

Schmiege D, Arredondo AMP, Ntajal J, Paris JMG, Savi MK, Patel K, Yasobant S and Falkenberg T, 2020. One Health in the context of coronavirus outbreaks: A systematic literature review. One Health, 10: 100170. doi: 10.1016/j.onehlt.2020.100170

Schultz M, 2008. Rudolf virchow. Emerg. Infect. Dis., 14(9): 1480–1481. doi: 10.3201/eid1409.086672

Seang S, Burrel S, Todesco E, Leducq V, Monsel G, Le Pluart D, Cordevant C, Pourcher V and Palich R, 2022. Evidence of human-to-dog transmission of monkeypox virus. The Lancet, 400(10353): 658–659. doi: 10.1016/S0140-6736(22)01487-8

Sekiguchi S, Wiratsudakul A and Nguyen VG, 2022. The Epidemiology, Diagnosis and Prevention of Infectious Diseases in Livestock. Front. Vet. Sci., 8: 840635. doi: 10.3389/fvets.2021.840635

Shepherd W, Beard PM, Brookes SM, Frost A, Roberts H, Russell K and Wyllie S, 2022. The risk of reverse zoonotic transmission to pet animals during the current global monkeypox outbreak, United Kingdom, June to mid-September 2022. Eurosurveillance, 27(39): 2200758.

Sironi VA, Inglese S and Lavazza A, 2022. The "One Health" approach in the face of Covid-19: how radical should it be?. Philos. Ethics, Humanit. Med., 17(1): 3. doi: 10.1186/s13010-022-00116-2

Soman Pillai V, Krishna G and Valiya Veettil M, 2020. Nipah virus: past outbreaks and future containment. Viruses, 12(4): 465. doi: 10.3390/v12040465

Song TZ and Zheng YT, 2022. Monkeypox, wild animals, and potential big problem. Zoo. Res., 43(4): 612. doi: 10.24272/j.issn.2095-8137.2022.217

Sooksawasdi Na Ayudhya S and Kuiken T, 2021. Reverse zoonosis of COVID-19: lessons from the 2009 influenza pandemic. Vet. Pathol., 58(2): 234–242. doi: 10.1177/0300985820979843

Steffen W, Richardson K, Rockström J, Cornell SE, Fetzer I, Bennett EM, Biggs R, Carpenter SR, De Vries W, De Wit CA and Folke C, 2015. Planetary boundaries: Guiding human development on a changing planet. science, 347(6223): 1259855. doi: 10.1126/science.1259855

Stephen C and Stemshorn B, 2016. Leadership, governance and partnerships are essential One Health competencies. One Health, 2: 161–163. doi: 10.1016/j.onehlt.2016.10.002

Sykes JE, 2022. A call for more evidence documenting human-to-dog transmission of monkeypox virus. The Lancet, 400(10357): 993. 10.1016/S0140-6736(22)01780-9

Tangwangvivat R, Boonyo K, Toanan W, Muangnoichareon S, Iamsirithaworn S and Prasarnphanich O, 2019. Promoting the One Health concept: Thai Coordinating Unit for One Health. Revue Sci Tech, 38(1): 271–278. doi: 10.20506/rst.38.1.2959

Tilak R and Kunte R, 2019. Scrub typhus strikes back: are we ready?. Med J Armed Forces India, 75(1): 8–17. doi: 10.1016/j.mjafi.2018.12.018.

Tiwari R, Dhama K, Sharun K, Iqbal Yatoo M, Malik YS, Singh R, Michalak I, Sah R, Bonilla-Aldana DK and Rodriguez-Morales AJ, 2020. COVID-19: animals, veterinary and zoonotic links. Vet. Quart., 40(1): 169–182. doi: 10.1080/01652176.2020.1766725

Trenovski B and Merdzan G, 2020. Lessons learned from the fourth industrial revolution for the global economy. Knowl. Int. J., 43(1): 89–95.

Tun YM, Charunwatthana P, Duangdee C, Satayarak J, Suthisawat S, Likhit O, Lakhotia D, Kosoltanapiwat N, Sukphopetch P and Boonnak K, 2022. Virological, serological and clinical analysis of chikungunya virus infection in Thai patients. Viruses, 14(8): 1805. doi: 10.3390/v14081805

Velavan TP and Meyer CG, 2022. Monkeypox 2022 outbreak: an update. Trop Med Int Health, 27(7): 604–605. doi: 10.1111/tmi.13785

Viana R, Moyo S, Amoako DG, Tegally H, Scheepers C, Althaus CL, Anyaneji UJ, Bester PA, Boni MF, Chand M and Choga WT, 2022. Rapid epidemic expansion of the SARS-CoV-2 Omicron variant in southern Africa. Nature, 603(7902): 679–686. doi: 10.1038/s41586-022-04411-y

Wang X, Rainey JJ, Goryoka GW, Liang Z, Wu S, Wen L, Duan R, Qin S, Huang H, Kharod G and Rao CY, 2021. Using a One Health approach to prioritize zoonotic diseases in China, 2019. PLoS One, 16(11): e0259706. doi: 10.1371/journal.pone.0259706

WHO 2017. Zika virus disease – India (2017). Available at: https://www.who.int/emergencies/disease-outbreak-news/item/26-may-2017-zika-ind-en#:~:text=The%20routine%20laboratory%20surveillance%20detected,Medical%20College%2C%20Ahmedabad%2C%20Gujarat, Accessed 02 September 2024

WHO 2021[a]. Nipah virus Infection-India (2021). Available at: https://www.who.int/emergencies/disease-outbreak-news/item/nipah-virus-disease---india#:~:text=In%20India%2C%20the%20first%20Nipah,in%202007%2C%20both%20in%20West, Accessed 2 September 2024

WHO 2021[b]. Human infection with Avian Influenza A (H5N1). Available at: https://www.who.int/emergencies/disease-outbreak-news/item/human-infection-with-avian-influenza-a(h5n1)-%EF%BD%B0-india#:~:text=On%2021%20July%202021%2C%20the,from%20Haryana%20state%2C%20northern%20India, Accessed on 1 September 2024

WHO 2022[a]. One Health Initiative. Available online at: https://www.who.int/teams/one-health-initiative/about-us, Accessed 13 August 2024

WHO 2022[b]. WHO Hub for Pandemic and Epidemic Intelligence. Available online at: https://pandemichub.who.int/publications/m/the-who-hub-for-pandemic-and-epidemic-intelligence-starts-up-annual-report-2022, Accessed 13 August 2024

Wimalasiri-Yapa BR, Stassen L, Huang X, Hafner LM, Hu W, Devine GJ, Yakob L, Jansen CC, Faddy HM, Viennet E and Frentiu FD, 2019. Chikungunya virus in Asia–Pacific: a systematic review. Emerg. Microbes Infect., 8(1): 70–79. doi: 10.1080/22221751.2018.1559708

Woolhouse M E, 2002. Population biology of emerging and re-emerging pathogens. Trends Microbiol., 10(10): S3–S7. doi: 10.1016/S0966-842X(02)02428-9

Yadana S, Valitutto MT, Aung O, Hayek LAC, Yu JH, Myat TW, Lin H, Htun MM, Thu HM, Hagan E and Francisco L, 2023. Assessing behavioral risk factors driving zoonotic spillover among high-risk populations in Myanmar. Eco Health, 20(1): 31–42. doi: 10.1007/s10393-023-01636-9

Yasobant S, Saxena D, Bruchhausen W, Memon FZ and Falkenberg T, 2019. Multi-sectoral prioritization of zoonotic diseases: One health perspective from Ahmedabad, India. PloS one, 14(7): e0220152. doi: 10.1371/ journal.pone.0220152

Yek C, Li Y, Pacheco AR, Lon C, Duong V, Dussart P, Young KI, Chea S, Lay S, Man S and Kimsan S, 2023. National dengue surveillance, Cambodia 2002–2020. Bulletin of the World Health Organization, 101(9): 605. doi: 10.2471/BLT.23.289713

Yinka-Ogunleye A, Aruna O, Ogoina D, Aworabhi N, Eteng W, Badaru S, Mohammed A, Agenyi J, Etebu EN, Numbere TW and Ndoreraho A, 2018. Reemergence of human monkeypox in Nigeria, 2017. Emerging infectious diseases, 24(6): 1149. doi: 10.3201/eid2406.180017

Yong SEF, Ng OT, Ho ZJM, Mak TM, Marimuthu K, Vasoo S, Yeo TW, Ng YK, Cui L, Ferdous Z and Chia PY, 2020. Imported Monkeypox, Singapore. Emerg. Infect. Dis., 26(8): 1826. doi: 10.3201/eid2608.191387

Yuan P, Tan Y, Yang L, Aruffo E, Ogden NH, Bélair J, Heffernan J, Arino J, Watmough J, Carabin H and Zhu H, 2023. Assessing transmission risks and control strategy for monkeypox as an emerging zoonosis in a metropolitan area. J Med. Virol., 95(1): e28137. doi: 10.1002/jmv.28137

Yuan S, Jiang SC, Zhang ZW, Yang XY, Fu YF, Li ZL and Hu J, 2022. Multi-origins and complex transmission paths of monkeypox viruses. Travel Med. Infect. Dis., 50: 102444. doi: 10.1016/j.tmaid.2022.102444

Yu J, Collier ARY, Rowe M, Mardas F, Ventura JD, Wan H, Miller J, Powers O, Chung B, Siamatu M and Hachmann NP, 2022. Neutralization of the SARS-CoV-2 Omicron BA. 1 and BA. 2 variants. New Eng. J. Med., 386(16): 1579–1580. doi: 10.1056/NEJMc2201849

Zangpo T, Phuentshok Y, Dorji K, Dorjee C, Dorjee S, Jolly P, Morris R, Marquetoux N and McKenzie J, 2023. Environmental, occupational, and demographic risk factors for clinical scrub typhus, Bhutan. Emerg. Infect. Dis., 29(5): 909. doi: 10/3201/eid2905.221430.

Zinsstag J, Kaiser-Grolimund A, Heitz-Tokpa K, Sreedharan R, Lubroth J, Caya F, Stone M, Brown H, Bonfoh B, Dobell E and Morgan D, 2023. Advancing one human-animal-environment health for global health security: what does the evidence say?. The Lancet, 401(10376): 591–604. doi: 10.1016/S0140-6736(22)01595-1

Zinsstag J, Schelling E, Waltner-Toews D and Tanner M, 2011. From "one medicine" to "one health" and systemic approaches to health and well-being. Prev Vet. Med., 101(3–4):148–156. doi: 10.1016/j.prevetmed.2010.07.003

Zumla A, Valdoleiros SR, Haider N, Asogun D, Ntoumi F, Petersen E and Kock R, 2022. Monkeypox outbreaks outside endemic regions: scientific and social priorities. Lancet Infect. Dis., 22(7): 929–931. doi: 10.1016/S1473-3099(22)00354-1 [illegible] L, Paccaud [illegible] R, Long [illegible], Lvong [illegible] Y, Thussu [illegible] and Kirschke S. 2022. [illegible] national defense convention [illegible] Geneva 2022 [illegible] Bulletin of the World Health Organization [illegible] doi:10.2471/BLT.22.[illegible]

Mbala-Kingebeni [illegible] A, [illegible] Q, [illegible] P, [illegible] N, [illegible] V, [illegible] L, Kenda [illegible] and Mbala [illegible] A. [illegible] monkeypox virus [illegible] 2017. [illegible] Emerging Infectious Diseases [illegible] doi:[illegible]

[illegible] Qu [illegible] H, [illegible] Martinez [illegible] M, [illegible] K, [illegible] Sears [illegible]. [illegible] imported monkeypox [illegible] Emerging [illegible] Diseases [illegible] doi:10.[illegible]

M [illegible] Y, [illegible] Z, [illegible] Ogden NH, [illegible] and [illegible] 2022. [illegible] transmission [illegible] and [illegible] as [illegible] emergent [illegible] in [illegible] Med. [illegible] doi:[illegible]

[illegible] Y, [illegible] Y, [illegible] Y. [illegible] and [illegible] 2022. [illegible] in [illegible] Travel Med. Infect. Dis. [illegible] doi:10.1016/j.tmaid.2022.[illegible]

[illegible] D, [illegible] M, [illegible] D, [illegible] and [illegible] 2022. [illegible] Emerging [illegible] and [illegible]

[illegible] L, [illegible] D, [illegible] R, [illegible] and [illegible] 2023. [illegible] and [illegible] for [illegible] Travel Med. Infect. Dis. [illegible] doi:10.1016/j.tmaid.2023.[illegible]

[illegible] Brown [illegible], [illegible] P, [illegible] and [illegible] 2023. [illegible] human-animal [illegible] health [illegible] The Lancet. [illegible] doi:10.1016/[illegible]

[illegible] Stehling [illegible] Weiler [illegible] and [illegible] 2011. [illegible] health and [illegible] approaches to health and well-being. Am. J. Prev. Med. [illegible] doi:10.1016/j.amepre.2011.07.001

[illegible] S, [illegible] D, [illegible] P, [illegible] and [illegible] 2022. Monkeypox [illegible] Infect. Dis. 22[illegible] doi:10.1016/S1473-3099(22)[illegible]

9

The Vaccine Development Against Covid-19: Public Health and Socioeconomic Impacts

***Sunita Panda*[1]*, Madhusmita Rout*[1]*, NS Manisha*[1]*, Jyotirmayee Turuk*[1*]*, Snehasish Mishra*[2*]**

[1]*ICMR-Regional Medical Research Centre, Bhubaneswar-751 023 Odisha, India*
[2]*School of Biotechnology, KIIT Deemed-to-be University Bhubaneswar-751 024, Odisha, India*

Abstract

The pandemic in 2019-2022 spread swiftly and became global in no time, caused by SARS-CoV-2. Vaccines were rapidly developed against the virus to restore public health and save global economy. Vaccines for immunisation drives were developed in a year of the pandemic becoming global and approved for 'emergency use' following expeditious development protocols. Vaccine development employed numerous nucleic acid, adenovirus and protein-based state-of-art molecular platforms, alongside the conventional attenuated and inactivated virus approaches. The majority of the attempts were successful and approved for use. All the approved vaccines were found safe and effective as per Phase I through Phase III clinical trials' results. Mass immunisation drives demonstrably led to reduced hospitalisation, low disease severity and less mortality. Yet, there were initial vaccination hesitation across the world due to associated safety concerns about its possible long-term negative consequences. A part of it was attributed to technical reasons (as clinical trials were not fully complete with sturdy and convincing outcomes), and a majority was due to the misinformation that floated on the social media and other digital communications. Vaccine deployment across the globe was far from being equitable. Thus, immunisation was rapid in higher income (developed) nations with access to innovative advanced vaccines while low immunisation rates were seen in the low and medium income countries accessing majorly the vaccines based on simple technology. Given the scale and spread of the pandemic, scaled-up vaccine production and equitable distribution to limit viral spread and improve global health and socioeconomy were critical. This chapter attempts to dissect these scenarios and lessons learnt from these to prepare better for any such pandemic in future.

***Keywords*:** Pandemic, COVID-19, SARS-CoV-2, Community health, Socioeconomy, Vaccinology, Vaccination drive

1. Introduction

Initially discovered and reported towards 2019 end, a novel coronavirus variant caused an infectious disease termed as COVID-19 by the World Health Organisation (WHO) (Mohapatra *et al.*, 2020a). The WHO named the virus as SARS-CoV-2 (severe acute respiratory syndrome coronavirus 2). The horrific situation of the lives lost and economic devastation worldwide by the viral spread became evident in almost the next half-a-year that ensued, in the first half of 2020, with over 761 million confirmed cases and over 7 million global deaths (Mohajan, 2021). The disease outcomes varied across age, gender, ethnicity and existing comorbidities. The COVID-19 infected asymptomatic individuals exhibiting mild to severe respiratory symptoms were also observed. Severe co-infections and associated deaths were most prominently encountered among particularly individuals with pre-existing medical conditions (comorbidity), the elderly, and the immunocompromised individuals. Pneumonia, acute respiratory distress syndrome (ARDS), respiratory failure, systemic inflammatory respiratory syndrome (SIRS), uncontrolled inflammation, hypercoagulation, dysfunctional immune system, liver malfunction and organs failure were among the major complications noticed among the infected subjects (Li *et al.*, 2020a). To decelerate the fast spread of the virus, the immediate community health control strategies that were imposed included lockdowns and shutdowns, face-masking, social distancing, isolation of the symptomatic patients and quarantine (Mohapatra *et al.*, 2021). However, the results of these were far from what was expected then (Mohapatra *et al.*, 2023). As vaccines seemed to be the most plausible solution to reduce morbidity and mortalities, thus vaccine research, vaccine design and formulation, mass production of vaccines and equitable distribution attempts were swiftly undertaken (Watson *et al.*, 2022; Mohapatra *et al.*, 2022; Satapathy *et al.*, 2023; Sarangi *et al.*, 2024; Dash et al., 2024).

1.1. Origin of the COVID Pandemic

Isolated pneumonia-like virus outbreaks were noticed in December 2019 in the Wuhan city of the mainland China. The ailment showed pneumonia like symptoms, like high-fever and dyspnoea. The virus was confirmed as a novel coronavirus similar to SARS-CoV-1 after testing of the samples obtained from the infected individuals, and was termed by the WHO as 'severe acute respiratory syndrome coronavirus 2' (SARS-CoV-2). It was later identified as the viral entity that was responsible for the 'coronavirus disease 2019' (COVID-19) global pandemic. Although the origin of this COVID-19 virus remains debatable, two theories put forward that are widely accepted in the scientific community are, 1) zoonotic origin or infection in humans through the infected and carrier food animals sold in the wet markets in Wuhan city, and 2) the coronavirus being studied in the Wuhan Institute of Virology that might have accidentally spilled to infect the contiguous population first which progressively infected others. The world witnessed two such occurrences of infections, one in 2002 by the MERS-CoV (Middle East Respiratory Syndrome Coronavirus) and the other in 2012 by SARS-CoV (Severe Acute Respiratory Syndrome Coronavirus) (Mohapatra *et al.*, 2020b). Both these instances involved contagious coronaviruses of zoonotic origin as the aetiological agent that caused fatal respiratory illnesses in humans and was a matter of concern and worry for the humanity and a critical challenge for the community healthcare institutions.

The existing evidences have suggested that SARS-CoV-2 might have most likely originated from a similar zoonotic transmission, originating from the fruit bats with a possible involvement of an intermediate animal host like pangolins (Zheng, 2020; Nie *et al.*, 2023). As the SARS-CoV-2 demonstrated to spread rapidly after it infected the human population, thus it led to the understanding that transmission of the virus from humans to humans was faster. Its generalist nature was also highlighted due to its ability to transmit across various mammalian species. The concerns about the reverse zoonosis or spillback (wherein there was the risk of the virus spreading from humans to the animals) became more critical with the swift transmission of the virus between the humans. The spillover risk from the bats to other susceptible wildlife emphasised on a revamped human-animal interface surveillance, and a strategy in similar lines to the 'One Health' approach. Collaborations at the global level were crucial to monitor the diversity of the coronavirus so as to minimise the threat of the constantly evolving vaccine-evading and highly-transmissive variants, and the risk of spillover and spillback events.

1.2. Pathophysiology

SARS-CoV-2 invades the body at the upper respiratory tract primarily through the respiratory droplets, typically inhaled by a healthy individual within the close proximity of an infected person or by getting in contact with a contaminated surface (fomites) and subsequently transferring the virus to the mouth, nose or the eyes by touching them (Cui *et al.*, 2020). The ciliated cells and the mucus-producing Goblet cells in the lungs were targeted by the virus as it reached inside the body, where it replicates and causes the symptomatic damage (Singhal, 2020). The mucus served to protect the lungs from the invading pathogens and the cilia helped to clear the airways by cleaning off the debris (or artefacts) and pathogens including the viruses. However, SARS-CoV-2 disrupted this process by invading these cells, leading to the accumulation of debris in the airways and its inflammation (Chen *et al.*, 2020; Wang *et al.*, 2020a).

Symptoms due to SARS-CoV-2 infection commonly included high fever, dry cough, dyspnoea, fatigue and muscle aches, but it could vary (Huang *et al.*, 2020). With some infected subjects experiencing heavy pneumonia where both the lungs were affected, the symptom severity ranged from mild to severe (Li *et al.*, 2020b). The elderly individuals and the ones with underlying health complications (comorbidities) were more susceptible to severe illnesses (Liu *et al.*, 2020; Kutikuppala *et al.*, 2022). The clinical management of the disease included global surveillance, early diagnosis and detection, isolation and supportive care of the confirmed cases to address complications like acute respiratory distress syndrome (ARDS) and septic shock (Burleson and Maki, 2005). The immune system mounted an inflammatory response as the infection progressed, which could further damage the parietal and visceral layers of the lungs tissue and a respiratory failure if not attended in time (Cowling and Leung, 2020). A severely affected patient could experience respiratory failure, permanent lung damage, or even death in very critical cases. Difficulties like venous thromboembolism and catheter-related bloodstream infections may also arise particularly in the high-risk hospitalised patients with pre-existing clinical conditions (Goossens, 2015). It can also further exacerbate respiratory distress and complicate patient management (Mehta *et al.*, 2020). At this point, an overactive immune response could trigger a cytokine storm, with widespread inflammation through the body and organ failure. Overall, SARS-CoV-2 infection could lead to numerous respiratory and systemic clinical complications. The impact on community health could be minimised and the viral spread be mitigated through early diagnosis, appropriate and timely medical interventions and effective preventive measures such as vaccinations (Pal *et al.*, 2022).

1.3. The Epidemiology

The physicians at Wuhan hospital in China observed uncommon occurrences of pneumonia in the late December 2019. Subsequent investigations revealed that the ailment originated from a wet food market in the same City of the

Hubei Province, Central China. The Chinese division of the Centres for Disease Control and Prevention (CDC) confirmed that the sickness was caused by a novel coronavirus on 2 January 2020, and named it as nCoV-2019. The WHO accepted the results of genome sequencing of the isolated nCoV-2019 on 11 February 2020 (Hoffmann *et al.*, 2020). The WHO renamed this enveloped virus as SARS-CoV-2, a positive single-stranded RNA beta-coronavirus belonging to Subfamily Coronavirinae, Family Coronaviridae, Order Nidovirales, Class Pisoniviricetes, Phylum Pisuviricota and Kingdom Orthornavirae of Realm Riboviria (Heiat *et al.*, 2021). It was never realised at that point in time that the virus could be so devastating and would be responsible for the world's worst-ever pandemic on record.

The first confirmed SARS-CoV-2 case was reported in early December 2019, associating it with the local seafood market. A significant proportion of the initial cases in the cluster were linked to this wet market. Reports later emerged suggesting a probable earlier onset of the disease, with a suspected reported case on 17 November 2019 (Chan *et al.*, 2020). With the fatality rate recorded at 2.3% and the cases peaking up by 12 February 2020, there could be unreported or misreported cases partly due to altered diagnosis and classifications. SARS-CoV-2 swiftly spread across the globe that affected over 185 countries. As the cases surged, it was declared as a global pandemic on 11 March 2020 by WHO (Cucinotta and Vanelli, 2020). COVID-19 testing data revealed that many infected individuals remained undetected and remained asymptomatic possibly due to a lower viral load during the testings, contributing further to the aggressive human-human transmissions (Melis and Littera, 2020). Serological studies indicated higher infection rates than what was reported, with varying rates across countries. The basic reproduction number (R_0) of COVID-19 virus was more than 1, which indicated its high transmissibility (Karimizadeh *et al.*, 2023). The situation became grimmer as the virus could infect across the various mammalian species.

While most of the infected human subjects recovered in 6–14 days, however there were deaths particularly among the elderly (individuals in the 60+ age group) with comorbid complications. The mortality rates also varied across nations, with some countries experiencing higher death rates attributed to the strained and fragile healthcare systems there. China confirmed the first death on 9 January 2020, with deaths reported globally subsequently peaking each passing day. The worldwide death rate due to SARS-CoV-2 infection rose to 7.05% at one time, although different WHO regions reported varying fatality rates. While the Eastern Mediterranean region reported 4.08%, the Western Pacific region accounted 4.12%, the South-East Asia region reported 3.86%, the African region reported 3.79%, the European region accounted 9.47%, and the American region recorded 5.23%. The WHO divided SARS-CoV-2 transmission into three categories as the pandemic progressed: community spread, sporadic cases and case clusters. While cases in certain geographic regions with similar exposure trends were categorised under cluster transmission, the community transmission was established when multiple instances with unlikable transmission chains were documented across various regions.

The nosocomial (infection within the hospital settings) death risk factors were also investigated, the risk factors identified behind the nosocomial deaths were old age patient, higher sequential organ failure assessment (SOFA) score, and high (more than 1μg/mL) d-dimer levels in the hospital-admitted patients (Zhou *et al.*, 2020). Comorbidities (like coronary diseases, diabetes and hypertension), ARDS (acute respiratory distress syndrome), shock (a condition when body does not get enough flow of healthy blood), respiratory failure, and multi-organ failure were the additional risk factors. With China as the epicentre the virus expanded throughout the world, and the United States reported the greatest number of cases by early April 2020 (Bergquist *et al.*, 2020). Italy had very high death rate too, particularly among the elderly (Ciminelli and Garcia-Mandicó, 2020; Gaythorpe *et al.*, 2021).

The gender and the severity correlation of a defined illness is a clear point of increasing concern. In case of COVID-19, the male folks tended to experience more severe illness and mortality despite the fact that both sexes had the same number of infection cases, and were similarly susceptible. The potential reasons behind such a scenario could be the varying protective behaviour (with women more likely to adopt the COVID-appropriate preventative measures better) and the gender-specific immunological variations (Tan *et al.*, 2022). Comorbidities such as hypertension, cardiovascular disorders and diseased lungs were also linked to any undue unfavourable outcome (dos Santos *et al.*, 2022). Due to the complex morbidity and mortality nature of COVID-19, thorough foolproof mitigation and prevention strategies were required to be ensured in order to reduce the disease burden. This was more imminent owing to the fact that many countries had a fragile and already-burdened healthcare system to cater to the ailing population there.

High coverage of the vaccinated population through immunisation drives and campaigns were experienced to be crucial in reducing the risk of COVID-19-related serious infections and deaths (Calabrò *et al.*, 2023). Public healthcare initiatives like face-masking, social distancing and frequent hand-sanitising continued to be the essential components of all-encompassing preventative measures in the 'new normal' era. Also, addressing the COVID-19-related morbidity and death disparities required dedicated actions on the surveillance, early detection and an enhanced access to the healthcare infrastructure. Beside the reported short-term acute illness and mortality, COVID-19 was associated with long-term health consequences in specific individuals. The PASC (post-acute sequelae of COVID-19 after being infected with SARS-CoV-2), also stated as the 'long-haul COVID', encompassed a series of persistent signs, symptoms and complications that could significantly impact the quality of life and functional ability. Symptoms like fatigue, cognitive impairment and respiratory issues might persist for weeks or months following the phase of acute infection, underscoring the importance of a truly comprehensive healthcare management approach and a support system for the convalescing individuals. The virus variants like Omicron and Delta also had varying effects on the death rates and long-haul COVID. Trends in mortality were impacted by the higher transmissibility and disease severity. Given the varying nature of COVID-19 morbidity and mortality, effective monitoring, mitigation and prevention strategies across the nations were essential to reduce the disease burden. All in all, the vaccination campaigns aimed at achieving high population coverage proved to be instrumental in preventing COVID-19-associated severe illness and mortality.

2. Global Race to Develop COVID-19 Vaccine

As the global pandemic unfolded, it sparked unparalleled efforts to counter SARS-CoV-2 by developing vaccines against the virus and its variants that were aggressive in infection and transmission. The governments, research institutions, pharmaceutical firms across nations and international organisations promptly pooled their resources, knowledge and cooperation to confront the pressing demand for a viable vaccine. Philanthropic organisations and non-government non-profit organisations also proactively involved themselves. The race to develop COVID-19 vaccine reached an unprecedented pace, reducing the timeline of the conventional vaccine development from years into months (at least for 'emergency use' approval). This section of the chapter discusses the global responses to the pandemic, scrutinising the multifactorial endeavours to expedite the vaccine research, its manufacturing, equitable distribution and dissemination at global scale. It also presents a chronological overview of key milestones achieved in COVID-19 vaccine research and development. Beginning with the identification of SARS-CoV-2 virus and its genome sequencing, the timeline tracks the progresses on preclinical studies, clinical trials, regulatory approvals and mass vaccination drives.

The remarkable achievements in vaccine development, while the world faced the seemingly never-ending COVID-19 pandemic challenges, served as a testament to scientific innovations and endeavours, international collaborations and collective determination to counter global health crises. The WHO granted 'emergency use' approval to several vaccines in various countries to administer to the general public in order to reduce the transmission and causalities that was peaking every passing day (Fig. 1). The figure depicts how fast the vaccines were developed in about nine months after the confirmation of global pandemic by the WHO followed the approval of these vaccines in principle by WHO during 2020 and 2021, at least for emergency use.

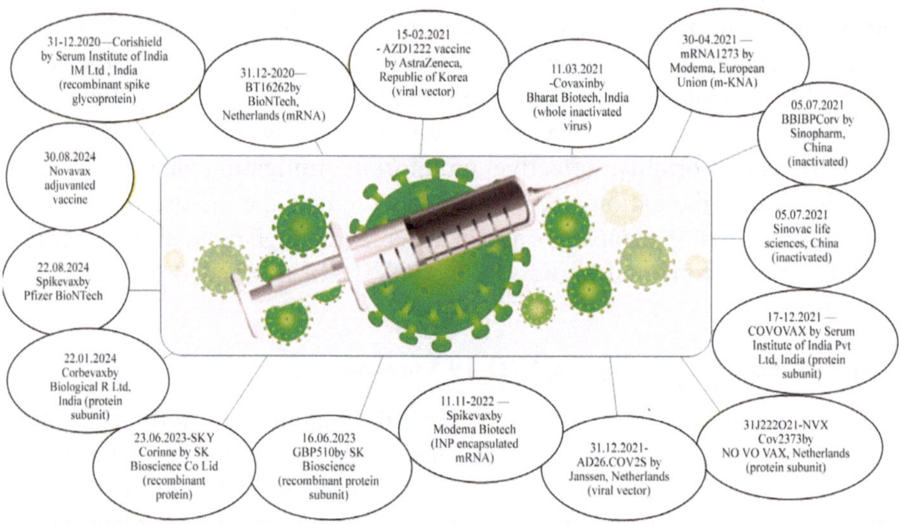

Fig. 1: A timeline of numerous WHO-approved COVID-19 vaccines developed worldwide

2.1. Viral biomaterials as Targets for the COVID-19 Vaccine Development

SARS-CoV-2 virus carries the largest single standed (ss) RNA genome. The manner in which the RNA genome is folded within the virus remains to be understood. The structural proteins of the SARS-CoV-2 virus, like the membrane (M), the envelope (E), the nucleocapsid (N) and the spike (S) are the suitable targets for the development of vaccines (Dai and Gao, 2021). SARS-CoV-2 genome also expresses nine auxiliary proteins and sixteen non-structural proteins (nsp1–16). The COVID-19 virus has two S protein components, S1 that binds to the angiotensin-converting enzyme II (ACE2), and S2 that is involved in the membrane fusion. These are necessary for the SARS-CoV-2 virus to successfully invade the human (host) body. S1 subunit comprises of two domains, the N-terminal domain (NTD) and the receptor-binding domain

(RBD). M protein is incorporated in the virion envelope which provides it the desired shape. E (Envelop) proteins are small polypeptides which are essential for the stability and infectivity of the viral particle.

The helical nucleocapsid of the virus (SARS-CoV-2) has the N protein which binds along the viral RNA genome. These viral proteins could be the targets for vaccine development to trigger immune responses (Dong *et al.*, 2020; Dai and Gao, 2021). Both the live-attenuated and inactivated vaccines are based on the whole virus cell, while nucleic acid based, viral vector and subunit vaccines utilise primarily the S protein of the virus (Dong *et al.*, 2020). The WHO has approved COVID-19 vaccines for clinical trials that were developed as either inactivated, live-attenuated, vector-based, nucleic acids (DNA or RNA) based, protein subunit or virus-like particle (VLP) forms. A schema of the same is presented in detail in Fig. 2. However, a framework to study the structure, function and dynamics is very necessary to carry the cause forward to counter the emerging deadly RNA viruses in future too.

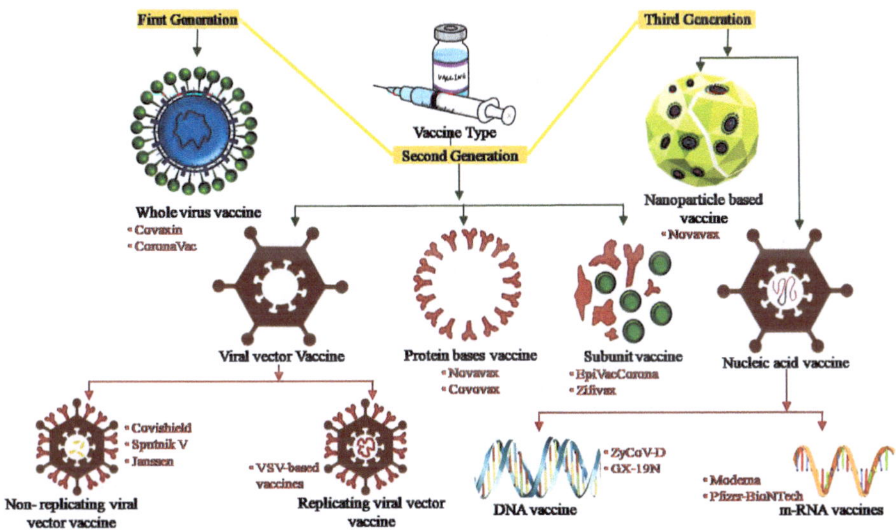

Fig. 2: Various platforms used to develop COVID-19 vaccines, with examples

2.2. Vaccine Development Platforms

As the article was drafted, 133 vaccines were being developed of which few were already in administration (for the purpose of 'emergency use' only) to combat the pandemic. Numerous conventional and advanced vaccine development platforms were implemented to develop the vaccines against COVID-19. However, each of these had its own distinct advantages and disadvantages over the other. There was a good chance that the world would need many authorised vaccines to combat the pandemic in future too, covering a wide range of diseases, for the target population with due diligent vaccine safety and efficacy. Designing and formulation of the vaccines for easy administration is only the preliminary endeavour. The endeavour also included expeditious manufacturing strategies, ideal storage conditions and seamless transportation channels for equitable distribution across nations. Various successfully developed vaccines against COVID-19 vary in the mechanisms of action too, as the underlying molecular mechanism differed from each other. Table 1 lists the many conventional and advanced vaccine technologies that were implemented in developing the various COVID-19 vaccines.

Table 1: Various COVID-19 vaccine development platforms and their mechanisms of action

Vaccine platform	Component for vaccine development	Mechanisms of antibody elicitation
Inactivated viral vaccine	Whole viruses are cultured *in vitro* and inactivated by chemical agents	The entire virus acted as immunogen to induce a wider range of antibodies production against different epitopes
Live attenuated vaccine	Whole virus is utilised but obtained by reverse genetics or by adaptation	Retained viral proteins induced extensive innate humoral and cellular immunity
Adenoviral vector vaccine	Non-replicating vectored vaccine expressing the full-length spike protein of SARS-CoV-2	Induced Th1 cell responses thus inducing strong protective effects
Protein subunit vaccine	Recombinant nanoparticle of full-length S protein with mutations at the S1/S2 cleavage sites to provide protease resistance and proline substitutions at two sites for protein stabilisation	Induced Th1 cell responses
DNA vaccine	Gene of SARS-CoV-2 spike protein was cloned into the pVAX-1 plasmid, or the same gene was cloned into pGX0001 expression vector	Induced neutral antibodies
m-RNA vaccine	mRNA-lipid nanoparticle expressing full-length spike protein with two proline substitutions for protein stabilisation in the pre-fusion conformation	Induced both Th1 and B-cell responses and generate plasma cells and memory cells to elicit neutral antibodies
VLP vaccine	Non infection particles consist of viral structural proteins and viral peptides	Induced neutralism antibodies against immune epitopes

2.2.1. Whole Virus as the Target

While an antiviral vaccine is often produced by the virus-infected cells, however an immediate alternative is inactivated vaccine. The first-ever flu vaccine was developed in 1940 using this technique, by using the embryonated eggs (Minor, 2015). The whole virus is used as the target to develop inactivated and live-attenuated viral vaccines as a conventional approach. A virus particle contains S, N, M and E proteins, and could create non-structural and auxiliary proteins *in vivo* (Minor, 2015). Consequently, such a whole-virus candidate vaccine might induce greater antibody and T-cell responses as compared to its vaccine counterpart that is based on a single viral protein or its fragment. As immunogens, inactivated vaccines could trigger an immune response while preserving the integrity of the virus.

Live-attenuated vaccine has a less-virulent form of an entire microbial (bacterial or viral) pathogen. Serial passaging is employed to attenuate the wild viral or bacterial entity. The target pathogen is introduced into a non-target host (wherein it is incapable of replicating properly) and is allowed to multiply randomly over an extended period of time. As a result, the less-virulent form thus obtained (live-attenuated vaccine) is capable of triggering almost exactly the same immune response as the reaction that an illness triggered by an actual infection shall trigger (Chaudhary *et al.*, 2021). Live-attenuated vaccine induces robust cellular and humoral immunity. COVI-VAC (trial number NCT04619628) and MV-014–212 (trial number NCT04798001) are examples of live-attenuated vaccine candidates against COVID-19, produced by Codagenix in collaboration with the Serum Institute of India (SII) and Meissa Vaccines Inc. (Nagy and Alhatlani, 2021).

Inactivated (or killed) vaccines are composed of culturable bacterial or viral pathogens wherein their genetic material were chemically (formalin, phenol) or physically (heat, radiation) destroyed. Owing to this, the immune system of the body identifies them while they are incapacitated to proliferate (Chaudhary *et al.*, 2021). Inactivated vaccines elicit the cellular immune response less effectively and persistently than their attenuated counterparts. These typically need numerous doses too, in addition to immunologic adjuvants. Beijing-based Sinovac Biotech developed an inactivated virus vaccine PiCoVacc (NCT04456595) that was approved for 'emergency use', and could efficiently generate high neutralising antibody. Sinopharm designed as an inactivated vaccine candidate (ChiCTR2000034780) for SARS-CoV-2 (Mathew *et al.*, 2020). The Indian Covaxin formulation developed by Bharat Biotech Ltd. is another example of inactivated viral vaccine, administered to elicit immunity against the SARS-Co-2 virus (Chakraborty *et al.*, 2023; Table 2).

2.2.2. Nucleic Acid as the Target

These contain the gene component (DNA or mRNA) of the targeted pathogen. The body cells receive the genetic code of the antigen that is translated into protein by using the transcription and translation machinery of the host cell. Then, the antigen-presenting cells (APCs) digest the generated protein and deliver it to the immune cells to generate the desired immune response. Nucleic acid (DNA or mRNA) vaccines are categorised under the next-generation vaccine platform that is readily adaptable to counter various emerging viral strains. DNA vaccine is made out of a synthetic DNA construct encoding the vaccine antigen (Acosta-Coley *et al.*, 2022). The plasmid DNA vaccine INO-4800 comprises of pGX001 expression vector expressing the spike protein from SARS-CoV-2, produced by Inovio Pharmaceuticals in collaboration with International Vaccine Institute (Bai *et al.*, 2021). ZyCoV-D by Zydus Cadila was the first authorised plasmid DNA vaccine approved for 'emergency use', wherein a non-replicating, non-integrating plasmid expressing coronavirus gene produced the vaccine.

The mRNA used in vaccine development programme encoded the antigen against a specific pathogen. Although RNA molecules are unstable however such vaccine design platforms are advantageous owing to increased stability and efficacy in translating the protein for an enhanced immune response (Acosta-Coley *et al.*, 2022). The mRNA vaccine m-RNA-1273 was developed by Moderna Inc. and the National Institute of Allergy and Infectious Diseases (NIAID) under the auspices of the National Institute of Health (NIH) of the US government. This vaccine candidate encoded the full-length S protein of SARS-CoV-2 that used lipid nanoparticle (LNP) capsule as the delivery vehicle. BioNTech of Germany and Pfizer of the US developed another mRNA-based vaccine, sold under the trade name Comirnaty (Bai *et al.*, 2021; Table 2).

Table 2. A list of the major WHO-approved COVID-19 vaccines with their performance efficacies

Sl. No.	Approved vaccine	Developer of vaccine	Vaccine type/ platform	Origin country	Storage temperature (°C)	Dosage	Efficacy	Source
1.	Pfizer-BioNTech vaccine	BioNTech SE, Pfizer Inc.	Nucleic Acid based vaccine modified mRNA	Germany, USA	–70±10	Two doses in three weeks apart	95%	Dighriri *et al.*, 2022
2.	Moderna vaccine	US National Institute of Allergy and Infectious Diseases, Moderna Inc., Biomedical Advanced Research & Development Authority, Coalition for Epidemic Preparedness Innovations	Nucleic Acid based vaccine modified mRNA	USA	–20±5	Two doses in three weeks apart	94.5%	Meo *et al.*, 2021
3.	Oxford-AstraZeneca vaccine	AstraZeneca Plc, University of Oxford and Coalition for Epidemic Preparedness Innovations	Modified adenovirus vector	Sweden, UK	2–8	Two doses given four to twelve weeks apart	Overall, 70% (64% after the 1st dose & 70.4% after the 2nd dose)	WHO, 2022a
4.	Sputnik V vaccine	Gamaleya Research Institute of Epidemiology and Microbiology	Modified adenovirus vector	Russia	$\leq$-18	Two doses given three weeks apart	91.6%	Forni and Mantovani, 2021
5.	Johnson & Johnson vaccine	Janssen Pharmaceuticals, Beth Israel Deaconess Medical Centre	Modified adenovirus vector	Belgium, Netherlands	2–8	Single dose	Overall, 66.3% (72% in the US)	Johnson & Johnson, 2021
6.	Ad5-nCoV vaccine	CanSino Biologics, Beijing Institute of Biotechnology	Modified adenovirus vector	China	2–8	Single dose	Overall, 92% against severe COVID-19	WHO, 2022b

Sl. No.	Approved vaccine	Developer of vaccine	Vaccine type/ platform	Origin country	Storage temperature (°C)	Dosage	Efficacy	Source
7.	BBIBP-CorV vaccine	Beijing Institute of Biological Products, Wuhan Institute of Biological Products, China National Pharmaceutical Group Corporation	Inactivated SARS-CoV-2	China	2–8	Two doses given 3–4 weeks apart	86–90% (in severe COVID-19)	Wang *et al.*, 2020b
8.	ZF2001 vaccine	Chinese Academy of Sciences, Anhui Zhifei Longcom Biologic Pharmacy Co., Ltd.	protein subunit with adjuvant	China	-	Three doses given 30 days apart	90–96%	Dai *et al.*, 2022
9.	CoronaVac vaccine	Sinovac Biotech Ltd.	Inactivated SARS-CoV-2	China	2–8	Two doses given two weeks apart	83.5% (after 2nd dose)	Fonseca *et al.*, 2022
10.	BBV152 vaccine	Bharat Biotech International Limited, Indian Council of Medical Research	Inactivated SARS-CoV-2	India	2–8	Two doses given four weeks apart	Overall 78% (93.4% in severe cases)	Luvira and Pitisuttithum, 2024
11.	EpiVacCorona vaccine	State Research Centre of Virology and Biotechnology VECTOR	Peptide subunit vaccine	Russia	2–8	Two doses in 3–4 weeks apart	70–75%	Luvira and Pitisuttithum, 2024
12.	CoviVac vaccine	Russian Academy of Sciences	Inactivated SARS-CoV-2	Russia	2–8	Two doses given two weeks apart	83% (after 2nd dose)	Chirico *et al.*, 2022

2.2.3. Viral Vector

The components of a viral vector vaccine include antigen-encoding recombinant virus that is cloned by employing recombinant DNA technology. A viral vector is often attenuated to reduce the pathogenicity of the virus. Viral vector vaccines are of two types, replicating and non-replicating. Vaccines using replicating vectors infect the new cells that subsequently produce the vaccine antigens while non-replicating vectors would first penetrate the cell and generate the vaccinating antigen without adding more new virus particles (as these are incapable of replicating). Viral vector vaccine boosts the humoral and cellular immune responses through which the body becomes capable to produce endogenous antigens. Thus, single dose viral vector vaccine is efficient to elicit the desired immune response (van Riel and de Wit, 2020).

The ChAdOx1 nCoV-19 vaccine (AZD1222) was developed by the University of Oxford, UK (Mercado *et al.*, 2020; Voysey *et al.*, 2021). It is a chimpanzee adenoviral vectored vaccine that expresses the full length SARS-CoV-2 spike protein. Sputnik V vaccine developed by Gamaleya Research Institute of Epidemiology and Microbiology is a heterologous recombinant adenovirus-based vaccine formulation that comprised the rAD type 26 and rAD type 5 which expressed the full length SARS-CoV-2 glycoprotein S. It was meant to be administered intramuscularly in double-dose with a 21-day interval. Another vaccine is the Janssen's COVID-19 vaccine which is a single-dose recombinant adenoviral vector vaccine that expressed the S protein of SARS-CoV-2 (Krammer, 2020). Adenovirus type-5-vectored coronavirus (Ad5-nCov) against SARS-CoV-2 was developed collaboratively by the Beijing Institute of Biotechnology and CanSino Biologics. It is a genetically modified vector that expressed the SARS-CoV-2 S protein which efficiently induced high immune response (Zhu *et al.*, 2020; Table 2).

2.2.4. Protein Subunit Vaccine

Subunit vaccine could be a protein nanoparticle or a virus like particle (VLP) that expresses a recombinant entity which is capable of expressing a particular piece of the viral antigen. Protein subunit (adjuvanted recombinant) vaccine has an antigen (a viral component) that could activate the human immune system without the direct involvement of the virus. Antigens alone often fail to induce long-term immunity, and hence adjuvants are added to trigger the immune response to the desired level and for the desired duration. Adjuvants necessarily elicit strong immune responses (Mathew *et al.*, 2020). S protein-expressing protein subunit vaccine expectedly activated the antibodies that blocked the binding and subsequent membrane fusion of the virus thereby hindering the process of the viral infection. Protein subunit vaccine was safe and it could be swiftly developed, easily scaled-up and efficiently stored to fulfil the demand at the global scale without logistics complications. Such vaccines could be efficiently tailored for potential epitope generation to trigger immune response by enhancing the process of neutralising antibody production and T-cell activation. EpiVacCorona is an approved vaccine against SARS-CoV-2 under this category (Acosta-Coley *et al.*, 2022; Table 2).

2.2.5. Virus-like Particles (VLPs)

Composed of one or more viral or nonviral proteins, VLPs are exceptionally small, non-infectious nanoparticles that could self-assemble. VLPs could self-assemble into various forms, including rod, circularised and helical. The VLPs resemble the structural configuration of the native viral particle. Upon administration, they are presented by antigen presenting cells to immune systems and become accessible to CD4+ and CD8+ T lymphocytes via the MHC proteins. Because of their molecular size and structural repetition, VLPs improve the B cell immunogenicity. VLP directly stimulates the B cells which significantly boost the humoral immune response and also could elicit the T-cell mediated immunity. The NVAX-CoV2372 (Nuvaxovid™, the adjuvanted Novavax COVID-19 vaccine) of the Novovax is the first COVID-19 vaccine that is protein-based, which was granted the EUA ('emergency use' authorisation) as a primary or a booster vaccine. It is a SARS-CoV-2 non-enveloped VLP-based vaccine candidate that expresses the S2P protein. It has proved to be highly immunogenic and safe, and has showed 89.7% efficacy against symptomatic COVID-19. ABNCoV2 is another vaccine developed by AdaptVac in collaboration with the Radboud University (Expres2ion Biotechnologies), is a neVLPs-based SARS-CoV-2 vaccine candidate that used proprietary capsid virus like particle (cVLP) (Prates-Syed *et al.*, 2021; Dhawan *et al.*, 2023).

3. Vaccine Development Phases and the Approval Process

An effective vaccine is designed and produced by using a right technology and the ideal vaccine development platform. After its successful design and formulation, the vaccine is evaluated for its safety initially through preclinical trials in mice and rabbits. After successful preclinical trials confirming that the vaccine does not elicit any major adverse immune response, the last phase (Phase III clinical trial) is initiated in human beings. Usually followed after the preclinical testing, a clinical trial has three defined phases. A limited number (10-100) of human volunteers are vaccinated in Phase I and the adverse immune responses are monitored. A larger number (100–1,000) of willing participants (volunteers) receive the candidate vaccine being tested in Phase II while an even bigger group (1,000–100,000) receives the same in Phase III. The objective behind involving a larger participation in the clinical trials is to get a closer look and foolproof clinical responses on how a vaccine works on a human body, and if the candidate vaccine adversely affects the volunteers. A placebo is also administered to a group alongside the group that is administered with the candidate vaccine being tested so as to observe any development in a volunteer that is not attributable to the vaccine.

The efficacy assessment usually takes several weeks to months for a preventive or therapeutic medical product, although the approval process could be shortened in the wake of a pandemic situation (as was observed during the COVID-19 pandemic). Clinical trial phases could be reduced and fast-forwarded. It could also partially overlap to counter the emergencies as was the situation during the recent pandemic. In either case, the monitoring of the thousands of vaccinated individuals for several months after they are vaccinated is crucial. After assessing the risk and evaluating the vaccine efficacy within the 'trial' population, the vaccine is approved by the authorised agencies for administration of the same to the general public (for vaccination drives and also to be available over-the-counter). For instance, the research ethics committees of the European Medicines Agency (EMA) and the US Food and Drug Administration (USFDA) review the clinical trial designs and the vaccine development regulations before the due approval of a vaccine that shall be available over-the-counter for public consumption.

4. Vaccine Rollout Strategies During COVID-19 and Challenges

Three steps were typically involved in vaccine development during the COVID-19 pandemic (Funk *et al.*, 2020). These were, identifying the target antigen, choosing the right platform to design the target antigen, formulating the vaccine for ease of administration, undertaking *in vitro* tests on cell lines and conducting studies in model animals *in vivo*. All these steps are important aspects of vaccine development leading to the preclinical trials. The Phase I, Phase II and Phase III clinical trials involving human volunteers testing are usually initiated in the event of a successful preclinical trial of the candidate vaccine. The recent pandemic due to the SARS-CoV-2 posed unprecedented global challenges, necessitating an engaging and effective vaccination campaign to save precious lives and mitigate the socioenomic impact owing to the global human health scenario that prevailed then.

In addition to the swift action to develop COVID-19 vaccines and assisting in expanding the manufacturing capacities, the WHO worked closely with the concerned countries, line researchers, regional healthcare professionals and other partnering stakeholders to develop necessary policies, bolster regulatory capabilities, provide trainings, and assisting nations in aligning their resources as necessary arrangements for the capacity building and distribution programmes for the COVID-19 vaccines. Resource-poor nations received ample of assistance from the WHO, the UNICEF and other such international agencies in preparing to launch the COVID-19 vaccination campaigns. A toolkit with workflow instructions, resources and trainings was created by the ACT (Access to COVID-19 Tools) accelerator that was made available worldwide for country-wise readiness and delivery. The ACT accelerator proved to be a successful global collaboration that ensured faster vaccines development, production and equitable access to testing, treatment and administration across the globe during the COVID-19 pandemic.

4.1. Implementing Vaccine Administration

A sizable global population was needed to be immunised through vaccination to block the further transmission of SARS-CoV-2 (direct protection) which would also provide herd immunity to the community (indirect protection) as an extended benefit to the population that could not be vaccinated. With seemingly limited resources and the need for an expeditious action, the situation that prevailed then put an enormous burden on the healthcare systems worldwide thereby exposing its underbelly. As SARS-CoV-2 virus transmitted and infected very rapidly, developing herd immunity through natural infection and recovery before immunisation programme could be established proved to have an opposite effect of what was expected (Randolph and Barreiro, 2020). Hence, vaccination was hoped to be the best and the most practical measure to achieve herd immunity with time. It meant that, 80–90% of the global population needed to be COVID-19 immunised to accomplish this (Nachega *et al.*, 2020). An estimated 6.3 billion COVID-19 vaccine doses were delivered globally by the end of September 2021, as per Our World in Data (OWID). By September 2022, the vaccination doubled that reached 12.8 billion doses (Yang *et al.*, 2023).

India undertook one of the largest COVID-19 immunisation global campaigns starting 16 January 2021, with a goal to immunise its large (1.38 billion) population in a planned and systematic manner with frontline workers identified as the first beneficiaries of it. The Indian government established a National Expert Group on Vaccine Administration for COVID-19 (NEGVAC) that offered assistance on all aspects of COVID-19 vaccine administration at the domestic level. Healthcare employees and staff received the vaccines (primarily Covaxin and Covishield and secondarily the Russian Sputnik versions) in the first phase. The aging population over 50 years (preferably over 60 years of age) were the next to receive the vaccine shots, followed by the individuals under 50 years with comorbidities, as per NEGVAC (Chirico *et al.*, 2022). As per the OWID database September 2022, 951.99 million had been COVID-19 vaccinated in India, the USA figures stood at 230.64 billion and China at 1.28 billion. France, Italy and Spain had completed vaccinating 53.19, 47.95, 40.74 million population till 12 June 2024, as per Our World in Data (OWID).

4.2. Vaccine Hesitancy

Vaccination is the most critical public health intervention to block the transmission of an infectious disease and diminish the harm it could otherwise significantly cause. However, concerns were frequently raised from numerous quarters and organisations claiming the conflicts that were majorly related to politics, science and religion that stalled the process to accomplish it. Due to misinformation that floated on the social media and other digital platforms, the public confidence became weak due to the low understandings on the epidemiology of COVID-19 virus, the associated immunology, and the unprecedented speed and global competition to develop the vaccines (Caceres *et al.*, 2022). However, the degree of vaccine reluctance varied across the various regions around the world. India too had such a difficult situation to address due to the floating misinformation, and mishandling of the public perception by several quarters including the politicians and the religious leaders.

Contingent on the severity of the health and socioeconomic consequences, the global COVID-19 pandemic varyingly affected the public confidence in the related vaccine research, healthcare institutions and the overall healthcare infrastructure (Verger and Dubé, 2020). Numerous approaches were used at various levels by the MoHFW of the government of India to raise awareness, increase the vaccination rates, decrease vaccine hesitancy and curb the virus from spreading throughout the nation. A survey on the acceptance and hesitancy of COVID-19 vaccine across 23 countries till 10 July 2022 revealed that there were 79.1% acceptance and 10.9% hesitancy among the population (Lazarus *et al.*, 2023). The rates varied across nations as depicted in Fig. 3.

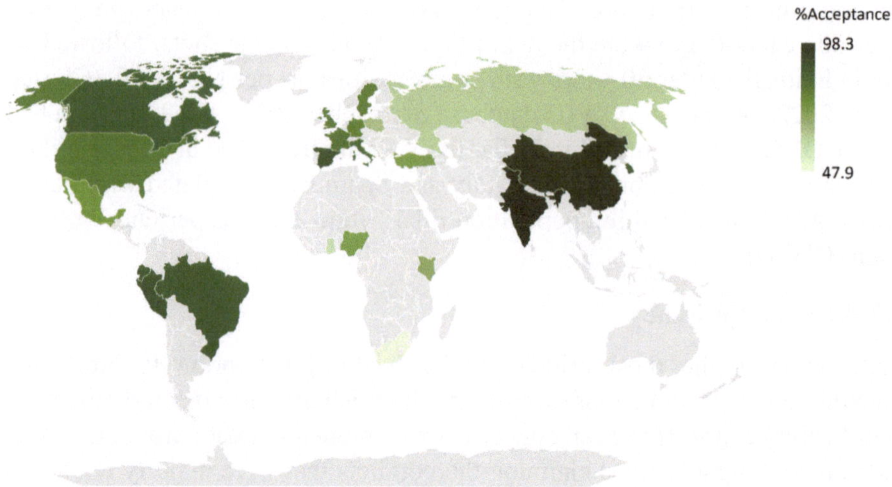

Fig. 3: The percent COVID-19 vaccine acceptance in 23 countries till 10 July 2022
Source: Lazarus *et al.* (2023)

5. Age Group and High-risk Category-wise Impact of COVID-19 on the GDP

As an immediate implication of lockdowns enforced at the onset of the pandemic, it brought an unprecedented economic recession globally along with healthcare and socioeconomic crises. Although isolation and quarantine measures were able to contain the transmission rate of the pathogen (SARS-CoV-2), it also led to a decline in even the basic economic activities, employment and businesses. As a result, numerous countries were hard hit with a drastically reduced growth rate in gross domestic product (GDP). The World Bank Global Economic Prospects Report issued on January 2020 which was before proclamation of the pandemic by the World Health Organisation (which was declared on 11 March 2000) did not include the implications of the COVID-19 pandemic. It the same report, the World Bank projected an increment of global GDP by 2.5%, from US$85 trillion in 2019 to US$87 trillion by 2020. However, there was a 3.1% drop in the global GDP due to the impact of the pandemic, accounting to about US$4.7 trillion less from the earlier predicted value (Reddy, 2020).

COVID-19 has had a significant and diverse influence on the economy across the various age groups, affecting employment, financial stability, education and general wellbeing. The pandemic highlighted the importance of specific economic measures to encourage recovery and resilience across countries and populations (Clemente-Suárez *et al.*, 2021). The second quarter of 2020 had an estimated 495 million job loss globally while it was estimated at 195 million in the third quarter (Clemente-Suárez *et al.*, 2021). In Japan, 85% of the population reported stable condition in employment while in China about 43% of the population has a temporary job loss. It was observed that, the middle aged (46-65) population were the least affected during the recession. About 18% of the population who were above 66 years were found to be more vulnerable to job loss than their 26 years old or younger counterparts. Further, the young and middle-aged population preferred teleworking than their senior counterparts. The economic recession had disproportionately affected the elderly population (in the 65–74 age groups), as also those beyond this age group who continued their active professional lives. This scenario might be attributed to the fact that the professionally active older people were susceptible to social insecurity, but the younger ones were likely burdened with mortgage down payments (Reddy, 2020). India also suffered the brunt in the overall GDP contribution and employment rate in several sectors including the international services, travel industry, trade and commerce, and the real estate. On the contrary, the agriculture sector remained as an exception with and observed increase in employment (Mizik, 2021). The population in the 15–39 years age groups was impacted the worst in terms of job loss. The population in the 25–29 years age groups accounted for about 46% of the overall job losses (Reddy, 2020).

The overall GDP losses were also attributed to the hospitalisation expenses, diagnosis and disease management. SARS-CoV-2 viral infection increasingly affected organ transplant recipients, cancer patient on chemotherapy, smokers and those on long-term steroids, diabetes, hypertension, lungs diseases, hepatic diseases and renal diseases (Chavda *et al.*, 2022). ICU-admitted COVID-19 patients were more likely subjected to high hospitalisation cost like extracorporeal membrane oxygenation and mechanical ventilation in comparison to the patients in regular ward facilities. This scenario was observed across nations, wherein the surveys found a substantial increase in medical expenses among the ICU admitted COVID-19 patients. Mechanical ventilation in the ICU-admitted patients resulted in an additional increase in expenses, from US$2082.65±345.04 to US$2990.76±545.98.9 (Chang *et al.*, 2021). Surveys in the US, Europe and Asia revealed that the patients with more severe COVID-19 symptoms used more resources and incurred more expenses than those with milder symptoms. Macroeconomically, the COVID-19 pandemic directly contributed to the overall GDP losses, primarily resulting from a decreased production and an increased use of non-pharmaceutical therapies (Chang *et al.*, 2021). The estimated smallest expenses figure across the surveyed nations regarding the healthcare during the pandemic was

US$1264 in India, while the figure was the highest in the United States at US$54,165. As per reports, the medical expenses ranged between US$5264 and US$79,315 in China (Faramarzi *et al.*, 2024).

All in all, the impact of COVID-19 pandemic on the GDP across the various age groups and the high-risk category were greatly influenced by the vaccination coverage. The countries that had reported varying vaccination rates, vaccine hesitancy and the extent of success of the immunisation programmes depended on an array of variables, including the public acceptance and preference, infrastructure and logistics limitations, and the purchasing capacity due to financial constraints. An effective immunisation programme and enhanced vaccination coverage have had positive and encouraging impacts on the health and socioeconomy of the nations across the globe.

5.1. Impact of COVID-19 Vaccination on Public Health and Socioeconomy

COVID-19 pandemic caused considerable morbidity and mortality worldwide, with declined social and financial health at individual (microeconomy) as well as community or national (macroeconomy) levels. Due to the high transmissibility and high infectivity of the pandemic, the majority of the population remained vulnerable to SARS-CoV-2 infection leading to devastating consequences. As a result of this, designing and developing vaccines became the matter of top priority and the primary objective across the globe. Thus, the scope, pace and efforts to develop vaccines were astounding, with highly safe and effective vaccines being developed and more-or-less equitably supplied around the world. The first vaccine trial was administered on 8 Dec 2020, *i.e.*, within a period of nine months of the formal declaration by the WHO of the COVID-19 disease as a pandemic.

As per the estimates, vaccination drive could successfully prevent 19.8 million deaths due to COVID-19 in a year of its initiation across 185 countries, representing 63% reduction in the global death cases (Watson *et al.*, 2022). Even though COVID-19 vaccine provided only a modest protection against the infection, it surely and certainly helped in significantly reducing the transmission and thereby helped curb future outbreaks, hospitalisation and ICU admission. Analysing the progress of the vaccination programmes was vital to ascertain their overall efficacy over time (Singh *et al.*, 2024). COVID-19 vaccination was projected to have prevented a median of 151 million illnesses and 620,000 global fatalities (Yang *et al.*, 2023). Vaccination was estimated to have saved medical expenses associated with outpatient treatment caused by the COVID-19 pandemic by US$155 billion (also accounting for the productivity loss). This overall savings figure would be far larger worldwide given the fact that a median reduction of US$21 billion due to inpatient expenditures alone was calculated among the 26 nations with related hospitalisation data. An estimated 1.6 million hospitalisation cases and 235,000 deaths among the US population could be prevented till September 2021 (Steele *et al.*, 2022). Analysing the US Research and Development Survey (RANDS) data, the weekly productivity or loss of earnings of individuals (or a family) affected by COVID-19 during May–June 2021 was US$588 for 45–64 years old adults and US$611 for adults above 65 years (Wang and Wang, 2022). The COVID-19 pandemic caused a considerable temporary loss of human capital owing to absenteeism and reduced efficiency of the staff members. COVID-19 vaccination prevented US$135.1 billion worldwide in terms of the productivity loss. It highlighted that vaccination coverage especially among the adults in the working age groups indirectly extended financial benefits as a guarantee of their physical wellbeing was crucial in determining their productivity and income (Yang *et al.*, 2023).

6. Challenges and Lessons Learnt

The COVID-19 pandemic inadvertently impacted diverse sectors of human life like health, social life, education and the economy. Vaccination remained the game-changer in alleviating the impact of pandemic and catalysing the human lives back to normal worldwide. The vaccination against COVID-19 was essential to attain herd immunity too (considering that few members in the population could not be vaccinated due to health condition, social, religious, financial or logistics reasons) that prevented viral transmission across the populations. Vaccination decreased the mortality attributed to COVID-19, reduced the cases of hospitalisation and induced herd immunity against SARS-CoV-2. In the wake of it, not only the rapid designing and scaled-up production of various successful vaccine candidates was challenging, but also their manufacturing within a limited timeframe and administering to the large population were major challenges to overcome.

The long-term efficacy concerns, immunoreactions and side-effects of the various formulated vaccines that were approved for 'emergency use' remained an issue with regard to their acceptance beyond the emergency period. The emerging and reemerging strains of the SARS-CoV-2 virus, as also the swiftly evolving variants, were also other major challenges that defied the vaccine efficacy and aggravated vaccine hesitancy even among the literate and informed citizens. The state-of-art technologically advanced platforms for the nucleic acids (DNA and m-RNA) based vaccines allegedly showed better efficacy against the COVID-19 virus than the conventionally formulated vaccines irrespective of the variant in question. Thus, innovative and effective technologies need to be researched and employed with early preparedness against such health and wellbeing emergencies in future.

Collaborative efforts and fund mobilisation from the governments, public and private sectors, dedicated research efforts by the scientific communities, strong practically-feasible policies and awareness building through digital revolution has had a positive impact on the vaccination drives across tiers worldwide. Vaccine inequity (noncompliance of the equitable distribution of the vaccines) was another critical challenge during the pandemic, and there is a strong lesson to learn from it. While the COVID-19 pandemic had grappled the globe completely, multinational pharmaceutical industries preferred to supply their cutting-edge technology vaccines to the higher income countries. As a result, the low- and medium-income countries (LMIC) which were left out from the benefits of these vaccines or were forced to continue with the conventional (like adenoviral, protein subunit and inactivated viral) vaccines developed through low-end technology platforms. It was crucial therefore to scale-up the production of the cutting-edge technology vaccines as well as the distribution of both the conventional and innovative vaccines irrespective of the financial status of individual nation as the pandemic spared none. India played an exemplary role with regard to this through its well-timed and well-orchestrated vaccine diplomacy.

7. Conclusion

Researchers had earlier attempted to develop vaccines against the coronavirus during the SARS-CoV-1 and MERS epidemics, but they faced several challenges and had little success. The severe and lethal coronavirus pandemic COVID-19 spread far more widely than SARS-CoV-1 and MERS. This situation forced many research organisations and vaccine firms worldwide to aggressively pursue their research to develop an efficient vaccine to combat SARS-CoV-2, with accelerated preclinical, clinical and human trials. Due to the rapid spread and severity of the COVID-19 pandemic, the social, economic and human capital suffered to a great extent.

The diverse state-of-art technology platforms adopted in developing SARS-CoV-2 vaccine was a significant step forward in vaccine research and development. While COVID-19 vaccines provided the much-needed public healthcare benefits, these had their associated economic and social fallouts too. Millions of mortalities and billion dollars of medical expenses could be averted owing to the administration of COVID-19 vaccines. Despite the mass vaccination and public health benefits, LMICs were still facing the vaccine inequity challenges. Studies have revealed that SARS-CoV-2 variants of concern (VOCs) could also be playing a critical role in compromising with the efficacy of the vaccines by escaping the neutralising antibodies and cell-mediated immunity. Albeit rare, long-term adverse effects have also been reportedly observed in the COVID-19 vaccinated individuals. Continued research and development of COVID-19 vaccinology, finding a clear link between the COVID-19 vaccine and the systemic adverse effects, up-scaling and decentralising the vaccine production capabilities and deployment (equitable distribution) of the vaccines remained some of the most critical aspects for pandemic preparedness and limiting the effects of future pandemic, containing the SARS-CoV-2 transmission, ensuring a better global community health, providing psychological support and upholding the socioeconomy.

8. References

Acosta-Coley I, Cervantes-Ceballos L, Tejeda-Benítez L, Sierra-Márquez L, Cabarcas-Montalvo M, García-Espiñeira M, Coronell-Rodríguez W and Arroyo-Salgado B, 2022. Vaccines platforms and COVID-19: what you need to know. Trop. Dis. Travel Med. Vaccines, 8: 1–19. doi: 10.1186/s40794-022-00176-4

Bai C, Quayson M and Sarkis J, 2021. COVID-19 pandemic digitization lessons for sustainable development of micro-and small-enterprises. Sustain. Prod. Consum., 27: 1989–2001. doi: 10.1016/j.spc.2021.04.035

Bergquist S, Otten T and Sarich N, 2020. COVID-19 pandemic in the United States. Health Policy Technol., 9(4): 623–638. doi: 10.2139/ssrn.3657404

Burleson BS and Maki ED, 2005. Acute respiratory distress syndrome. J. Pharm. Pract., 18: 118–131. doi: 10.1177/0897190004273595

Caceres MMF, Sosa JP, Lawrence JA, Sestacovschi C, Tidd-Johnson A, Rasool MHU, Gadamidi VK, Ozair S, Pandav K, Cuevas-Lou C and Parrish M, 2022. The impact of misinformation on the COVID-19 pandemic. AIMS Public Health, 9(2): 262. doi: 10.3934/publichealth.2022018

Calabrò GE, Pappalardo C, D'Ambrosio F, Vece M, Lupi C, Lontano A, Di Russo M, Ricciardi R and de Waure C, 2023. The impact of vaccination on COVID-19 burden of disease in the adult and elderly population: A systematic review of italian evidence. Vaccines, 11. doi: 10.3390/vaccines11051011

Chakraborty C, Bhattacharya M and Dhama K, 2023. SARS-CoV-2 vaccines, vaccine development technologies, and significant efforts in vaccine development during the pandemic: The lessons learned might help to fight against the next pandemic. Vaccines, 11: 1–19. doi: 10.3390/vaccines11030682

Chang R, Elhusseiny KM, Yeh YC and Sun WZ, 2021. COVID-19 ICU and mechanical ventilation patient characteristics and outcomes—A systematic review and meta-analysis. PloS One, 16(2): e0246318. doi: 10.1371/journal.pone.0246318

Chan JFW, Yuan S, Kok KH, To KKW, Chu H, Yang J, Xing F, Liu J, Yip CCY, Poon RWS and Tsoi HW, 2020. A familial cluster of pneumonia associated with the 2019 novel coronavirus indicating person-to-person transmission: a study of a family cluster. Lancet, 395: 514–523. doi: 10.1016/S0140-6736(20)30154-9

Chaudhary JK, Yadav R, Chaudhary PK, Maurya A, Kant N, Rugaie OA, Haokip HR, Yadav D, Roshan R, Prasad R and Chatrath A, 2021. Insights into covid-19 vaccine development based on immunogenic structural proteins of sars-cov-2, host immune responses, and herd immunity. Cells, 10. doi: 10.3390/cells10112949

Chavda VP, Patel AB, Pandya A, Vora LK, Patravale V, Tambuwala ZM, Aljabali AA, Serrano-Aroca Á, Mishra V and Tambuwala MM, 2022. Co-infection associated with SARS-CoV-2 and their management. Future science OA, 8(9): FSO819. doi: 10.2144/fsoa-2022-0011

Chen WH, Strych U, Hotez PJ and Bottazzi ME, 2020. The SARS-CoV-2 Vaccine Pipeline: an Overview. Curr. Trop. Med. Reports, 7: 61–64. doi: 10.1007/s40475-020-00201-6

Chirico F, da Silva JAT, Tsigaris P and Sharun K, 2022. Safety & effectiveness of COVID-19 vaccines: A narrative review. Indian J. Med. Res., 155(1): 91–104. doi: 10.4103/ijmr.IJMR_474_21

Ciminelli G and Garcia-Mandicó S, 2020. COVID-19 in Italy: An analysis of death registry data. J. Public Heal. (United Kingdom), 42: 723–730. doi: 10.1093/pubmed/fdaa165

Clemente-Suárez VJ, Rodriguez-Besteiro S, Cabello-Eras JJ, Bustamante-Sanchez A, Navarro-Jiménez E, Donoso-Gonzalez M, Beltrán-Velasco AI and Tornero-Aguilera JF, 2022. Sustainable development goals in the COVID-19 pandemic: A narrative review. Sustainability, 14(13): 7726. doi: 10.3390/su14137726

Cowling BJ and Leung GM, 2020. Epidemiological research priorities for public health control of the ongoing global novel coronavirus (2019-nCoV) outbreak. Eurosurveillance, 25. doi: 10.2807/1560-7917.ES.2020.25.6.2000110

Cucinotta D and Vanelli M, 2020. WHO declares COVID-19 a pandemic. Acta Biomed., 91: 157–160. doi: 10.23750/abm.v91i1.9397

Cui P, Chen Z, Wang T, Dai J, Zhang J, Ding T, Jiang J, Liu J, Zhang C, Shan W and Wang S, 2020. Severe acute respiratory syndrome coronavirus 2 detection in the female lower genital tract. Am. J. Obstet. Gynecol., 223: 131–134. doi: 10.1016/j.ajog.2020.04.038

Dai L, Gao L, Tao L, Hadinegoro SR, Erkin M, Ying Z, He P, Girsang RT, Vergara H, Akram J and Satari HI, 2022. Efficacy and safety of the RBD-dimer–based COVID-19 vaccine ZF2001 in adults. N. Engl. J. Med., 386(22): 2097–2111. doi: 10.1056/nejmoa2202261

Dai L and Gao GF, 2021. Viral targets for vaccines against COVID-19. Nat. Rev. Immunol., 21: 73–82. doi: 10.1038/s41577-020-00480-0

Dash R, Sahoo RN, Pattnaik G, Sarangi AK, Kandi V, Mishra S, Verma S and Mohapatra RK, 2024. An open call for nano-based therapy to address COVID-19 and oncological clinical conditions. Int. J. Surg., 110(4):2430-2. DOI: 10.1097/JS9.0000000000000071

Dhawan M, Saied AA and Sharma M, 2023. Virus-like particles (VLPs)-based vaccines against COVID-19: Where do we stand amid the ongoing evolution of SARS-CoV-2? Heal. Sci. Rev., 9: 100127. doi: 10.1016/j.hsr.2023.100127

Dighriri IM, Alhusayni KM, Mobarki AY, Aljerary IS, Alqurashi KA, Aljuaid FA, Alamri KA, Mutwalli AA, Maashi NA, Aljohani AM and Alqarni AM, 2022. Pfizer-BioNTech COVID-19 vaccine (BNT162b2) side effects: a systematic review. Cureus, 14(3). doi: 10.7759/cureus.23526

Dong Y, Dai T, Wei Y, Zhang L, Zheng M and Zhou F, 2020. A systematic review of SARS-CoV-2 vaccine candidates. Signal Transduct. Target. Ther. 5. doi: 10.1038/s41392-020-00352-y

dos Santos NC, Miravitlles M, Camelier AA, de Almeida VDC, Tosta Maciel RRB and Rosa Camelier FW, 2022. Prevalence and Impact of Comorbidities in Individuals with Chronic Obstructive Pulmonary Disease: A Systematic Review. Tuberc. Respir. Dis. (Seoul). 85: 205–220. doi: 10.4046/trd.2021.0179

Faramarzi A, Norouzi S, Dehdarirad H, Aghlmand S, Yusefzadeh H and Javan-Noughabi J, 2024. The global economic burden of COVID-19 disease: a comprehensive systematic review and meta-analysis. Syst. Rev., 13(1): 68. doi: 10.1186/s13643-024-02476-6

Fonseca MHG, de Souza TDFG, de Carvalho Araújo FM and de Andrade LOM, 2022. Dynamics of antibody response to CoronaVac vaccine. J. Med. Virol., 94(5): 2139–2148. doi: 10.1002/jmv.27604

Forni G and Mantovani A, 2021. COVID-19 vaccines: where we stand and challenges ahead. Cell Death Differ., 28(2): 626–639. doi: 10.1038/s41418-020-00720-9

Funk CD, Laferrière C and Ardakani A, 2020. A snapshot of the global race for vaccines targeting SARS-CoV-2 and the COVID-19 pandemic. Front. Pharmacol., 11: 937. doi: 10.3389/fphar.2020.00937

Gaythorpe KA, Bhatia S, Mangal T, Unwin HJT, Imai N, Cuomo-Dannenburg G, Walters CE, Jauneikaite E, Bayley H, Kont MD and Mousa A, 2021. Children's role in the COVID-19 pandemic: a systematic review of early surveillance data on susceptibility, severity, and transmissibility. Sci. Rep., 11(1): 13903. doi: 10.1038/s41598-021-92500-9

Goossens GA, 2015. Flushing and Locking of Venous Catheters: Available Evidence and Evidence Deficit. Nurs. Res. Pract., 2015: 1–12. doi: 10.1155/2015/985686

Heiat M, Hashemi-Aghdam MR, Heiat F, Rastegar Shariat Panahi M, Aghamollaei H, Moosazadeh Moghaddam M, Sathyapalan T, Ranjbar R and Sahebkar A, 2021. Integrative role of traditional and modern technologies to combat COVID-19. Expert Rev. Anti Infect. Ther., 19(1): 23–33. doi: 10.1080/14787210.2020.1799784

Hoffmann M, Kleine-Weber H, Schroeder S, Krüger N, Herrler T, Erichsen S, Schiergens TS, Herrler G, Wu NH, Nitsche A and Müller MA, 2020. SARS-CoV-2 cell entry depends on ACE2 and TMPRSS2 and is blocked by a clinically proven protease inhibitor. Cell, 181(2): 271–280. doi: 10.1016/j.cell.2020.02.052

Huang C, Wang Y, Li X, Ren L, Zhao J, Hu Y, Zhang L, Fan G, Xu J, Gu X and Cheng Z, 2020. Clinical features of patients infected with 2019 novel coronavirus in Wuhan, China. The Lancet, 395(10223): 497–506. doi: 10.1016/S0140-6736(20)30183-5

Johnson & Johnson (2021), Johnson & Johnson COVID-19 Vaccine Authorized by U.S. FDA For Emergency Use - First Single-Shot Vaccine in Fight Against Global Pandemic. Available online at: https://www.jnj.com/media-center/press-releases/johnson-johnson-covid-19-vaccine-authorized-by-u-s-fda-for-emergency-usefirst-single-shot-vaccine-in-fight-against-global-pandemic, Accessed on 20th October 2024.

Karimizadeh Z, Dowran R, Mokhtari-azad T, and Shafiei-Jandaghi NZ, 2023. The reproduction rate of severe acute respiratory syndrome coronavirus 2 different variants recently circulated in human: a narrative review. Eur. J. Med. Res., 28: 1–10. doi: 10.1186/s40001-023-01047-0

Krammer F, 2020. SARS-CoV-2 vaccines in development. Nature, 586: 516–527. doi: 10.1038/s41586-020-2798-3

Kutikuppala LS, Kandi V, Sarangi AK, Mishra S and Mohapatra RK, 2022. COVID-19 era and the constantly reemerging novel SARS-CoV-2 variants calls for special attention for the geriatrics: a real challenge. Geriatrics. 7(6):143.

Lazarus JV, Wyka K, White TM, Picchio CA, Gostin LO, Larson HJ, Rabin K, Ratzan SC, Kamarulzaman A and El-Mohandes A, 2023. A survey of COVID-19 vaccine acceptance across 23 countries in 2022. Nat. Med., 29(2): 366–375. doi: 10.1038/s41591-022-02185-4

Li K, Wu J, Wu F, Guo D, Chen L, Fang Z and Li C, 2020. The clinical and chest CT features associated with severe and critical COVID-19 pneumonia. Investig. Radiol., 55(6): 327–331. doi: 10.1097/RLI.0000000000000672

Liu K, Chen Y, Lin R, and Han K, 2020. Clinical features of COVID-19 in elderly patients: A comparison with young and middle-aged patients. J. Infect., 80: e14–e18. doi: 10.1016/j.jinf.2020.03.005

Li X, Sridhar S, and Chan JFW, 2020a. The Coronavirus Disease 2019 pandemic: How does it spread and how do we stop it? Curr. Opin. HIV AIDS, 15: 328–335. doi: 10.1097/COH.0000000000000650

Luvira V and Pitisuttithum P, 2024. Effect of homologous or heterologous vaccine booster over two initial doses of inactivated COVID-19 vaccine. Expert Rev. Vaccines, 23(1): 283–293. doi: 10.1080/14760584.2024.2320861

Mathew S, Faheem M, Hassain NA, Benslimane FM, Al Thani AA, Zaraket H and Yassine HM, 2020. Platforms exploited for SARS-CoV-2 vaccine development. Vaccines, 9: 1–24. doi: 10.3390/vaccines9010011

Mehta P, McAuley DF, Brown M, Sanchez E, Tattersall RS and Manson JJ, 2020. COVID-19: consider cytokine storm syndromes and immunosuppression. Lancet, 395(10229): 1033–1034. doi: 10.1016/S0140-6736(20)30628-0

Melis M and Littera R, 2021. Undetected infectives in the Covid-19 pandemic. Int. J. Infect. Dis., 104: 262–268. doi: 10.1016/j.ijid.2021.01.010

Meo SA, Bukhari IA, Akram J, Meo AS and Klonoff DC, 2021. COVID-19 vaccines: comparison of biological, pharmacological characteristics and adverse effects of Pfizer/BioNTech and Moderna Vaccines. Eur. Rev. Med. Pharmacol. Sci., 25(3).

Mercado NB, Zahn R, Wegmann F, Loos C, Chandrashekar A, Yu J, Liu J, Peter L, McMahan K, Tostanoski LH and He X, 2020. Single-shot Ad26 vaccine protects against SARS-CoV-2 in rhesus macaques. Nature, 586: 583–588. doi: 10.1038/s41586-020-2607-z

Minor PD, 2015. Live attenuated vaccines: Historical successes and current challenges. Virology, 479: 379–392. doi: 10.1016/j.virol.2015.03.032

Mizik T, 2021. The performance of the agri-food sector in the recent economic crisis and during Covid-19 pandemic. HighTech Innov. J., 2(3): 168–178. doi: 10.28991/HIJ-2021-02-03-02

Mohajan HK, 2021. Global COVID-19 pandemic: prevention and protection techniques. J. Econ. Dev. Environ. People, 10(1): 51–72.

Mohapatra RK, Das PK and Kandi V, 2020a. Challenges in controlling COVID-19 in migrants in Odisha, India. Diabetes Metab. Syndr., 14(6):1593-9. doi: 10.1016/j.dsx.2020.08.024

Mohapatra RK, El-Shall NA, Tiwari R, Nainu F, Kandi V, Sarangi AK, Mohammed TA, Desingu PA, Chakraborty C and Dhama K, 2022. Need of booster vaccine doses to counteract the emergence of SARS-CoV-2 variants in the context of the Omicron variant and increasing COVID-19 cases: An update. Hum. Vaccin. Immunother., 18(5):2065824. https://doi.org/10.1080/21645515.2022.2065824

Mohapatra RK, Mishra S, Azam M and Dhama K, 2021. COVID-19, WHO guidelines, pedagogy, and respite. Open Med., 16(1):491-3. doi: 10.1515/med-2021-0266

Mohapatra RK, Pintilie L, Kandi V, Sarangi AK, Das D, Sahu R and Perekhoda L, 2020b. The recent challenges of highly contagious COVID-19, causing respiratory infections: Symptoms, diagnosis, transmission, possible vaccines, animal models, and immunotherapy. Chem. Biol. Drug Des., 96(5):1187-208. doi: 10.1111/cbdd.13761

Mohapatra RK, Verma S, Kandi V, Sarangi AK, Seidel V, Das SN, Behera A, Tuli HS, Sharma AK and Dhama K, 2023. The SARS-CoV-2 Omicron variant and its multiple sub-lineages: transmissibility, vaccine development, antiviral drugs, monoclonal antibodies, and strategies for infection control–a review. ChemistrySelect., 8(9):e202201380. https://doi.org/10.1002/slct.202201380

Nachega JB, Mbala-Kingebeni P, Otshudiema J, Zumla A and Tam-Fum JJM, 2020. The colliding epidemics of COVID-19, Ebola, and measles in the Democratic Republic of the Congo. Lancet Glob. Health, 8(8): e991–e992. doi: 10.1016/S2214-109X(20)30281-3

Nagy A and Alhatlani B, 2021. An overview of current COVID-19 vaccine platforms. Comput. Struct. Biotechnol. J., 19: 2508–2517. doi: 10.1016/j.csbj.2021.04.061

Nie Y, Mou L, Long Q, Deng D, Hu R, Cheng J and Wu J, 2023. SARS-CoV-2 ORF3a positively regulates NF-κB activity by enhancing IKKβ-NEMO interaction. Virus Res., 328: 199086. doi: 10.1016/j.virusres.2023.199086

Pal M, Parija S, Mohapatra RK, Mishra S, Rabaan AA, Al Mutair A, Alhumaid S, Al-Tawfiq JA and Dhama K, 2022. Symptom-Based COVID-19 Prognosis through AI-Based IoT: A Bioinformatics Approach. BioMed Research International. 2022(1):3113119.

Prates-Syed WA, Chaves LC, Crema KP, Vuitika L, Lira A, Côrtes N, Kersten V, Guimarães FE, Sadraeian M, Barroso da Silva FL and Cabral-Marques O, 2021. VLP-based COVID-19 vaccines: An adaptable technology against the threat of new variants. Vaccines, 9(12): 1409. doi: 10.3390/vaccines9121409

Randolph HE and Barreiro LB, 2020. Herd immunity: understanding COVID-19. Immunity, 52(5): 737–741. doi: 10.1016/j.immuni.2020.04.012

Reddy SG, 2020. Population health, economics and ethics in the age of COVID-19. BMJ Glob. Health, 5(7): e003259. doi: 10.1136/bmjgh-2020-003259

Sarangi AK, Salem MA, Younus MD, El-Haroun H, Mahal A, Tripathy L, Mishra R, Shabil M, Alhumaydhi FA, Khatib MN and Bushi G, 2024. Advanced biomaterials for regenerative medicine and their possible therapeutic significance in treating COVID-19: a critical overview. Int. J. Surg., 110(12):7508-27. doi: 10.1097/JS9.0000000000002110

Satapathy BS, Pattnaik G, Sahoo RN, Pattanaik S, Sarangi AK, Kandi V, Mishra S, Rabaan AA, Mohanty A, Sah R and Mohapatra RK, 2023. COVID-19 vaccines and their underbelly: Are we going the right way?. Health Sci. Rep., 6(9):e1540. doi: 10.1002/hsr2.1540

Singhal T, 2020. A Review of Coronavirus Disease-2019 (COVID-19). Indian J. Pediatr., 87: 281–286. doi: 10.1007/s12098-020-03263-6

Singh P, Anand A, Rana S, Kumar A, Goel P, Kumar S, Gouda KC and Singh H, 2024. Impact of COVID-19 vaccination: a global perspective. Front. Pub. Health, 11: 1272961. doi: 10.3389/fpubh.2023.1272961

Steele MK, Couture A, Reed C, Iuliano D, Whitaker M, Fast H, Hall AJ, MacNeil A, Cadwell B, Marks KJ and Silk BJ, 2022. Estimated number of COVID-19 infections, hospitalizations, and deaths prevented among vaccinated persons in the US, December 2020 to September 2021. JAMA Network Open, 5(7): e2220385–e2220385. doi: 10.1001/jamanetworkopen.2022.20385

Tan J, Yoshida Y, Sheng-Kai Ma K, Mauvais-Jarvis F, and Lee CC, 2022. Gender differences in health protective behaviours and its implications for COVID-19 pandemic in Taiwan: a population-based study. BMC Pub. Health, 22. doi: 10.1186/s12889-022-14288-1

van Riel D and de Wit E, 2020. Next-generation vaccine platforms for COVID-19. Nat. Mater., 19: 810–812. doi: 10.1038/s41563-020-0746-0

Verger P and Dubé E, 2020. Restoring confidence in vaccines in the COVID-19 era. Expert Rev. Vaccines, 19: 991–993. doi: 10.1080/14760584.2020.1825945

Voysey M, Clemens SAC, Madhi SA, Weckx LY, Folegatti PM, Aley PK, Angus B, Baillie VL, Barnabas SL, Bhorat QE and Bibi S, 2021. Single-dose administration and the influence of the timing of the booster dose on immunogenicity and efficacy of ChAdOx1 nCoV-19 (AZD1222) vaccine: a pooled analysis of four randomised trials. Lancet, 397: 881–891. doi: 10.1016/S0140-6736(21)00432-3

Wang F, Kream RM, and Stefano GB, 2020b. An evidence based perspective on mRNA-SARScov-2 vaccine development. Med. Sci. Monit., 26. doi: 10.12659/MSM.924700

Wang F and Wang J Der, 2022. Estimating US Earnings Loss Associated with COVID-19 Based on Human Capital Calculation. Int. J. Environ. Res. Public Health, 19. doi: 10.3390/ijerph19021015

Wang H, Zhang Y, Huang B, Deng W, Quan Y, Wang W, Xu W, Zhao Y, Li N, Zhang J and Liang H, 2020b. Development of an inactivated vaccine candidate, BBIBP-CorV, with potent protection against SARS-CoV-2. Cell, 182(3): 713-721. doi: 10.1016/j.cell.2020.06.008

Watson OJ, Barnsley G, Toor J, Hogan AB, Winskill P, and Ghani AC, 2022. Global impact of the first year of COVID-19 vaccination: a mathematical modelling study. Lancet Infect. Dis. 22, 1293–1302. doi: 10.1016/S1473-3099(22)00320-6

WHO, 2022a. The Oxford/AstraZeneca (ChAdOx1-S [recombinant] vaccine) COVID-19 vaccine: what you need to know. Available online at: https://www.who.int/news-room/feature-stories/detail/the-oxford-astrazeneca-covid-19-vaccine-what-you-need-to-know, Accessed on 13th September 2024.

WHO, 2022b. The CanSino Biologics Ad5-nCoV-S [recombinant] COVID-19 vaccine: What you need to know. Available online at: https://www.who.int/news-room/feature-stories/detail/the--cansino-biologics-ad5-ncov-s--recombinant---covid-19-vaccine--what-you-need-to-know, Accessed on 10th August 2024.

Yang J, Vaghela S, Yarnoff B, De Boisvilliers S, Di Fusco M, Wiemken TL, Kyaw MH, McLaughlin JM and Nguyen JL, 2023. Estimated global public health and economic impact of COVID-19 vaccines in the pre-omicron era using real-world empirical data. Expert Rev. Vaccines, 22: 54–65. doi: 10.1080/14760584.2023.2157817

Zheng J, 2020. SARS-coV-2: An emerging coronavirus that causes a global threat. Int. J. Biol. Sci., 16: 1678–1685. doi: 10.7150/ijbs.45053

Zhou F, Yu T, Du R, Fan G, Liu Y, Liu Z, Xiang J, Wang Y, Song B, Gu X and Guan L, 2020. Clinical course and risk factors for mortality of adult inpatients with COVID-19 in Wuhan, China: a retrospective cohort study. Lancet, 395: 1054–1062. doi: 10.1016/S0140-6736(20)30566-3

Zhu FC, Li YH, Guan XH, Hou LH, Wang WJ, Li JX, Wu SP, Wang BS, Wang Z, Wang L and Jia SY, 2020. Safety, tolerability, and immunogenicity of a recombinant adenovirus type-5 vectored COVID-19 vaccine : Lancet, 395: 1845–1854. doi: 10.1016/S0140-6736(20)31208-3

Index